OXFORD MEDICAL PUBLICATIONS

Emergencies in Oncology

Emergencies in Oncology

Edited by

Martin Scott-Brown MBiochem, MA, MB, BCh, MRCP
Specialist Registrar in Clinical Oncology,
Oxford Radcliffe Trust

Roy A.J. Spence OBE, JP, MA, MD, FRCS
Consultant Surgeon, Belfast City Hospital,
Honorary Professor, Queen's University Belfast and
Honorary Professor, University of Ulster

Patrick G. Johnston MD, PhD, FRCP, FRCPI
Professor of Oncology, Belfast City Hospital and
Queen's University Belfast and
Director of the Centre for Cancer Research and
Cell Biology, Queen's University Belfast

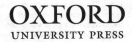

OXFORD
UNIVERSITY PRESS

OXFORD
UNIVERSITY PRESS

Great Clarendon Street, Oxford OX2 6DP

Oxford University Press is a department of the University of Oxford.
It furthers the University's objective of excellence in research, scholarship,
and education by publishing worldwide in

Oxford New York

Auckland Cape Town Dar es Salaam Hong Kong Karachi
Kuala Lumpur Madrid Melbourne Mexico City Nairobi
New Delhi Shanghai Taipei Toronto

With offices in

Argentina Austria Brazil Chile Czech Republic France Greece
Guatemala Hungary Italy Japan Poland Portugal Singapore
South Korea Switzerland Thailand Turkey Ukraine Vietnam

Oxford is a registered trade mark of Oxford University Press
in the UK and in certain other countries

Published in the United States
by Oxford University Press Inc., New York

© Oxford University Press, 2007

First published 2007

British Library Cataloguing in Publication Data

Data available

Library of Congress Cataloging in Publication Data

Data available

Typeset by Newgen Imaging Systems (P) Ltd., Chennai, India
Printed in Italy
on acid-free paper by
Legoprint S.p.A.

ISBN 978–0–19–9215–638

10 9 8 7 6 5 4 3 2 1

Preface

One in three of the population of the UK will be diagnosed with cancer in their lifetime. Many of these become acutely ill and require emergency treatment. Also, patients with undiagnosed cancer can present with oncological emergencies and therefore, as doctors in specialist oncology units, emergency departments and indeed almost any medical and surgical speciality, we need to be aware of the specific challenges presented by the acutely ill patient with cancer.

Patients with cancer may present with emergencies caused by their underlying malignancy, for example spinal cord compression or hypercalcaemia, or because of the side effects of their treatment, such as neutropenic sepsis following chemotherapy. Cancer may predispose the patient to certain emergencies (e.g. pulmonary embolism), whilst cancer patients may also be at increased risk of many other medical and surgical emergencies by virtue of their lifestyle choice (e.g. smoking), that increase the risk of many cancers and e.g. myocardial infarction and stroke.

In this book we have sought to provide an easily accessible evidence-based guide to the diagnosis and management of acutely ill patients with cancer. We have limited the scope to those emergencies directly caused by the cancer or by its treatment and those conditions where there is a strong predisposition caused by the cancer. Many of these emergencies will be familiar to non-oncologists; however, others will not. Any delay caused by unfamiliarity can have disastrous results; for example, irreversible neurological deficit in unrecognized spinal cord compression. Not all the emergencies covered in this book require immediate recognition and treatment to prevent potential fatal outcomes. However, all these conditions require urgent action to reduce morbidity and distressing symptoms for our patients. We, therefore, provide practical guidance on the management of the acute and distressing symptoms that often arise in the ill cancer patient

As cancer treatments improve many people diagnosed with cancer can look forward to a cure and a life after cancer. For others the outlook is not so optimistic and many oncological emergencies increase in frequency as the patient approaches the terminal phase of their life. Therefore similar emergencies may need very different treatments in patients at different stages of their disease. Patients with potentially curable disease should be managed aggressively with the full benefit of modern medical expertise, including admission to intensive care units if necessary. For patients entering the terminal phase of their life we must sometimes accept that, even with aggressive management, we will be unable to return the patient to a quality of life that is acceptable to them. We need to be open with our patients as to the likely outcome and listen to their wishes for their future management.

The book is designed for any doctor coming into contact with cancer patients, including general practitioners, emergency department doctors, acute medical teams and those specialities with a high cancer load. It will be of great use for oncology units, for nursing staff and doctors in training to improve the management of acute oncological problems. The book will also be of interest to senior medical students.

Acknowledgements

We would like to thank all the contributors for their hard work in producing this book. We would also like to thank Clare Rahemtulla and Michelle Maxwell (Radiotherapy Specialist Nurses) for their advice on the practical management of radiotherapy-related side effects, and also to Zoë Traill (Consultant Radiologist) for radiological advice.

MS-B is indebted to Frances, Thomas, and Jonty for their support and patience during the writing of this book.

Contents

Contributors

Joss Adams
Consultant Clinical Oncologist,
Berkshire Cancer Centre, Royal
Berkshire NHS Foundation Trust,
Reading, UK

Gerard Andrade
Locum Consultant
Clinical Oncologist,
Churchill Hospital,
Oxford, UK

Charlie Bond,
Locum Consultant
Palliative care, Severn Hospice,
Shrewsbury, UK

Phillip Camilleri
Consultant Clinical Oncologist,
Northampton General Hospital,
Northampton, UK

Graham Collins
Lymphoma Research Foundation
Lymphoma Research Registrar,
John Radcliffe Hospital,
Oxford, UK

Matthew Croucher
Consultant Old Age Psychiatrist,
Canterbury District Health Board,
Christchurch, New Zealand

David Cutter
Specialist Registrar in Clinical
Oncology, Oxford Regional
Rotation, Chuchill Hospital,
Oxford, UK

Stephen Dorman
Specialist Registrar in Cardiology,
South West Regional Rotation,
North Bristol NHS Trust,
Bristol, UK

Nishan Guha
Specialist Registrar in Chemical
Pathology, Oxford Radcliffe
Hospitals NHS Trust,
Oxford, UK

Jon-Paul Meyer
Specialist Registrar in Urology,
Oxford Regional Rotation,
Churchill Hospital, Oxford, UK

Michael Puttick
Specialist Registrar in General
Surgery, Oxford Regional Rotation,
Oxford, UK

Jonny Seymour
Specialist Registrar in
Respiratory Medicine,
London Deanery,
Clinical Research Fellow,
King's College, London, UK

Symbols and abbreviations

[]	Concentration
>	Greater than
<	Less than
≥	Greater than or equal to
≤	Less than or equal to
°C	Degrees centigrade
↑	Increased
↓	Decreased
#	Fraction of radiotherapy
α-FP	Alpha-fetoprotein
A₁	Adrenergic receptor 1
A–a gradient	Alveolar–arterial oxygen gradient
Ab	Antibody
ABG	Arterial blood gas
ACE	Angiotensin-converting enzyme
ACh	Acetylcholine receptor
ACTH	Adrenocorticotrophic hormone
ADH	Antidiuretic hormone
AF	Atrial fibrillation
AHTR	Acute haemolytic transfusion reaction
ALP	Alkaline phosphatase
ALT	Alanine aminotransferase
ANA	Antinuclear antibodies
ANC	Absolute neutrophil count
ANCA	Antineutrophil cytoplasmic antibodies
aPC	Activated protein C
APTT	Activated partial thromboplastin time
ARDS	Adult respiratory distress syndrome
ARF	Acute renal failure
AST	Aspartate aminotransferase
ATN	Acute tubular necrosis
ATP	Adenosine triphosphate
AUC	Area under the curve
AV	Atrioventricular
AVM	Arteriovenous malformation
AXR	Abdominal X-ray

β-HCG	β-human chorionic gonadotrophin
bd	*bis die* (twice a day)
BEP	Bleomycin, etoposide, cisplatin chemotherapy regimen
BMI	Body mass index
BP	Blood pressure
bpm	Beats per minute or breaths per minute
BSO	Bilateral salpingo-oophorectomy
BTS	British Thoracic Society
Ca^{2+}	Calcium
CBD	Common bile duct
CCF	Congestive cardiac failure
CDT	*Clostridium difficile* toxin
CEA	Carcinoembryonic antigen
CHART	Continuous hyperfractionated accelerated radiotherapy
CLL	Chronic lymphocytic leukaemia
cm	Centimetre
CMV	Cytomegalovirus
CNS	Central nervous system
CO_2	Carbon dioxide
COPD	Chronic obstructive pulmonary disease
CPAP	Continuous positive airway pressure
CPR	Cardiopulmonary resuscitation
CR	Complete response
CRP	C-reactive protein
CSF	Cerebrospinal fluid
CT	Computed tomography
CTPA	Computed tomography pulmonary angiography
CTU	Computed tomography urography
CTZ	Chemoreceptor trigger zone
CVAD	Central venous access device
CVD	Cerebrovascular disease
CVP	Central venous pressure
CVS	Cardiovascular
CXR	Chest X-ray
D	Day
D_2	Dopamine receptor 2
DIC	Disseminated intravascular coagulation
DKA	Diabetic ketoacidosis
dl	Decilitre
DMSO	Dimethyl sulfoxide
DNAR	Do not attempt resuscitation
DVLA	Driver and vehicle licensing agency

EBV	Epstein–Barr virus
ECG	Electrocardiogram
Echo	Echocardiogram
ECT	Electroconvulsive therapy
EGFR	Epidermal growth factor receptor
EMD	Electromechanical dissociation
ENT	Ear, nose and throat
EPS	Extrapyramidal syndromes
ERCP	Endoscopic retrograde cholangiopancreatography
ESR	Erythrocyte sedimentation rate
EUA	Examination under anaesthesia
EUS	Endoscopic ultrasound
FBC	Full blood count
FEC	5-Fluorouracil, epirubicin, cyclophosphamide chemotherapy regimen
FEIBA	Factor VIII inhibitor bypassing fraction
FEV_1	Forced expiratory volume in first second
FFP	Fresh frozen plasma
FiO_2	Partial pressure of oxygen in inspired air
FSH	Follicle-stimulating hormone
fT_3	Free tri-iodothyronine
fT_4	Free thyroxine
5-FU	5-Fluorouracil
FVC	Forced vital capacity
γ-GT	Gamma-glutamyl transpeptidase
g	Gram
GA	General anaesthetic
GABA	Gamma-aminobutyric acid
GBM	Glomerular basement membrane
GCS	Glasgow Coma Scale
G-CSF	Granulocyte colony stimulating factor
GFR	Glomerular filtration rate
GI	Gastrointestinal
GPC	Gastric parietal cell
G6PD	Glucose-6 phosphate dehydrogenase
GTN	Glyceryl trinitrate
GU	Genitourinary
GvHD	Graft-versus-host disease
Gy	Gray
h	Hour
H_1	Histamine receptor 1
Hb	Haemoglobin
HCO_3^-	Bicarbonate

HDU	High dependency unit
5-HIAA	5-hydroxyindoleacetic acid
HIT	Heparin-induced thrombocytopenia
HIV	Human immunodeficiency virus
HLA	Human leukocyte antigens
H_2O	Water
HPA	Human platelet alloantigen
HR	Heart rate
HRCT	High resolution computed tomography
HRT	Hormone replacement therapy
HSV	Herpes simplex virus
HT	Hypertension
5-HT_2, 5-HT_3, 5-HT_4	Serotonin receptor 2/3/4
HUS	Haemolytic uraemic syndrome
IBD	Inflammatory bowel disease
ICP	Intracranial pressure
ICU	Intensive care unit
IF	Intrinsic factor
IFN	Interferon
Ig	Immunoglobulin
IGF-1	Insulin-like growth factor 1
IHD	Ischaemic heart disease
IL-2	Interleukin-2
IM	Intramuscular
IMCA	Independent mental capacity advocate
INR	International normalized ratio
ITP	Idiopathic thrombocytopenic purpura
IU	International units
IV	Intravenous
IVC	Inferior vena cava
IVHP	Intravenous high potency
IvIg	Intravenous immunoglobulin
IVU	Intravenous urography
JVP	Jugular venous pressure
K^+	Potassium
kcal	Kilocalorie
KCl	Potassium chloride
kg	Kilogram
KUB	Kidneys, ureters, and bladder
l	Litre
LA	Local anaesthetic
LBO	Large bowel obstruction

LDH	Lactate dehydrogenase
LFTs	Liver function tests
LH	Luteinizing hormone
LIF	Left iliac fossa
LMN	Lower motor neurone
LMWH	Low molecular weight heparin
LV	Left ventricle
LVEF	Left ventricular ejection fraction
LVF	Left ventricular failure
µg	Microgram
µmol	Micromole
m	Metre
MAOIs	Monoamine oxidase inhibitors
MBq	Megabecquerels
MC&S	Microscopy, culture, and sensitivities
mcg	microgram
MCV	Mean cell volume
mg	Milligram
Mg^{2+}	Magnesium
MGUS	Monoclonal gammopathy of undetermined significance
MI	Myocardial infarction
ml	Millilitre
mmHg	Millimetres of mercury
mmol	Millimole
MMP	Matrix metalloproteinase
MMSE	Mini-mental state examination
mOsm	Milliosmole
mPa	Millipascal
MR	Modified release
MRCP	Magnetic resonance cholangiopancreatography
MRI	Magnetic resonance imaging
MRSA	Methicillin-resistant *Staphylococcus aureus*
MSU	Midstream urine
MUGA	Multigated acquisition scan
M–W	Mallory–Weiss
N	Normal
$NaHCO_3^-$	Sodium bicarbonate
Na^+	Sodium
NBM	Nil by mouth
Nd:YAG	Neodymium-doped yttrium aluminium garnet
NG	Nasogastric
NHL	Non-Hodgkin's lymphoma

NICE	National Institute for Health and Clinical Excellence
nocte	At night
NR	Normal release
NSAIDs	Non-steroidal anti-inflammatory drugs
NSCLC	Non-small cell lung cancer
N&V	Nausea and vomiting
O_2	Oxygen
OAR	Organ at risk
od	*omni die* (once daily)
OGD	Oesophagogastroduodenoscopy
P_2	Pulmonary component of second heart sound
PAI-1	Plasminogen activator inhibitor-1
PAN	Polyarteritis nodosa
PCA	Patient-controlled analgesia
pCO_2	Partial pressure of CO_2
PCP	*Pneumocystis carinii* pneumonia
PCR	Polymerase chain reaction
PCV	Packed cell volume
PDT	Photodynamic therapy
PE	Pulmonary embolus
PEA	Pulseless electrical activity
PEFR	Peak expiratory flow rate
PEG	Percutaneous endoscopic gastrostomy
PET	Positron emission tomography
PFTs	Pulmonary function tests
pH	*pouvoir hydrogène*, measure of the acidity of a solution
PICC	Peripherally inserted central catheter
PNET	Primitive neuroectodermal tumour
PNH	Paroxysmal nocturnal haemoglobinuria
PO	*Per os* (by mouth)
pO_2	Partial pressure of O_2
PO_3^-	Phosphate
PPE	Palmar–plantar erythrodysaesthesia
PPI	Proton pump inhibitor
prn	*pro re nata* (as required)
PS	Performance status
PSA	Prostate specific antigen
PSVT	Paroxysmal supraventricular tachycardia
PT	Prothrombin time
PTC	Percutaneous transhepatic cholangiography
PTH	Parathyroid hormone
PTH-rp	Parathyroid hormone-related peptide

PTP	Post-transfusion purpura
PTU	Propylthiouracil
qds	*quarter die sumendus* (to be taken 4 times a day)
q4h	*quaque 4 hora* (every 4 hours)
RBC	Red blood cell
RIF	Right iliac fossa
RR	Response rate or respiratory rate
RSV	Respiratory syncytial virus
RUQ	Right upper quadrant
RV	Right ventricle
s	Second
S_1, S_2, S_3, S_4	First, second, third, fourth heart sounds
SAAG	Serum ascites albumin gradient
SaO_2	Oxygen saturation of haemoglobin
SBO	Small bowel obstruction
SBP	Systolic blood pressure
SC	Subcutaneous
SCC	Spinal cord compression
SCLC	Small cell lung cancer
SCT	Stem cell transplant
SIADH	Syndrome of inappropriate ADH secretion
SLE	Systemic lupus erythematosus
SNRI	Selective noradrenaline re-uptake inhibitor
SSRI	Selective serotonin re-uptake inhibitor
stat	*statim* (immediately; at once)
STIR	Short T1 inversion recovery
SVCO	Superior vena cava obstruction
TAC	Docetaxel, doxorubicin, cyclophosphamide chemotherapy regimen
TAH	Total abdominal hysterectomy
TB	Tuberculosis
TBI	Total body irradiation
TCA	Tricyclic antidepressant
TCC	Transitional cell carcinoma
tds	*ter die sumendus* (to be taken 3 times a day)
TED	Thromboembolism deterrent
TENS	Transcutaneous electrical nerve stimulation
TFTs	Thyroid function tests
TIPS	Transjugular intrahepatic portocaval shunt
TLS	Tumour lysis syndrome
TNF	Tumour necrosis factor
TOE	Transoesophageal echocardiogram
TPN	Total parenteral nutrition

TRALI	Transfusion-related acute lung injury
TSH	Thyroid stimulating hormone
TT	Thrombin time
TTP	Thrombotic thrombocytopenic purpura
TURBT	Transurethral resection of bladder tumour
TURP	Transurethral resection of prostate
U	Units
U&Es	Urea and electrolytes
UGI	Upper gastrointestinal
UO	Urine output
UMN	Upper motor neurone
USS	Ultrasound scan
UTI	Urinary tract infection
VATS	Video-assisted thoracic surgery
VEGF	Vascular endothelial growth factor
VF	Ventricular fibrillation
VIP	Vasoactive intestinal polypeptide
VOD	Veno-occlusive disease
V/Q	Ventilation:perfusion ratio
VRE	Vancomycin-resistant *Enterococci*
VT	Ventricular tachycardia
VTE	Venous thromboembolic disease
VZV	Varicella zoster virus
WBRT	Whole brain radiotherapy
WCC	White cell count
WHO	World Health Organisation
ZN	Ziehl–Nielsen

Symptoms

⑦ **Pain**

Three-quarters of cancer patients experience pain at some point in their illness. Acute, severe pain produces intense fear and anxiety for the patient and their carers. Chronic, unrelieved pain is extremely debilitating, is associated with depression, and impairs a patient's ability to cope with ongoing treatment.

Pain at a particular site may lead to the first diagnosis of cancer. It is also frequently the first sign of metastatic spread from a known primary cancer so a new pain always warrants thorough assessment. Multiple, concurrent pains are common, particularly in advanced cancer, and it is important to consider the cause and appropriate management of each pain separately.

The experience of pain is modified by physical, psychological, social, and spiritual factors. Pain threshold will vary not only between patients but in the same patient over time depending on other factors in their life and illness. It is important to consider the meaning of pain to the patient. Increasing pain levels may lead to fear that the cancer is spreading or enlarging.

Types of pain

Nociceptive pain

- This is 'normal' pain resulting from stimulation of peripheral nerves in an undamaged nervous system. It includes visceral, bone, and soft tissue pain.
- It is usually opioid-responsive.

Neuropathic pain

- This refers to pain initiated or caused by a primary lesion or dysfunction in the nervous system (peripheral or central).
- Nerves may be damaged by compression or infiltration from tumour or by inflammatory processes:
  - spinal cord compression   • post-herpetic neuralgia
  - chemotherapy-induced neuropathy
- Neuropathic pain is always associated with abnormal sensory features in the distribution of the affected nerve.
- Neuropathic pain may respond incompletely to opioids and may require the use of adjuvant analgesics.

Episodic pain

- This is pain that occurs on an intermittent rather than a continuous basis and may be an exacerbation of more constant 'baseline pain' at the same site.
- It can be divided into three categories:
  - Predictable
    — pain is associated with a particular position or activity
      - weightbearing on bony metastases
      - oesophageal pain on swallowing
      - dressing changes over a painful wound

- Unpredictable
  - pain is spontaneous and not related to predictable factors
    - bowel colic
    - some forms of neuropathic pain
- End of dose failure
  - pain recurs before the next dose of analgesia is due. In the context of opioids this is usually a sign that the dose is inadequate

Assessment of pain

Assessment of pain requires careful history-taking and examination which should be carried out in the light of the known sites and spread of malignant disease. It requires a holistic and multidisciplinary approach. Carers, nursing staff, and physiotherapists may gather valuable information from hands-on care and observation of a patient over a period of time.

In acute pain there is acute anxiety and adrenergic activation, causing pallor, sweating, pupillary dilatation, tachycardia, and tachypnoea.

In chronic pain there may be little adrenergic activation but instead more negative symptoms commonly associated with depression such as sleep disturbance, anorexia, loss of interest, and low mood.

History

- Number and location of pain sites.
- Radiation of pain.
- Character of the pain.
  - This is important in the diagnosis of:
    - 'colicky' abdominal pain associated with constipation or bowel obstruction
    - neuropathic pain where the pain may be described as 'burning', 'shooting', 'electric shocks' or strange sensations such as 'water trickling under the skin'
- Does the pain feel deep or superficial?
- Is the pain continuous or episodic?
- Is the pain related to posture or movement?
- Does the pain disturb sleep?
- Pain that is only there during the day may be associated with movement or daytime stresses.
- Pain that is only there at night may be related to posture or increased anxiety at night.

Examination

Painful areas should be examined gently and carefully to avoid exacerbating pain or causing further tissue damage.

- Tumour masses and lymphadenopathy.
- Organomegaly in the area of pain.
- Areas of local tenderness in bone or soft tissue related to pain sites.
- Tenderness and mobility of joints in areas of pain.

- Evidence of nerve damage related to spinal level or peripheral innervation.
  - Sensory changes
    - numbness   — paraesthesia
    - hyperaesthesia
  - Motor deficits
  - Hypo/hyperreflexia
- Evidence of non-malignant pathology which could be causing pain.

Causes of pain in the cancer patient

- Headache and facial pain
  - leptomeningeal metastases   • retro-orbital metastases
  - raised intracranial pressure from tumour/metastases
  - bony metastases of skull and cervical spine
- Back pain
  - vertebral metastases   • spinal cord compression
- Chest pain
  - lung tumour   • pulmonary embolism
  - rib metastases   • mediastinal tumour
  - malignant infiltration of pleura or chest wall
- Abdominal pain
  - bowel obstruction   • liver metastases
  - constipation   • renal/adrenal metastases
  - invasion/pressure on coeliac plexus
  - tumour in bowel, mesentery or peritoneum
  - involvement of retro-peritoneal lymph nodes
- Pelvic/perineal pain
  - constipation   • pelvic metastases
  - rectal tenesmus   • urinary retention
- Limb/joint pain
  - bony or soft tissue metastases
  - venous thrombosis
  - nerve compression by tumour
  - neuropathy
    - chemotherapy   — paraneoplastic effect

Pain management

General principles

- Look for and treat reversible causes for the pain:
  - constipation   • infection
- Consider whether pain may be helped by disease-modifying treatment:
  - radiotherapy   • chemotherapy
- Give the patient an explanation for the cause of their pain.
- Give analgesics on a regular basis to maintain an analgesic effect.
- Always have additional analgesia written up for pain that breaks through the regular analgesic regimen ('breakthrough pain').
- New analgesics should usually be added one at a time, to be able to assess the efficacy of each drug.

- Drugs that have not been effective or that are no longer making a significant contribution to analgesia should be stopped.
- Opioids should generally be titrated to effect or tolerance before adding in additional drugs to avoid unnecessarily complicated regimes.
- In difficult cancer pain, combinations are often necessary to achieve adequate analgesia with minimum side effects.
  - non-opioid analgesics
  - opioids
  - adjuvants

The **WHO** analgesic ladder

The WHO analgesic ladder (See Fig. 1.1) provides a systematic approach to pain management in cancer.
- An adjuvant:
  - is a drug which is not analgesic in its prime function but has analgesic actions in particular types of pain and can enhance pain control in combination with analgesics;
  - may be appropriate at any stage of the ladder;
  - examples:
    — corticosteroids
    — tricyclic antidepressants
    — anticonvulsants

In practice this is a guideline; the choice of analgesic should be determined by the cause and nature of the pain, and the significance of potential adverse effects for a particular patient.

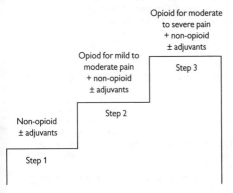

Fig. 1.1 The WHO analgesic ladder.

Non-opioid analgesics

Paracetamol

- Paracetamol is analgesic and antipyretic but has no peripheral anti-inflammatory effect.
- It acts in the CNS to inhibit prostaglandin synthesis but may also interact with other systems.
- It is metabolized mainly by the liver and can cause hepatotoxicity if taken above the maximum recommended dose of 4 g/day.
- Inside the recommended dose range it is generally well tolerated.
- It is available in combination with codeine or dihydrocodeine.

NSAIDs

- NSAIDs are effective analgesics for most pains associated with cancer, especially if there is an inflammatory component to the pain. They are also antipyretic.
- NSAIDs inhibit prostaglandin synthesis peripherally and in the CNS by the inhibition of cyclo-oxygenase (COX). They also have another as yet uncharacterized central analgesic action (not COX-dependent).
- COX exists in two forms:
  - COX-1 (constitutive)
  - COX-2 (inducible by inflammation)
- There is some evidence that NSAIDs with greater selectivity for COX-2 (e.g. celecoxib) may show less gastroduodenal toxicity but may also be more pro-thrombotic (↑ risk of myocardial infarction and stroke) than NSAIDs with more balanced COX inhibition.
- The use of NSAIDs is limited by their side effects and interactions. In debilitated patients or those with additional risk factors for gastro-duodenal ulceration it is recommended that they are prescribed with the gastric protection of a proton pump inhibitor.
  - Adverse effects
    - salt and water retention
    - thrombotic events
    - renal failure
      - particularly in the presence of dehydration/hypovolaemia.
    - GI ulceration
  - Cautions
    - dyspeptic symptoms
    - hypovolaemia
    - renal impairment
    - age >60
    - history of peptic ulceration
    - debilitated patient
    - ischaemic heart disease
    - cerebrovascular disease
    - ↑ risk of GI ulceration and haemorrhage if patient also on
      - steroids
      - aspirin
      - anticoagulants
      - SSRIs
    - NSAIDs decrease renal excretion and increase toxicity of methotrexate.
- Administration
  - NSAIDs should be prescribed regularly rather than prn to maximize analgesic effect.
  - There are many oral preparations available.
  - Diclofenac may be given IM/SC but is painful by injection.
  - Tenoxicam is available as a once-daily injection (IV/IM).
  - Diclofenac and ibuprofen are available as topical gels which are effective for superficial soft tissue pain.

Opioids

Table 1.1 Potency ratios of commonly used opioids

Opioid	Potency ratio with oral morphine
Codeine PO	1/10
Dihydrocodeine PO	1/10
Tramadol PO	1/5
Morphine PO	1
Morphine SC/IV	2
Diamorphine SC/IV	3
Oxycodone PO	2
Hydromorphone PO	7.5
Fentanyl transdermal	100–150

Codeine
- Codeine is an opioid for mild to moderate pain and exerts its analgesia principally as a pro-drug of morphine.
- Conversion is reduced:
  - in poor CYP2D6 metabolisers (5–10% of Caucasians).
  - by the SSRIs
    - — fluoxetine   — paroxetine
- Codeine tablets are 15 mg, 30 mg, maximum dose 260 mg/day (morphine equivalent 24 mg).
- It is often given in combination with paracetamol as co-codamol.
  - This comes in three strengths.
    - — 8 mg codeine/500 mg paracetamol
    - — 15 mg codeine/500 mg paracetamol
    - — 30 mg codeine/500 mg paracetamol
  - At maximum dosage these are given as two tablets qds.
  - This equates to a daily morphine equivalence of 6 mg and 24 mg respectively.

Dihydrocodeine
- Dihydrocodeine is of equivalent strength to codeine orally although it is twice as strong parenterally.
- If a patient's pain is not controlled on codeine there will be no benefit in switching to dihydrocodeine.
- Dihydrocodeine tablets are 30 mg, 40 mg or 60 mg, maximum dose 240 mg/day (morphine equivalent 24 mg).
- It can be given in combination with paracetamol as co-dydramol
  - This comes in three strengths:
    - — paracetamol 500 mg/dihydrocodeine 10 mg
    - — paracetamol 500 mg/dihydrocodeine 20 mg
    - — paracetamol 500 mg/dihydrocodeine 30 mg

- At maximum dosage these are given as two tablets qds.
- This equates to a daily morphine equivalence of 8 mg, 16 mg and 24 mg respectively.

Tramadol

- Tramadol is an opioid analgesic but also exerts analgesia via central serotonergic and adrenergic effects in a similar way to tricyclic antidepressants, and may therefore have slightly more efficacy in neuropathic pain.
- Like codeine it has little effect in poor CYP2D6 metabolizers.
- It is also an opioid for mild to moderate pain, but is twice as potent as codeine.
- It causes less constipation and less respiratory depression than morphine.
- Standard dosing is 50–100 mg qds PO although there are also 100–200 mg MR bd preparations available. The maximum daily dose is 400 mg (morphine equivalent 80 mg).

Morphine

- Morphine is generally the first line opioid for moderate to severe cancer pain.
- Morphine is effective and widely available in oral and parenteral preparations.

Oral morphine preparations

- Morphine (normal release) is available as liquid (Oramorph) or tablets (Sevredol).
- Onset of action is 20–30 minutes and duration of action is 3–6 hours.
- Oral morphine (NR) preparations are therefore given q4h to maintain analgesia.
- If there is renal impairment give at 6–8-hourly intervals or switch to an alternative opioid.

Modified release morphine

- This is most commonly prescribed as the 12-hourly preparations MST Continus or Zomorph.
- It is important that these are taken at 12-hourly intervals to avoid peaks and troughs of analgesia.
- Morphine (MR) preparations should be avoided if there is any degree of renal impairment as morphine and its metabolites will accumulate.

Breakthrough doses of morphine

- Patients on regular morphine should have additional doses of morphine (NR) available q4h prn for pain that 'breaks through' the regular dose.
- The breakthrough dose is calculated as one-sixth of the total daily dose of regular morphine whether this is being given as NR or MR morphine.

Patients often express concerns about starting morphine
- They may be concerned that they may become addicted.
  - Although morphine causes a physiological dependency with chronic use, psychological addiction is not a problem when it is used appropriately as an analgesic.
- They may be concerned that morphine will shorten their prognosis.
  - There is no evidence for this if morphine is correctly titrated, in which case patients can take morphine safely for months or years.

Morphine titration
- If the patient is still in pain, increase the total daily morphine dose by 30–50% daily.
- Alternatively, a new total daily dose of morphine can be calculated by adding the total of prn morphine required over the previous 24 hours to the old total daily dose.
- The prn 'breakthrough' dose must then be recalculated as one-sixth of the new total daily dose.
- Titration can continue until either:
  - the patient is free of pain
  - a ceiling of unacceptable side effects is reached
- There is no maximum limit to titration of morphine but it is rare to reach a total daily dose above 600 mg.
- If rapid titration is needed or pain levels are very unstable it is safer to titrate on NR morphine and switch to 12-hourly MR morphine only when pain has stabilized and morphine needs are established.

Parenteral morphine and diamorphine
The SC route is generally preferable to IV for stat parenteral doses as it is safer and gives more sustained analgesia. The IV route may occasionally be necessary for patients in acute severe pain.
- Morphine
  - Parenteral morphine is twice as potent as oral morphine so when converting from oral to parenteral morphine divide the dose by two.
  - Like oral morphine (NR), parenteral morphine needs to be given 4-hourly to maintain analgesia.
    — In practice it is usually given as a continuous SC infusion via a syringe driver or as an IV infusion via a PCA pump.
      – In a syringe driver it can be mixed with many of the drugs used for symptom control.
- Diamorphine
  - Parenteral diamorphine is three times as potent as oral morphine so when converting from oral morphine to parenteral diamorphine divide the dose by three.
  - It is often preferred when available in the UK because of its greater solubility.
    — This allows larger doses to be given in smaller volumes and facilitates mixing with combinations of other drugs in a SC syringe driver.

Side effects of morphine

- Constipation
  - This is an almost invariable side effect of strong opioids unless the patient has an ileostomy or fast bowel transit (see Constipation p54)
- Dry mouth
  - Occurs in most patients
  - Advise regular drinks or chewing gum
- Nausea
  - Opioids may precipitate nausea and vomiting by two routes
    — Gastric stasis
    — 'chemical nausea' acting via the chemoreceptor trigger zone
  - A regular antiemetic such as metoclopramide or haloperidol is often needed when morphine is started but can usually be stopped after 1 week (see Nausea and vomiting p38)
- Pruritus and sweating
  - Consider an alternative strong opioid
  - Pruritus may respond to a 5-HT$_3$ antagonist
  - Refer to specialist palliative care if persistent
- Sedation
  - This is common on first starting morphine or after an increase in dose
  - It usually resolves after a few days
  - Persistent sedation is a sign of
    — central toxicity
    — poor tolerance
  - The morphine dose may be too high or a switch to an alternative strong opioid should be considered
  - Check renal function to ensure that morphine is not accumulating
  - Consider other causes of sedation
    — hypercalcaemia
    — deranged liver function
- Central morphine toxicity
  - Clinical features
    — cognitive impairment
    — hallucinations
    — myoclonus
  - These may occur if:
    — The morphine dose is too high
      - a level of morphine that was previously tolerated may now cause toxicity if pain levels have dropped after
        - nerve block
        - radiotherapy
        - chemotherapy
    — There is accumulation of morphine or its metabolites
      - renal impairment
    — The patient is poorly tolerant of morphine.

- Management
  - Check for renal impairment and dehydration
  - Reduce morphine dose
  - Consider other causes of cognitive impairment (see Drowsiness and decreased GCS 📖 p70)
  - Haloperidol 1.5–5 mg PO/SC nocte may help confusion and hallucinations
  - Myoclonus can be helped by a regular benzodiazepine if severe
  - Consider an alternative strong opioid
- Respiratory depression
  - Pain is a physiological antagonist to the respiratory depressant effects of morphine
  - Effects on respiration will usually be preceded by sedation and/or central toxicity
  - It is rare to encounter this problem in the management of cancer pain if opioids are appropriately titrated
  - Management
    - Indications for naloxone (see p14)
    - Check for renal impairment and dehydration
    - Reduce or stop morphine
      - A level of morphine that was previously tolerated may now cause respiratory depression if pain levels have dropped after
        - nerve block
        - radiotherapy
        - chemotherapy

Alternative opioids for moderate to severe pain

- Opioids differ in their receptor profile, their distribution, and their metabolism.
- There is no evidence that one opioid causes any less sedation or central toxicity than another. There is, however, extensive experience that if one opioid is effective but poorly tolerated then a switch to an alternative opioid may give equivalent analgesia with less sedation or central toxicity.

Fentanyl transdermal patches

- Fentanyl is a synthetic and highly lipophilic opioid.
- It appears to be less constipating than morphine at analgesic equivalence.
- Fentanyl is converted to an inactive metabolite in the liver and does not appear to accumulate or cause toxicity in renal failure.
- Fentanyl transdermal patches are designed to release fentanyl at a steady rate and to be replaced every 72 hours. When started plasma levels take 36–48 hours to achieve steady state and after removal of the patch the elimination half life is 13–22 hours.
- Patches are available in five strengths:
  - 12 μg/hour
  - 25 μg/hour
  - 50 μg/hour
  - 75 μg/hour
  - 100 μg/hour
  - Intermediate doses and doses >100 μg/hour can be obtained by combining patches of different strengths.

- Changing from morphine to fentanyl patches.
  - Fentanyl takes 12 hours to reach analgesic levels.
    — morphine will need to continue during this time to keep the patient free of pain. This is often achieved by putting the first fentanyl patch on at the same time as the last dose of morphine MR is given (usually at night).
  - Some patients may experience opioid withdrawal symptoms when converting from morphine to fentanyl patches.
    — these last only a few days and are helped by prn doses of morphine.
  - Patients on fentanyl patches will still need morphine for breakthrough pain, at a dose of one-sixth of the equivalent total daily dose of morphine (see Table 1.2).
  - Fentanyl should be titrated cautiously due to its long half life; toxicity may continue for up to 24 hours or longer after a patch has been removed.
- Indications for switching from morphine to fentanyl patches:
  - Constipation with morphine in spite of high dose laxatives.
  - Partial/subacute bowel obstruction.
  - Loss of the oral route.
  - Impaired renal function or renal failure.
  - Pain is morphine-responsive but titration is limited by sedation or central toxicity.
- Contraindications to the use of fentanyl patches:
  - Unstable pain
    — including recent treatment such as radiotherapy that could lower pain levels.
  - Severe pain requiring rapid opioid titration.
- Cautions:
  - Sweating may prevent patch adherence and reduce effective dose.
  - Fever or close external heat sources (hot water bottles and electric blankets) will increase rate of fentanyl absorption from patch and increase dose.

Oral transmucosal fentanyl citrate (OTFC)
- This is a lozenge preparation designed to be absorbed by rubbing against the buccal mucosa.
- Onset of analgesia is 5–10 minutes and its duration is 1–3 hours.
- It is indicated for episodic pain of short duration and may be tried if oral morphine (NR) has too slow an onset or is poorly tolerated.
- There is no relationship between the background opioid level and the required dose of OTFC.
  - It must always therefore be titrated up from the lowest dose lozenge (200 µg).

Table 1.2 Conversion of regular morphine to fentanyl patches

Total daily dose morphine (mg)	Fentanyl patch (µg/hour)
30	12
60–90	25
120	37
180	50
240	75
300	100

The patch size (in µg/hour) is approximately one-third of the total daily dose of morphine (mg). Conversions are approximate and vary between individuals. Patients need to be carefully monitored for inadequate analgesia or toxicity.

Oxycodone
- Oxycodone has similar properties to morphine and is available in equivalent preparations.
- Oxycodone (Oxynorm) is given 4–6-hourly and is available as capsules or liquid.
- Oxycodone MR (Oxycontin) is given 12-hourly as tablets.
- As with morphine the MR preparation should be avoided in patients with renal impairment and the NR preparation should be used at 8-hourly intervals.
- Breakthrough doses are calculated as for morphine.
- When converting from oral morphine to oral oxycodone, divide the dose by two.
- Parenteral oxycodone is also available and can be given as a SC infusion.
  - The manufacturers recommend dividing the dose by two when changing from oral to parenteral oxycodone.
    - this may represent an underdosing for some patients.
- Indications for switching from morphine to oxycodone
  - Pain responds to morphine but titration is limited by sedation or central toxicity.

Hydromorphone
- Hydromorphone also has similar properties to morphine and is available in 4-hourly and 12-hourly MR preparations.
- To convert from oral morphine to hydromorphone divide the dose by 7.5
  - The strength of tablets available reflects this conversion ratio.
- Hydromorphone is less widely used than oxycodone and the parenteral preparation is not generally available in the UK.
- Hydromorphone clearance is not changed in renal impairment although its metabolites may accumulate.

- Indications for switching from morphine to hydromorphone:
  - Pain responds to morphine but titration is limited by sedation or central toxicity.
  - Used by some units in renal failure (seek specialist palliative care advice).

Methadone

- Methadone has a high volume of distribution and a variable half life of 8–75 hours. It accumulates with repeated dosing and conversion from morphine is complex. It should only be started under the supervision of a specialist palliative care or pain team.
- Possible indications for switching from morphine to methadone:
  - Pain responds to morphine but titration is limited by sedation or central toxicity.
  - Renal failure.

Management of iatrogenic opioid overdose

- Patients stabilized on strong opioids for severe cancer pain should not be given large IV boluses of naloxone (0.4 mg to 2 mg as in the treatment of an overdose for an addict) as they may be plunged directly into severe pain plus symptoms of opioid withdrawal.
- If the symptoms of opioid toxicity are not severe then they can be managed by reducing or stopping the opioid.
  - If respiratory rate >8 bpm, the patient is easily rousable and not cyanosed then the opioid should be stopped and the patient carefully monitored for recurrence of pain. The opioid can then be re-titrated with a NR preparation when pain returns (see opioid titration p9).
- IV naloxone for iatrogenic opioid overdose.
  - Indications
    - Respiratory rate <8 bpm.
    - Patient barely rousable/unconscious.
    - Patient cyanosed or SaO_2 <90% on pulse oximeter.
  - Administration
    - Give oxygen.
    - Dilute a 400 µg ampoule of naloxone to 10 ml with 0.9% saline.
    - Give naloxone 40 µg (1 ml) increments every 2 minutes until respiratory function is satisfactory and the patient is rousable.
    - Flush with 0.9% saline between doses.
    - The duration of action of naloxone is 15–90 minutes.
      - return to the patient every 15 minutes and give additional bolus if necessary.
    - Anticipate the possible duration of opioid toxicity according to the duration of action of the preparation of opioid that has been given. This may be lengthened in renal impairment.
    - If a MR preparation of opioid has been given or a fentanyl patch is present it may be necessary to set up an IV infusion of naloxone based on the patient's requirements over the first 30–60 minutes.

Management of acute severe pain

Oral morphine

- Give morphine doses at regular 4-hourly intervals; give prn doses up to every 30 minutes.
  - If the patient is opioid-naive start at 5–10 mg PO (2.5–5 mg SC/IM).
    - 2.5–5 mg PO (1.25–2.5 mg SC/IM) in the very frail/elderly.
  - If already on an opioid, use the current prn breakthrough dose.
  - If the patient has been on codeine/dihydrocodeine/tramadol and is still in pain then the starting dose of morphine should represent an increase on the morphine equivalence that they have been taking (see Table 1.1).
    - a patient on codeine 60 mg qds should start on morphine 10 mg q4h.
- Monitor for sedation, confusion, and respiratory compromise.
- Convert to a regular 4-hourly dose or syringe driver once opioid needs are established.
- Avoid MR opioids until the pain has stabilized and opioid needs are established.
- Once the pain has settled on regular morphine doses consider switching to a MR preparation for convenience of dosing, if morphine is well tolerated.
  - total the doses given over 24 hours and give as two divided MR doses 12 hours apart.
- Warn the patient that they may feel sedated for a few days after starting morphine.
  - therefore advise caution with driving although there is no legal restriction on driving whilst on opioids.
- Start the patient on a laxative:
  - senna 7.5–15 mg *nocte*
  - co-danthrusate 1–3 capsules *nocte*
  - increase the dose of any laxatives they are already taking (see Constipation 📖 p54)
- Prescribe an anti-emetic on a prn basis:
  - metoclopramide 10 mg tds
  - haloperidol 1.5 mg *nocte*

Intravenous morphine

- Consider using morphine IV if very rapid analgesia is needed.
  - Have naloxone 400 µg, oxygen, and resuscitation equipment available.
  - If not on an anti-emetic, give metoclopramide 10 mg IV.
  - Dose:
    - for opioid-naive patients: diamorphine 5 mg or morphine 10 mg.
    - for patients on opioids: diamorphine or morphine dose equivalent to their breakthrough dose.
    - draw up dose into 10 ml water for injection.
    - give 1 ml/minute IV until there is a significant reduction in pain or there are signs of opioid toxicity.
      - maximum 10 ml in 10 minutes.

- Monitor
  - conscious level
  - respiratory rate
- Check for
  - confusion
  - myoclonus
- Multiply the dose of diamorphine or morphine required in 10 minutes by six and give this as a continuous SC infusion over 24 hours.
- If the pain is not controlled and there are no signs of opioid toxicity, increase the dose of regular morphine (see morphine titration p9).

NSAIDs

- NSAIDs may also be useful in acute severe pain if there are no contraindications.

Other

- Try to establish the cause of pain and consider:
  - Does the patient need surgical referral?
    - acute abdomen
    - pathological fracture
  - Is there a role for a specific adjuvant?

Management of specific pains

Neuropathic pain

- This is pain associated with nerve compression or injury.
- Nerve damage may result in neuronal hyperexcitability at the site of injury and/or central sensitization of central pain pathways.
- A neuropathic component to pain may be suggested by:
  - Cancer in an anatomical area that could result in nerve compression or damage.
  - An area of skin numbness, paraesthesia or hyperaesthesia in the vicinity of the pain.
- Neuropathic pain usually responds to standard analgesics.
  - NSAIDs may help especially if there is also an inflammatory component to the pain.
  - Opioids are often effective and should be titrated up to the maximal tolerated dose.
  - In neuropathic pain there may, however, be a ceiling of unacceptable side effects with opioids before complete analgesia is achieved.
  - Adjuvants may be necessary.

Adjuvants for neuropathic pain

- Corticosteroids.
  - If nerve compression is caused by a tumour mass in a confined space (e.g. spinal canal, axilla or groin) then high dose steroids may relieve pressure and help with pain.
  - Dexamethasone 8 mg/PO/IM/IV/od.
    - Stop after 1 week if no benefit.
    - If there is a reduction in pain then gradually reduce to the lowest effective dose.

- Tricyclic antidepressants.
  - These drugs probably exert analgesia via the descending inhibitory pathways by blocking re-uptake of serotonin and noradrenaline.
  - Amitriptyline is the most widely used but analgesia is a class effect.
  - Doses for neuropathic pain are generally lower than for depression and onset of action is faster for analgesia (3–7 days) than depression (>2 weeks).
  - They are sedative and are best given at night.
  - Amitriptyline
    — Start at 10 mg *nocte*, titrate dose up to 50–100 mg *nocte*.
    — Beneficial effect will become apparent within 4–7 days.
    — Side effects are commonly a limiting factor.
    — Side effects:
      - sedation   – dry mouth
      - hypotension   – blurred vision
      - arrhythmia   – constipation
      - cognitive impairment   – urinary retention
- Anticonvulsants.
  - Different anticonvulsants have various actions in the pain pathways.
    — inhibition of excitatory systems.
    — enhancement of inhibitory systems.
    — reduction in the hyperexcitability of damaged nerves.
  - Gabapentin and carbamazepine are well supported by trial evidence for neuropathic pain but other anticonvulsants such as valproate have also been found to be effective in practice.
  - They are all used in standard anticonvulsant doses and, as in epilepsy, should be gradually withdrawn (over at least 1 week) rather than stopped abruptly.
  - Gabapentin
    — Fast titration
      - Day 1: 300 mg *nocte*, day 2: 300 mg bd, day 3: 300 mg tds
    — In frail or elderly patients
      - Day 1: 100 mg tds, day 7: 300 mg tds
    — Subsequently titrate according to response to a maximum of 3.6 g daily.
    — Decrease dose and frequency in renal impairment.
    — Side effects:
      - sedation   – ataxia
      - dizziness
  - Pregabalin
    — Start with 75 mg bd; titrate over next 7–10 days to maximum dose of 600 mg in 2–3 divided doses.
- Trial evidence shows similar effectiveness and tolerability for tricyclic antidepressants and anticonvulsants.
- It is reasonable to start with the class of drug whose side effect profile is likely to be better tolerated by the individual patient. If there is only a partial response to tricyclic antidepressants then anticonvulsants can be added in and vice versa.

- In difficult neuropathic pain consider referral to the pain team for consideration of:
  - ketamine
  - regional nerve block
    — local anaesthetic +/− corticosteroid
      - femoral block, e.g. fractured neck of femur
      - intercostal block, e.g. rib fracture
    — alcohol/phenol neurolysis
      - coeliac plexus block, e.g. pancreatic pain
  - epidural analgesia
    — opioid
    — local anaesthetic
    — corticosteroid
  - intrathecal analgesia
    — opioid
    — local anaesthetic
  - radiofrequency ablation
    — cordotomy for chest wall pain, e.g. mesothelioma

Bone pain
See Bone pain and pathological fracture 🕮 p220

Abdominal colic
- Colic arises from smooth muscle spasm.
- Treat any constipation present.
  - See Constipation 🕮 p54
  - Constipation will be worsened by opioids or anticholinergic drugs.
- Colic may respond poorly to opioids when it is secondary to:
  - bowel obstruction
  - bladder spasm
  - biliary spasm
    — may respond to NSAIDs SC/IM.
- Adjuvants for abdominal colic
  - Anticholinergic drugs
    — Bladder spasm
      - Oxybutinin PO 2.5–5 mg tds
      - Tolterodine PO 2 mg bd
    — Intestinal or biliary colic
      - Hyoscine butylbromide (Buscopan)
        • 20–40 mg SC qds
        • 20–80 mg/24 hours SC infusion via syringe driver.
        • Hyoscine butylbromide is poorly absorbed and is of limited effect orally.

Liver pain
- Multiple liver metastases or involvement of the liver capsule may cause intense RUQ abdominal pain which may be exacerbated by inspiration.
- There may be a palpable, tender liver and intercostal tenderness over the liver.
- Liver pain may respond to NSAIDs and opioids but a corticosteroid may be highly effective as an adjuvant and reduce the need for opioids.
  - Dexamethasone 8 mg od/IV/IM/PO.
    - Stop after 1 week if no benefit.
    - If there is a reduction in pain then gradually reduce to the lowest effective dose.
- Patients can present with acute severe liver pain secondary to a bleed into a liver metastasis (see Hepatic bleeding 📖 p262).
  - This may require rapid titration of opioids to achieve analgesia and prompt reduction of opioids once the acute episode has settled.

Rectal pain
- Rectal pain is associated with pelvic cancer (especially rectal cancer) and can be difficult to treat because it often has components of neuropathic pain and smooth muscle spasm.
- Patients may describe a sensation of rectal fullness (tenesmus).
- Constipation should always be excluded.
- If it is not controlled by standard analgesics then it can be managed as a neuropathic pain.
- Calcium channel blockers can be useful adjuvants in relieving smooth muscle spasm.
  - Nifedipine MR 10–20 mg bd.
    - Side effects:
      - headache
      - hypotension.

Somatization
- Some patients can become so overwhelmed by distress associated with psychological, social or spiritual factors that they present this distress as physical pain. In this situation, titrating up analgesics without addressing these other factors may lead to increasing side effects without apparent resolution of the pain.
- Consider early referral to:
  - psychology
  - psychiatry
  - palliative care team
  - hospital chaplaincy team.

When pain management is difficult

- Is there a problem with the absorption of oral analgesics?
  - Vomiting
  - Diarrhoea
- Check for and treat hypercalcaemia which may precipitate or exacerbate pain.
- Check for and treat hypomagnesaemia which may interfere with management of neuropathic pain.
- Check that a strong opioid has been maximally titrated.
- Consider whether there may be a neuropathic component to the pain.
- Is the patient anxious or depressed?
- Is there a component of psychological, social or spiritual distress to the pain?
- Consider referral to the palliative care or pain team.

Further reading

Davis, M., Glare, P. and Hardy, J.R. (eds) (2005). *Opioids in Cancer Pain*. Oxford: Oxford University Press.

Twycross, R.G., Wilcock, A. and Toller, C.S. (2007). *Symptom Management in Advanced Cancer*, 4th edn. palliativedrugs.com Ltd.

Twycross, R.G., Wilcock, A., Mortimer, J., Howard, P. and Charlesworth, S. (2007). *Palliative Care Formulary*, 3rd edn. palliativedrugs.com Ltd.

Watson, M., Lucas, C., Hoy, A. and Back, I. (eds) (2005). *Oxford Handbook of Palliative Care*. Oxford: Oxford University Press.

ⓘ **Dyspnoea**

Shortness of breath is an all too common and distressing symptom in the cancer patient.

The differential diagnosis is broad and must be narrowed down by detailed history-taking, examination, and further investigations.

Causes

Malignancy-related
- PE
- Pleural effusion
- Airway obstruction
- SVCO
- Pericardial effusion
- Lymphangitis carcinomatosis
- Ascites and abdominal distension
- Gross pleural thickening
- Wasting of respiratory muscles from cachexia
- Widespread pulmonary masses
  - Lung primary
  - Multiple metastases
- Diaphragm weakness owing to phrenic nerve palsy (mediastinal disease)

Treatment-related
- Radiation pneumonitis
- Pulmonary drug toxicity
- Hypersensitivity reaction
- Pneumothorax
- CCF
  - Cardiomyopathy
  - Arrhythmia
  - IV fluids/blood transfusion

Malignancy and treatment-related
- Pneumonia
  - Bacterial
  - Fungal
  - Viral
  - PCP
  - Mycobacterial
- Acute renal failure
  - Fluid overload
  - Metabolic acidosis
- Anaemia

Co-morbidity
- CCF
  - IHD
  - Arrhythmia
  - Decompensated valve disease
- Asthma
- Fibrosing lung disease
- Acute exacerbation of COPD
- Anxiety

Clinical features
Symptoms
- Speed of onset
  - Minutes/hours
  - Hours/days
  - Days/weeks
  - Weeks/months
- Cough
  - Dry
  - Productive
- Haemoptysis
- Chest pain
- Fever

Signs
- Stridor
- Wheeze
- Tracheal deviation
- Dull percussion
- Decreased air entry
- Crepitations
- Pleural rub
- Vocal resonance
- Unilateral reduced expansion
- Gallop rhythm, ↑ JVP, peripheral oedema

Investigations
Bloods
- FBC
  - Anaemia
  - Pneumonia
- U&Es
  - Acute renal failure
- CRP
  - Pneumonia
  - Metastatic disease
  - Radiation pneumonitis
  - PE
- ABG
  - To assess severity and CO_2 retention (COPD)
- Cardiac enzymes
  - IHD
- D-dimers
  - PE
- Blood culture
  - Pneumonia
- Atypical serology
  - Atypical pneumonia

Sputum
- MC&S
  - Pneumonia
- Cytology
  - Lung malignancy

ECG
- Ischaemia
  - IHD
  - CCF
- Abnormal rhythm
  - Arrhythmia
- Sinus tachycardia, $S_IQ_{III}T_{III}$, RV strain pattern
  - PE
- Small complexes
  - Pericardial effusion

CXR
- Unremarkable
  - SVCO
  - Pericardial effusion
  - Ascites
  - PE
  - Asthma
  - IHD
  - Hypersensitivity reaction
  - Upper airway obstruction
  - Anaemia
  - Metabolic acidosis
  - Acute exacerbation of COPD
- Multiple pulmonary masses
  - Pulmonary abscesses
  - Metastatic malignancy
- Collapse
  - Airway obstruction
- Consolidation
  - Malignancy
  - PE
  - Pneumonia
  - Pulmonary abscess
  - Encysted effusion
- Interstitial shadowing
  - CCF
  - Fibrosing lung disease
  - Radiation pneumonitis
  - Opportunistic infection
  - Lymphangitis carcinomatosis
  - Pulmonary drug toxicity
- Pleural effusion
- Pneumothorax

Further investigations
- CT scan
  - HRCT
- CTPA
- Respiratory function tests
  - PEFR
  - FEV_1, FVC, FEV_1/FVC
  - Gas transfer
  - Flow-volume loops
  - Lung volumes
- Bronchoscopy
  - Biopsy
  - Bronchoalveolar lavage
- V/Q scan
- Echo
- Mediastinoscopy and biopsy
- Pleural aspirate
- PET scan
- Pleural biopsy

Initial management
- Rapid assessment of Airway/Breathing/Circulation.
- Sit patient up and provide high flow oxygen (Take early ABG if possibility of COPD and reduce O_2 flow if evidence of CO_2 retention).
- Treat underlying cause:
  - SVCO (see Superior vena cava obstruction 📖 p92.)
  - PE (see Venous thromboembolism 📖 p98.)
  - Pericardial effusion (see Pericardial effusion and tamponade 📖 p110.)
  - Pleural effusion (see Malignant pleural effusion 📖 p128.)
  - Pneumothorax (see Pneumothorax 📖 p156.)
  - Airway obstruction (see Airway obstruction 📖 p140.)
  - Lymphangitis carcinomatosis (see Lymphangitis carcinomatosis 📖 p152.)
  - Ascites and abdominal distension (see Malignant ascites 📖 p244.)
  - Pulmonary drug toxicity (see Chemotherapy-related pulmonary toxicity 📖 p350.)
  - Radiation pneumonitis (see Radiation pneumonitis 📖 p382.)
  - A dying patient who is breathless (see The distressed dying patient 📖 p30.).

ⓘ *Widespread pulmonary malignancy*
- Oral morphine
  - if on morphine increase dose by 50%; if opioid-naive start with 2.5 mg q4h and increase to 5 mg q4h if necessary.
- Diazepam (if anxious)
  - 5–10 mg stat, 5–20 mg *nocte* (↓ dose in the elderly).
  - diazepam has a long therapeutic action (up to 36 hours) and accumulates (particularly in the elderly). Can consider a shorter acting benzodiazepine, e.g. lorazepam 0.5–1 mg bd.
- Refer to oncologist for consideration of treatment of underlying malignancy.

① *Pneumonia*
- Ensure patient is not neutropenic (see Infections in the neutropenic patient 🕮 p326).
- Assess severity (CURB-65 score) at time of admission (see Table 1.3).
  - **C**onfusion (MMSE <8)
  - **U**rea >7 mmol/l
  - **R**espiratory rate ≥30 bpm
  - **B**lood pressure
    — systolic <90 mmHg or diastolic ≤60 mmHg
  - **A**ge ≥**65** years

Table 1.3 CURB-65 score and mortality or ICU admission (%)

Score	Mortality or ICU admission (%)
0	0.7
1	3.2
2	13.0
3	17.0
4	41.5
5	57.0

- Patients with a CURB-65 score ≥2 require hospital admission for IV antibiotics and may require fluid resuscitation.
- Refer to local guidelines for choice of antibiotic,
  - CURB-65 0–1
    — Amoxicillin 500 mg tds PO for 7 days.
    — Clarithromycin 500 mg bd PO if penicillin-allergic.
  - CURB-65 2
    — Amoxicillin 500 mg to 1g tds PO/IV +/− clarithromycin 500 mg bd PO for 7 days.
    — Penicillin-allergic
      - Ceftriaxone 2 g od IV +/− clarithromycin 500 mg bd PO.
  - CURB-65 ≥3
    — Co-amoxiclav 1.2 g tds IV + clarithromycin 500 mg bd IV/PO.
    — Change to PO antibiotics after 3 days if clinically improving.
    — Penicillin-allergic
      - Ceftriaxone 2 g od IV + clarithromycin 500 mg bd IV/PO.
- Non-invasive ventilation or CPAP may be beneficial in patients with severe pneumonia.
- In patients who fail to improve with antibiotics consider:
  - Alternative diagnosis
    — PE   — progressive malignancy
    — pleural effusion   — lymphangitis carcinomatosis
  - Resistant pathogen
    — seek advice from microbiology team

- Complication of pneumonia
  - Empyema
  - ARDS
  - lung abscess
  - parapneumonic effusion

☼ CCF

- Furosemide IV 40–80 mg.
- Diamorphine IV 2.5–5 mg with metoclopramide IV 10 mg.
- Consider GTN infusion if SBP >90 mmHg.
- Accurate fluid balance
  - consider urinary catheter insertion and fluid restriction.
- Treat underlying cause for the acute deterioration in cardiac function.

⑦ Anaemia

- Blood transfusion if symptomatic.
- See Anaemia 🕮 p282.

☼ Acute exacerbation of COPD

- Nebulized bronchodilators
  - 5 mg salbutamol prn + 0.5 mg ipratropium qds.
- If the pCO_2 is raised, further retention can often be prevented by adjusting the FiO_2 (Venturi adaptor 24%/28%/35%) to give an SaO_2 of 88–92% (pO_2 >7.5 kPa) with verification of pCO_2 by ABG.
- Consider aminophylline infusion (0.5 mg/kg/h) if patient is not improving. Omit IV loading dose (5 mg/kg over 20 minutes) if patient on oral aminophylline.
- Corticosteroids
  - prednisolone 30 mg PO or hydrocortisone 100 mg IV.
- Treat cause for acute exacerbation
  - antibiotics for infective exacerbation if ↑sputum volume, purulent sputum or fever.
- Consider non-invasive ventilation if pH <7.26 with rising pCO_2 if patient is not responding to maximal medical therapy.
- Consider doxapram infusion only if the patient is failing to improve with non-invasive ventilation and the patient is hypoventilating.

☼ Asthma

- Assess severity (British Thoracic Society guidelines).
- Nebulized bronchodilators
  - 5 mg salbutamol prn +/– ipratropium 0.5 mg qds
- Corticosteroids
  - prednisolone 30 mg PO or hydrocortisone 100 mg IV
- Consider magnesium sulphate (1.2–2 g IV over 20 minutes) if acute severe asthma without good initial response to bronchodilator therapy.
- Refer to ICU if failing to respond to treatment (if appropriate).
- Whilst awaiting ICU support give IV loading dose (5 mg/kg over 20 minutes) of aminophylline, and then commence aminophylline infusion (0.5 mg/kg/h).

⑦ *Fibrosing lung disease*

- The therapeutic window for opioid use may be narrow in advanced hypoxic fibrosing lung disease.
- Oral morphine
  - If advanced lung disease and hypoxic, start with 1.25–2.5 mg q4h in opioid-naive patients or increase morphine dose by 25%.
  - If less advanced and not hypoxic, start with 2.5 mg q4h in opioid-naive patients and increase to 5 mg q4h if necessary; if already on morphine increase dose by 50%.
- Diazepam (if anxious)
  - 5–10 mg stat, 5–20 mg *nocte* (↓ dose in the elderly).
  - diazepam has a long therapeutic action (up to 36 hours) and accumulates (particularly in the elderly). Can consider a shorter acting benzodiazepine, e.g. lorazepam 0.5–1 mg bd.
- Refer to chest physician for assessment and treatment.

⑦ *Anxiety*

- Reassurance/calming presence/breathing exercises/relaxation therapy.
- Diazepam
  - 5–10 mg stat, 5–20 mg *nocte* (↓ dose in the elderly)
  - diazepam has a long therapeutic action (up to 36 hours) and accumulates (particularly in the elderly). Can consider a shorter acting benzodiazepine, e.g. lorazepam 0.5–1 mg bd.

Further reading

British Guideline on the Management of Asthma (2005) *A National Clinical Guideline*. British Thoracic Society. Scottish Intercollegiate Guidelines Network. www.brit-thoracic.org.uk
Chronic Obstructive Pulmonary Disease. (2004). *Management of Chronic Obstructive Pulmonary Disease in Adults in Primary and Secondary Care*. Clinical Guideline 12. www.nice.org.uk

ⓘ **The distressed dying patient**

In medical emergencies death is an outcome that we are usually trying to avoid. Death is, however, an inevitable outcome when cancer is recurrent or metastatic although treatment may delay it by some years. In advanced cancer there comes a point when aggressive management does not improve prognosis or prolong life that is of such poor quality that it is not valued by the patient. It is important to recognize this stage and to keep the patient and family as informed as they will allow.

For patients whose condition is deteriorating with advanced cancer the following questions should be considered before initiating treatment aimed at prolonging life:

- Is this an acute event or the final stage of a progressive deterioration?
- Are the causes of this deterioration reversible?
  - ICU is not appropriate for the majority of patients with advanced cancer.
- Are there any therapeutic options left that may improve the prognosis from the cancer?
  - this should be discussed with a senior oncologist.
- What is the patient's perception of his or her quality of life?
- Is there a realistic chance of return to a quality of life that will be of value to the patient?
- Is the patient dying?

Complications such as hypercalcaemia, renal failure, and chest infection may be correctable in the short term but treatment may not be in the patient's best interests if they recover only to face a period of further deterioration and distressing symptoms before they die. Honest and sensitive communication is necessary to assess how patients perceive their quality of life and to set realistic goals and expectations.

The diagnosis of dying

The diagnosis of dying is not always easy but it is important in order to avoid inappropriate treatment and investigations which may cause distress to the patient and their family. If there is any doubt it is always better to seek the opinion of more experienced colleagues. Experienced nurses frequently make this diagnosis before doctors as they are usually less focused on pathology and investigations and more aware of the global deterioration of the patient. It is essential for medical and nursing staff to be involved together in this decision.

The following can be helpful indicators in the context of advanced cancer:

- The patient is profoundly weak and bed-bound.
- They are semi-comatose.
- They are unable to take oral medication.
- They are unable to take more than sips of water.

Management of the dying patient

The priorities at this stage are:
- Comfort
- Good symptom control
- Clear, sensitive communication with the patient and their family

A patient dying with distress is a medical emergency. It is not just the patient who suffers but also the attending family, friends, nursing, and medical staff who may be deeply affected psychologically. A 'bad death' can contribute to difficult bereavement issues that may last for years.

General management

- If the hospital has a care pathway for dying patients then it should be initiated (e.g. The Liverpool Care Pathway).
- The patient should be designated 'Do Not Attempt Resuscitation'.
- If the hospital palliative care team are not involved then they should be contacted
  - if symptom control is complex or difficult.
  - if there are difficult communication issues with the patient or family.
  - if the medical or nursing team are not adequately skilled to manage the situation.
- Cancel investigations, including blood tests that are not going to alter management.
- Discontinue nursing interventions that are now inappropriate
  - monitoring vital signs.
- Discontinue medication that will have no impact on the patient's symptoms
  - this may include antibiotics.
- Convert essential medication where possible to the SC route
  - set up a syringe driver if necessary.
- Consider urinary catheterization.

Communication

- If the patient is still responsive and lucid then insight into their condition should be assessed and they should be sensitively offered the opportunity to discuss prognosis and plan of care as far as they wish.
- The patient should be given the opportunity to express any religious or spiritual needs and offered the support of the chaplaincy team or representative of their own faith as appropriate.
- If deterioration is unexpected or the family is not aware of it then they should be contacted as a matter of priority.
- The family should be given the opportunity to discuss the patient's condition and plan of care with medical and nursing staff in a quiet, private, and uninterrupted environment.
- Patients and families will often ask 'how long?' It is usually not possible to give an exact time but this question can be answered in general terms from the speed of deterioration.
  - If the patient is deteriorating every
    — week the prognosis is probably 'weeks'.
    — day the prognosis is probably 'days'.
    — hour the prognosis is probably 'hours'.

- When the patient is 'minutes' or 'hours' away from death it becomes easier to anticipate because of:
  - deepening coma
  - variable respiratory pattern
  - poor peripheral circulation.
- It is good practice to inform the patient's general practitioner and any consultant who has been recently involved in the patient's care that they are now dying.

Symptom control
Pain
- Assessment
  - If the patient is responsive, pain should be assessed in the usual way.
  - Once they become unresponsive you have to rely on non-verbal cues.
  - The most useful indicators are:
    — grimacing
    — groaning
    — muscle tension in areas of pain.
  - If there is any doubt, give a breakthrough dose of SC morphine and monitor the apparent level of distress.
- Management
  - See also Pain 🕮 p2.
  - If there is any difficulty with oral medication, regular PO opioids should be converted to a SC infusion of diamorphine (see Pain 🕮 p2 for conversion).
  - If the patient is dying of renal failure, the opioid level may need to be reduced.
    — Myoclonus can be managed with a SC midazolam infusion.
  - If the patient has a fentanyl patch, leave the patch in place as taking it off will result in unpredictable opioid levels for the next 24 hours.
    — Give any additional regular opioid that is required as a SC infusion of diamorphine.
    — When calculating the breakthrough dose of prn SC diamorphine required, the total daily dose of opioid will include the fentanyl patch and the SC diamorphine infusion.
  - Patients who have not had significant pain and are opioid-naive may develop a generalized musculoskeletal pain when they are bed-bound and dying.
    — This usually responds well to low dose diamorphine SC 10–20 mg/24 hours.
  - If oral NSAIDs have been important for pain control, they can be converted to:
    — Tenoxicam SC 20 mg od   — Diclofenac PR 50 mg bd
    — Alternatively the dose of opioid can be increased to compensate.

- If the patient is using co-analgesics such as tricyclic antidepressants or anticonvulsants, the opioid levels may need to be increased once the levels of these drugs have significantly reduced.
  - Increased sedation with midazolam or levomepromazine may be necessary.
- Dexamethasone can be continued as a SC stat dose in the morning on a 1:1 conversion ratio but is usually not necessary in the terminal phase unless the patient has been symptomatic with headache from raised intracranial pressure.

Breathlessness

- To die with severe breathlessness is often an overriding fear for patients with any kind of lung disease.
- Patients must be reassured that this symptom can be relieved when they are dying but they may have to be sedated to achieve adequate relief.
- Slowly progressive breathlessness:
  - This can be managed with a SC infusion of morphine 10–20 mg/24 hours plus midazolam 10–20 mg/24 hours.
    - If the patient is already taking morphine, increase the dose by 25%.
    - If breathlessness worsens increase the morphine in increments of 50% and the midazolam titrated up to 60 mg/24 hours.
- Rapidly progressive breathlessness:
  - Patients who are dying consequent to rapidly deteriorating respiratory function are in severe distress and need urgent attention.
  - Sedation is usually the only way to provide relief and midazolam needs to be titrated rapidly.
    - Midazolam SC 5–10 mg stat doses should be repeated until the patient is comfortable, at half hour intervals if necessary.
    - Morphine SC 5–10 mg can be given with the midazolam and will help to reduce respiratory distress.
    - Midazolam IV 5–10 mg may be needed in severe cases.
  - If the patient lives long enough to require a SC infusion then it can be given as above but with midazolam doses of 30–60 mg/24 hours.

Vomiting

- See Nausea and vomiting 📖 p38.
- Medication needed for the control of nausea and vomiting should be continued by the SC route in the terminal phase.

Restlessness and agitation

- There are many potential causes of restlessness, agitation, and cognitive failure in the terminal phase of cancer.

  - sepsis
  - renal failure
  - accumulation of drugs
    - opioid toxicity
  - liver failure
  - cerebral metastases
  - hypoxia

- It is not usually possible at this stage to single out or treat a specific cause.
  - It is important to exclude urinary retention.
  - It is worth considering a reduction in opioids if the patient is not in pain and there are signs of opioid toxicity (see Pain 📖 p2).
- The priority is to use appropriate drugs to gain control of the symptoms (see Table 1.4).
- Attention to the patient's surroundings is also important, with familiar faces, and a peaceful quiet environment.
- If symptoms do not settle, seek specialist palliative care advice.
- Occasionally agitation is resistant to midazolam 20–100 mg/24 hours and levomepromazine 12.5–200 mg/24 hours and may require a SC infusion of phenobarbital.

Table 1.4 Drugs for terminal restlessness and agitation

Drug and action	Dose	Indication
Midazolam Sedative Muscle relaxant Anticonvulsant	2.5–5 mg SC stat 20–100 mg/24 hours SC infusion Titrate to 20–40 mg/24 hours if necessary Higher doses will be required with previous regular use of benzodiazepines or alcohol	Restlessness Muscle stiffness Seizures If given alone with cognitive failure it may worsen agitation
Haloperidol Antipsychotic Anti-emetic	1–3 mg PO/8 hours 5–15 mg/24 hours SC infusion or regular *nocte* dose	Agitation and cognitive failure Use with midazolam to avoid stiffness Effective anti-emetic
Levomepromazine Sedative Antipsychotic Anti-emetic Analgesic	25–50 mg SC stat 12.5–200 mg/24 hours SC infusion or regular *nocte* dose Titrate to 200 mg/24 hours if necessary	Restlessness and agitation second line Use with midazolam to avoid stiffness Effective anti-emetic

Upper respiratory tract secretions ('death rattle')
- These can be reduced using anticholinergic drugs, but they are usually difficult to control completely.
- The family may need to be reassured that, if the patient is unconscious, they will not be distressed by the secretions.
- Better control is often achieved if they are treated early.
- They may be helped by positioning the patient on the side.

- Suction is best avoided except in severe cases.
- Drugs for upper respiratory tract secretions.
  - Hyoscine butylbromide
    — 20 mg SC stat and 20–60 mg/24 hours by SC infusion.
  - Glycopyrronium
    — 200 µg SC stat and 0.6–1.2 mg/24 hours by SC infusion.
  - Hyoscine hydrobromide
    — 400 µg–600 µg SC stat and 0.6–2.4 mg/24 hours by SC infusion.
    — The disadvantage of hyoscine hydrobromide is that it crosses the blood–brain barrier and may contribute to cognitive failure and agitation (unlike hyoscine butylbromide and glycopyrronium).

Nutrition and hydration

- If nutrition and hydration need to be given by a non-oral route then, under UK law, they constitute medical treatments rather than basic human rights.
- For patients and families, however, they remain deeply symbolic of survival and this area often needs very sensitive communication.
- If the patient is still responsive and competent, then his or her wishes are paramount.
- At this stage, comfort is the primary goal and this can usually be achieved without recourse to artificial nutrition or hydration.
- The following guidelines are appropriate in the context of a patient who is dying in a matter of a few hours or days.
  - It is normal for patients who are dying to lose interest in food and fluid.
  - Artificial nutrition will not affect the outcome in this context.
  - Artificial nutrition that has already been started can be stopped unless the patient or family remains against this in spite of adequate explanation.
  - Symptoms of thirst can usually be alleviated by sips of water from a cup or sponge and good mouth care.
  - If patients remain symptomatically thirsty in spite of these measures then intravenous or subcutaneous fluids can be considered.
  - If they are bed-bound and dying, the infusion rate need not be more than 1–2 litres/24 hours.
  - If parenteral fluids do not help with thirst, they can be stopped.
  - If the family cannot accept that parenteral fluids are not necessary then it may be appropriate to continue them rather than provoke conflict and risk a complicated bereavement.

Syringe drivers and the SC route
- Most dying patients will not be able to manage oral medication.
- If medication is needed then a continuous SC infusion via a syringe driver has several advantages over the IV and IM routes.
  - Once established it maintains fairly constant blood levels of drugs and avoids peaks and troughs.
  - It is not painful and avoids the need for repeated injections.
  - The syringe driver usually only needs to be changed every 24 hours.
- The patient may well continue to require 'breakthrough' medication for pain and other symptoms.
  - Repeated SC doses can be given without repeat injections by placing a second SC butterfly needle for this purpose.
- Combinations of drugs can be safely and effectively given in the same syringe driver.
- No more than three drugs should be given in the same syringe unless under the supervision of the palliative care team.
- Haloperidol and levomepromazine have a 24-hour action and can be effectively given as a single SC dose at night.

Further reading

Ellershaw, J. and Wilkinson, S. (2003). *Care of the Dying — A Pathway to Excellence*. Oxford: Oxford University Press.
The Liverpool Care Pathway. www.lcp-mariecurie.org.uk

⑦ **Nausea and vomiting**

Nausea and vomiting is very common in cancer patients (up to 50%), especially those receiving chemotherapy (70–80%). Nausea and vomiting contributes significantly to the morbidity of cancer and its treatment. It is important to determine the underlying cause for the vomiting as this guides treatment. In many cases the causes of vomiting are multifactorial. This requires an understanding of the sites of action of the anti-emetics and a logical approach to their use to achieve control of this distressing symptom.

Causes

Chemical/metabolic
- Characteristics
  - Nausea may be continuous
  - Nausea is often not relieved by vomiting
- Chemotherapy
- Radiotherapy
  - Abdominal/pelvic
  - Cranial
  - TBI
- Opioids
- High serum digoxin or carbamazepine
- Uraemia
- Hypercalcaemia
- Infection
- Carcinomatosis
- Antibiotics
- Antifungals

Gastric stasis/gastric outlet obstruction
- Characteristics
  - Abdominal distension
  - Abdominal fullness/bloating after eating
  - Intermittent nausea
  - Nausea relieved by vomiting
- Opioids
- Anticholinergic drugs
- Peptic ulceration/gastritis
  - NSAIDs
- Carcinoma of gastrointestinal tract
- Previous gastric surgery
- Autonomic failure
- Hepatomegaly
- Corticosteroids

Bowel obstruction
See Gastrointestinal obstruction 📖 p238.

Regurgitation
- Characteristics
  - Dysphagia
  - Regurgitation of food after swallowing
- Oesophageal tumour/stricture
- Mediastinal tumour/lymphadenopathy
- Pharyngeal/oesophageal candidiasis

Cranial disease/treatment

- Characteristics
  - Nausea and vomiting often worse in morning
  - Headache
  - Neurological signs (sometimes)
- Raised intracranial pressure
- Brainstem/meningeal disease
- Cranial radiotherapy

Movement-related

- Characteristics
  - Exacerbated by movement
- Vestibular disease
- Base of skull tumour

Clinical features

History

- Is the patient troubled principally by nausea or vomiting?
- Is the nausea relieved by vomiting?
- How soon after ingestion does vomiting occur?
- Is there dysphagia or dyspepsia?
- Any recent chemotherapy or radiotherapy?
- Any recent drug changes?
  - 30% of patients feel nauseated when starting opioids.
- Any changes in bowel habit?
- Associated symptoms
  - Colicky abdominal pain may suggest obstruction.
  - Sedation and confusion may suggest hypercalcaemia or renal failure.
  - Headache and neurological symptoms may suggest an intracerebral cause.
  - Vertigo may suggest vestibular disease.

Examination

- Check mucous membranes and skin turgor for dehydration.
- Oral *Candida*
  - There may be oesophageal candidiasis with no signs in the mouth.
- Enlarged or tender liver
- Abdominal distension or masses
- Bowel sounds
- Consider rectal examination for faecal impaction
- Neurological examination and fundoscopy

Investigations

Bloods

- U&Es
  - dehydration
  - renal failure
  - hypokalaemia
  - hyponatraemia
- Ca^{2+}
  - hypercalcaemia
- LFTs
- Digoxin or carbamazepine levels

Imaging
- AXR
  - bowel obstruction
  - constipation
- CT brain
  - cerebral metastases
  - base of skull metastases
- Upper GI endoscopy
  - oesophageal stricture
  - gastritis
  - gastric outlet obstruction
  - peptic ulceration
- Gastrografin swallow/meal
  - upper GI obstruction
  - gastric dysmotility

Management

- Most patients with nausea and vomiting can be managed as an outpatient.
  - Adequate oral intake to maintain hydration status.
  - Not hypotensive.
  - No electrolyte imbalance.
- If the patient is severely dehydrated, drowsy or confused then start IV rehydration and perform blood tests immediately.
- If the patient is distressed by severe nausea and/or vomiting consider giving a broad spectrum anti-emetic such as cyclizine 50 mg SC/IV prior to further assessment.
- Rehydrate patient
  - If patient is hypotensive or tachycardic give IV fluids.
  - If patient is oliguric give IV fluids and insert a urinary catheter to monitor urinary output (aim >0.5 ml/kg/h) (see Acute renal failure 📖 p268).
- Correct hypokalaemia
  - 20–40 mmol KCl in each litre of IV fluid.
- In persistent vomiting
  - Absorption by oral route may be poor.
  - Give essential medication by SC/IV routes.
- Review current medications
  - Consider stopping drugs which may be causative.
  - Do not stop opioids if the patient has been in pain but add an anti-emetic.
- Treat correctable causes
  - Hypercalcaemia
  - Uraemia
  - Candidiasis
  - Peptic ulceration/gastritis
  - Raised intracranial pressure
  - Constipation
  - Infection
- Anti-emetics
  - Anti-emetics should be given on a regular basis, and with a prn dose.
  - If oral absorption is poor because of continuous vomiting give SC/IV/PR.
  - If there is little response to the first anti-emetic after 24 hours:
    — Optimize the dose, taking account of prn doses used.
    — Change to an alternative anti-emetic
      – with a different receptor profile.

— Add in a second anti-emetic
  – with a different receptor profile.
  – antimuscarinic drugs (e.g. cyclizine) block the cholinergic pathway through which prokinetic drugs (e.g. metoclopramide, domperidone) act. Although the central effects of metoclopramide are not inhibited, a combination of cyclizine and metoclopramide is best avoided.
- If nausea/vomiting remains difficult to control, seek advice from the palliative care team.

Anti-emetics

Appropriate prescription of anti-emetics relies on identifying the underlying cause(s) for the nausea and vomiting. Anti-emetics are classified according to their receptor profile and their site of action depends on the distribution of receptors in the vomiting pathways (see Fig. 1.2 and Table 1.5). All causes of vomiting eventually pass through the vomiting centre.

Acting on gastrointestinal tract

- Prokinetic drugs
  - metoclopramide
  - domperidone
- Antisecretory drugs
  - hyoscine butylbromide
  - octreotide
- Anti-inflammatory
  - dexamethasone
- 5-HT_3 antagonists
  - granisetron
  - ondansetron

Chemoreceptor trigger zone (CTZ)

- D_2 antagonist
  - haloperidol
  - metoclopramide
- 5-HT_3 antagonists
  - ondansetron
  - granisetron

Vestibular nuclei

- Antihistamines/anticholinergic
  - cyclizine

Cerebral cortex

- Benzodiazepines
  - lorazepam
- Corticosteroids
  - dexamethasone

Vomiting centre

- Antihistamines/anticholinergic
  - cyclizine
- Anticholinergic
  - hyoscine hydrobromide
- 5-HT_2 antagonists
  - levomepromazine

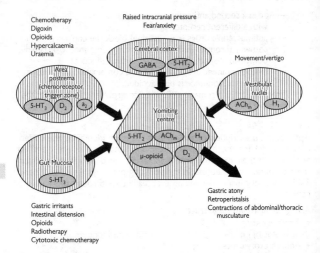

Fig. 1.2 Schematic of the vomitting pathways showing distribution of relevant receptors. (Adapted from Twycross, R.G., Wilcock, A. and Toller, C.S (2007). *Symptom Management in Advanced Cancer*, 4th edn. Palliativedrugs.com Ltd.)

Table 1.5 Common anti-emetics

Anti-emetic	Receptor profile and site of action	Clinical indication
Metoclopramide	Prokinetic UGI tract	Gastric stasis
10–20 mg qds PO/SC (pre-meal)	D_2 antagonist	Functional GI obstruction
30–100 mg/24 hour SC infusion	5-HT$_4$ agonist	
	5-HT$_3$ >100 mg/24 hour	
	CTZ	Chemical/metabolic
	D_2 antagonist	Cytotoxic chemotherapy
	5-HT$_3$ >100 mg/24 hour	Hypercalcaemia
		Uraemia
		Opioids
Domperidone	Prokinetic UGI tract	Gastric stasis
10–20 mg qds PO (pre-meal)	D_2 antagonist	
60 mg bd PR	No action inside blood–brain barrier so no extrapyramidal side effects	
Haloperidol	CTZ	Chemical/metabolic
2.5–10 mg/24 hours PO/SC	D_2 antagonist	Cytotoxic chemotherapy
		Hypercalcaemia
		Uraemia
		Opioids
Cyclizine	Vomiting centre	Mechanical GI obstruction
50 mg tds PO/SC	ACh	↑ ICP
150 mg/24 hour SC infusion	H_1	
	Vestibular nuclei	
	ACh	Movement-related
	H_1	
Granisetron	CTZ	Cytotoxic chemotherapy
1–2 mg od PO/SC	5-HT$_3$	Radiotherapy
Ondansetron	GI tract	GI obstruction (2nd line)
8 mg bd PO/SC	5-HT$_3$	
Levomepromazine	Vomiting centre	Broad spectrum 2nd line
5–25 mg/24 hours SC	D_2	
6–25 mg/24 hours PO	5-HT$_2$	
	α_1	
	ACh	
Dexamethasone	Cerebral cortex	Cytotoxic chemotherapy
8–16 mg/daily PO	Mechanism unknown	Radiotherapy
	Anti-inflammatory	↑ ICP
	Adjunct in difficult emesis	Functional GI obstruction

Chemotherapy-associated nausea and vomiting

Effective anti-emetic therapy is vital for patients undergoing chemotherapy. Nausea and vomiting can lead to significant morbidity, delaying further cycles of treatment and may even lead to withdrawal from treatment.

Emetic risk

- High (>80%)
  - Cisplatin (>50 mg/m^2)
  - Dacarbazine
  - Cyclophosphamide (>1.5 g/m^2)
  - Methotrexate (>250 mg/m^2)
  - Carmustine (>250 mg/m^2)
- Moderate (30–80%)
  - Cisplatin (<50 mg/m^2)
  - Carboplatin
  - Lomustine
  - Doxorubicin
  - Liposomal doxorubicin
  - Cyclophosphamide (<1.5 g/m^2)
  - Epirubicin
  - Ifosfamide
  - Irinotecan
  - Oxaliplatin
  - Temozolamide
- Low (10–30%)
  - Mitomycin C
  - Mitoxantrone
  - Capecitabine
  - Cetuximab
  - Cyclophosphamide (oral)
  - Docetaxel
  - Etoposide
  - Procarbazine
  - Methotrexate (50–250 mg/m^2)
  - 5-FU
  - Gemcitabine
  - Paclitaxel
  - Permetrexed
  - Topotecan
  - Trastuzumab
  - Cytarabine (>1.0 g/m^2)
- Minimal (<10%)
  - Bleomycin
  - Bevacizumab
  - Chlorambucil
  - Fludarabine
  - Methotrexate (<50 mg/m^2)
  - Rituximab
  - Vinblastine
  - Vincristine
  - Vinorelbine
  - Hydroxycarbamide
  - Melphalan

Phases of nausea and vomiting

Acute

- <24 hours after administration.
- Incidence and severity depends on:
  - Drug
    - — emetogenic potential
    - — dose
    - — route of administration
    - — schedule
    - — infusion rate
    - — combination of drugs
  - Patient characteristics

Delayed

- >24 hours after administration.
- Particularly associated with highly emetogenic drugs.
- It can occur even when anti-emetics are effective in preventing acute nausea and vomiting.

Anticipatory
- Experiencing symptoms in the hours before receiving another chemotherapy treatment.
- It is a conditioned response to previous effects from chemotherapy and associated environmental stimuli.
- The most effective way to prevent the development of anticipatory nausea and vomiting is optimal prophylaxis against acute and delayed nausea and vomiting from the first cycle of chemotherapy.
- 20–65% of patients.
- Risk factors:
  - Moderate/severe post-chemotherapy nausea and vomiting.
  - High anxiety levels.
  - History of motion sickness.
  - High number of previous cycles of chemotherapy.
  - Younger age.

Management
Moderate and high emetic risk
- $5-HT_3$ antagonist PO/IV pre-chemotherapy and for 24 hours PO
  - granisetron 1–2 mg od
  - ondansetron 4–8 mg bd
- Dexamethasone 8–16 mg/24 hours
- Dopamine antagonist
  - domperidone 10–20 mg PO qds for 3 days and then prn
  - metoclopramide 10–20 mg PO qds for 3 days and then prn

Low emetic risk
- Dexamethasone 8–16 mg/24 hours
- Dopamine antagonist
  - domperidone 10–20 mg PO qds prn
  - metoclopramide 10–20 mg PO qds prn

Minimal emetic risk
- No routine prophylaxis
- Dopamine antagonist
  - domperidone 10–20 mg PO qds prn
  - metoclopramide 10–20 mg PO qds prn

Anticipatory nausea and vomiting
- Lorazepam PO 1–2 mg on morning of chemotherapy
- Behavioural and cognitive therapy

Not all patients will receive adequate control of nausea and vomiting on the above regimes. Individualization of anti-emetic prescribing is then required.

- Additional dexamethasone, for up to 1 week after chemotherapy, is the most useful agent for delayed emesis.

Radiotherapy-associated nausea and vomiting

The degree of nausea and vomiting depends on:
- Dose
  - per fraction
  - total dose
- Site
  - common sites
    - upper abdomen
    - whole abdomen
    - brain
    - TBI
- Size of field

Acute emesis usually occurs 30 minutes to 4 hours after radiotherapy treatment. Acute emesis is caused by release of 5-HT by cell death in the GI mucosa.

Management

- Oral 5-HT$_3$ antagonist 30 minutes before each fraction of abdominal radiotherapy.
  - Granisetron 1–2 mg PO od.
  - Ondansetron 4–8 mg PO od.
  - If nausea and vomiting remains a problem consider adding in dexamethasone 8–16 mg/24 hours.
- If nausea and vomiting occurs during radiotherapy to the brain
  - Examine patients for signs of raised intracranial pressure and treat accordingly (see Raised intracranial pressure 📖 p206).
- Patients receiving radiotherapy to other sites may develop nausea and vomiting; this can be managed with metoclopramide 10–20 mg PO qds.

Further reading

5-HT$_3$ receptor antagonists as anti-emetics in cancer. (2005). *Drug Ther. Bull.* **43**(8): 57–62.

Kris, M.G., Hesketh, P.J., Somerfield, M.R., Feyer, P., Clark-Snow, R., Koeller, J.M., Morrow, G.R., Chinnery, L.W., Chesney, M.J., Gralla, R.J. and Grunberg, S.M. (2006). *American Society of Clinical Oncology Guidelines for Antiemetics in Oncology: Update 2006.* www.asco.org

Twycross, R.G., Wilcox, A. and Toller, C.S. (2007). *Symptom Management in Advanced Cancer*, 4th edn. palliativedrugs.com Ltd.

⑦ **Diarrhoea**

Diarrhoea is the frequent passage of unformed liquid stools (>250 g/day). An accurate description of the patient's bowel habit is necessary as 'diarrhoea' has different meanings for different people.

The causes of diarrhoea in the cancer patient are often multifactorial.

Diarrhoea may be caused by any process which leads to:
- Malabsorption of food or fluid
- Inflammation of the GI mucosa
- Increased GI motility

Paradoxically it can also result from the impaired bowel motility of:
- Partial obstruction
- Faecal impaction

Diarrhoea may be the presenting symptom of rectal or colonic tumours.

Chemotherapy-induced diarrhoea is classified as:
- An increase of at least 2–3 more stools per day
- Causing waking at night
- An increase in loose, watery stoma output compared with before treatment

Causes
- Drugs
  - Laxatives
  - Chemotherapy
    - Any cytotoxic chemotherapy, especially
      - 5-FU/capecitabine   – Irinotecan
    - Tyrosine kinase inhibitors
      - Erlotinib (Tarceva)   – Gefitinib (Iressa)
  - Antibiotics
    - Macrolides (e.g. erythromycin) have a pro-motility action.
    - Broad spectrum antibiotics may predispose to *Clostridium difficile* infection
  - NSAIDs
  - Iron preparations
  - Sorbital as sweetener in drinks or sugar-free elixirs
  - Abrupt opioid withdrawal or switch from morphine to fentanyl
  - Antacids
- Abdominal/pelvic radiotherapy
  - Onset is usually after the first or second week of radiotherapy (10–20 Gy)
  - Resolution usually occurs within 4 weeks of completing radiotherapy
  - Damage to mucosa can result in:
    - release of prostaglandins   — malabsorption of bile salts
    - bacterial overgrowth   — lactose intolerance
    - alterations in GI motility
  - Increased risk if patient has IBD

- Malignancy
  - Partial bowel obstruction
  - Blood loss from GI tumour
  - Mucus secretion from colonic or rectal tumour
  - Enterocolic fistula
  - Pancreatic enzyme deficiency
    — pancreatic carcinoma
  - Biliary tract obstruction
  - Paraneoplastic visceral autonomic neuropathy
  - Hormone secretion by tumour
    — carcinoid tumours may secrete
      – serotonin   – bradykinin
      – prostaglandins   – VIP
    — medullary carcinoma of the thyroid
    — Zollinger–Ellison syndrome
    — VIPoma
- Infective
  - Bacterial or viral gastroenteritis
  - *Clostridium difficile* (pseudomembranous colitis)
    — usually associated with broad spectrum antibiotic therapy
    — can occur with low immunity and general debility
  - Bacterial overgrowth in bowel with no isolated pathogen
  - Typhlitis (see Gastrointestinal perforation 📖 p252)
- Constipation with faecal impaction and overflow
- Surgery resulting in malabsorption
  - Gastrectomy   • Ileal resection
  - Total or subtotal colectomy
  - Pancreaticoduodenectomy
- IBD

Clinical features

History
- Stool frequency   • Duration of diarrhoea
- Description of stool
  - steatorrhoea
    — pancreatic insufficiency   — biliary tract obstruction
  - bloody
    — infective cause
    — severe mucositis
      – radiotherapy   – chemotherapy
  - melaena
    — GI bleed
- Recent constipation   • Fever/sweats
  - faecal impaction   • infective cause
- Faecal incontinence   • Recent chemotherapy
- Drug history   • Recent radiotherapy

Examination
- Dehydration
  - dry mucous membranes   • postural hypotension
  - ↓ skin turgor   • oliguria

- Pyrexia
  - infective cause
- Jaundice
  - biliary tract obstruction
- Hepatomegaly
- Rectal examination
  - stool
    — fresh blood
    — melaena
    — steatorrhoea

- Tumour masses

  - faecal impaction
  - tumour

Investigations

Investigations are usually only necessary when diarrhoea is severe or persists for more than a few days.

Bloods

- FBC
  - infection
  - neutropenia if recent chemotherapy
- U&Es
  - dehydration
- LFTs
  - if there is steatorrhoea

- GI bleed

- hypokalaemia

Stool

- MC&S
- *Clostridium difficile* toxin

Urine

- 24-hour 5-HIAA
  - carcinoid tumour

Imaging

- AXR
  - high faecal impaction

- partial bowel obstruction

Management

- Most patients with diarrhoea can be managed as an outpatient
  - adequate oral intake (3 l/day) to maintain hydration status
  - not hypotensive
  - no electrolyte imbalance
- Rehydrate
  - oral route is more effective than intravenous if the patient can tolerate it. Aim for 3 l/day of fluid.
  - glucose/electrolyte drinks increase water absorption
    — dioralyte   — lucozade
  - if patient is hypotensive or tachycardic give IV fluids.
  - if patient is oliguric give IV fluids and insert a urinary catheter to monitor urinary output (aim >0.5 ml/kg/h) (see Acute renal failure 📖 p268)
- Correct hypokalaemia
  - 20–40 mmol KCl in each litre of IV fluid

- Give an anti-emetic if there is vomiting (see Nausea and vomiting 📖 p38)
- Consider stopping or reducing drugs that could be implicated
  - laxatives
  - NSAIDs
  - antibiotics
  - chemotherapy
- Consider route of essential drugs
  - absorption by oral route may be poor
  - modified release opioids can be switched to standard preparations or an equivalent dose by SC infusion (see Pain 📖 p2)
- Exclude faecal impaction or partial bowel obstruction before giving a drug that will slow bowel transit

Infective diarrhoea

Many hospitals will have local guidelines.
- *Clostridium difficile*
  - see Infections in the non-neutropenic patient 📖 p336
  - Metronidazole 400 mg PO tds 14 days
  - Vancomycin 125 mg PO qds 7–10 days
- *Salmonella/Shigella/Campylobacter*
  - Ciprofloxacin 500 mg PO bd 7 days
- Bacterial overgrowth (empirical treatment)
  - Metronidazole 400 mg PO tds 7 days
- If the patient meets the criteria for neutropenic sepsis give appropriate antibiotics (see Neutropenic sepsis 📖 p326) and consider adding in metronidazole.
- The use of antidiarrhoeal drugs may prolong symptoms and should be avoided

Faecal impaction
See Constipation 📖 p54

Chemotherapy
- Irinotecan
  - Early onset (<24 hours)
    — reduced gut transit time owing to cholinergic effect
    — atropine 250 μg SC
    — premedicate with atropine for future cycles of irinotecan
  - Late onset (>24 hours)
    — mucosal damage
    — Loperamide PO
      - 4 mg stat, then 2 mg every 2 hours until 12 hours after last episode of diarrhoea (i.e. do not exceed usual maximum daily dose of 16 mg/24 hours)
    — prophylactic ciprofloxacin 500 mg bd PO if diarrhoea persists for >24 hours
    — if diarrhoea continues for >48 hours admit patient to ward
      - give IV fluids   - investigate for infection
- Other cytotoxic drugs and tyrosine kinase inhibitors
  - ensure adequate hydration, especially when regimen contains a platinum drug that may cause renal impairment if the patient becomes dehydrated

- exclude infective cause
- symptomatic relief of diarrhoea
- Consideration must be given to chemotherapy dose reduction for future cycles according to clinical judgement and local protocols

Radiotherapy

- Adjusting fibre content of diet may improve symptoms
  - diet should not be adjusted prior to development of symptoms
  - reduce insoluble fibre, e.g. nuts, pulses, and raw vegetables
  - increasing soluble fibre (e.g. fybogel) may improve diarrhoea
- Symptomatic relief of diarrhoea
- Cholestyramine
  - useful if symptoms are caused by deficient bile salt absorption
  - 4 g PO qds, up to a maximum dose of 36 g/day
- Rectal steroids for rectal pain and rectal bleeding
  - Predfoam enemas 20 mg bd for 2 weeks
  - Proctofoam HC bd-tds

Pancreatic enzyme deficiency

- Pancreatic enzyme replacement
  - Creon 10 000–25 000 EC 1–2 capsules with each meal.
- Proton pump inhibitor

Biliary tract obstruction

- Consider referral for stenting (see Jaundice 📖 p62)

Bleeding from GI tumour

- See Gastrointestinal bleed 📖 p230
- Consider whether tumour is amenable to:
  - surgery
  - local radiotherapy
  - endoscopic treatment
- Tranexamic acid
  - 15–25 mg/kg 2–3 times daily if fibrinolysis is local
  - procoagulant
  - weigh beneficial effect against increased risk of thrombosis
- Etamsylate
  - 500 mg PO qds
  - no effect on normal coagulation
  - may increase platelet adhesiveness

Discharge from rectal tumour

- Radiotherapy or surgical intervention to reduce tumour size
- Rectal steroids to reduce local inflammation
  - Prednisolone suppositories 5 mg bd
  - Predfoam enemas every 2–3 days
- Octreotide

Symptomatic relief of diarrhoea

- Loperamide
  - Loperamide is a potent Mu opioid receptor agonist but it is almost completely metabolized by the liver and is actively excluded from the CNS. It therefore acts locally in the GI tract and does not cause significant central effects.
  - It reduces motility and also has some antisecretory action.

- It may have additional effect if the patient is already on a strong opioid
- Dose
  - Maximum dose 16 mg/24 hours
  - Acute diarrhoea
    - 4 mg PO stat and 2 mg after each loose stool
  - Chronic diarrhoea
    - 2–4 mg PO bd, titrate up to 8 mg bd if necessary
- May cause abdominal cramps and bloating
- Opioids
  - Codeine
    - PO 30–60 mg qds
    - if the patient is already on a strong opioid there is little rationale for adding codeine and the opioid dose may be increased by 25–50%
  - Morphine
    - if diarrhoea is severe and oral absorption of drugs unreliable, morphine may be given by SC infusion at a starting dose of 10 mg/24 hours
- Octreotide
  - Octreotide is a somatostatin analogue
  - It reduces GI hormone secretion
  - It has antisecretory and antimotility actions on the bowel
  - It is effective in:
    - the symptomatic relief of inoperable bowel obstruction (see Gastrointestinal obstruction 📖 p238)
    - chronic diarrhoea
      - intractable chemotherapy-associated diarrhoea
      - diarrhoea from hormone-secreting tumours
      - high output diarrhoea following ileostomy or colostomy
      - excess mucus secretion from colonic and rectal tumours
      - enterocolic fistula
  - Octreotide can be given by SC injection tds or SC continuous infusion
  - Dose range 150–1500 µg/24 hours.

Hyoscine butylbromide
  - Anticholinergic drug which does not cross the blood–brain barrier and is free of central side effects
  - Poor oral absorption means it must be given by SC infusion
  - Reduces bowel motility and secretions
  - Can provide symptomatic relief in:
    - inoperable bowel obstruction (see Gastrointestinal obstruction 📖 p238)
    - chronic high volume diarrhoea
  - Dry mouth may limit dose titration
  - Dose range 20–60 mg/24 hours.

Surgery
  - For intractable chronic diarrhoea or faecal incontinence, formation of a colostomy may relieve symptoms and improve quality of life in selected patients

⑦ **Constipation**

Constipation is the passage of hard faecal material less frequently and with more difficulty than is normal for each individual patient. Constipation is a common problem in patients with cancer. Constipation is not only uncomfortable for the patient but can lead to significant complications if not addressed.

- Faecal impaction
- Overflow diarrhoea
- Faecal incontinence
- Bowel obstruction
- Urinary retention or frequency
- Confusion and restlessness
  - particularly in the elderly

Causes

- Drugs
  - Opioids
    - including loperamide
  - Antimuscarinic action
    - cyclizine
    - tricyclic antidepressants
    - hyoscine
  - 5-HT$_3$ antagonists
    - ondansetron
    - granisetron
  - Vinca alkaloids
    - autonomic neuropathy
- Debility
  - Inactivity and immobility
  - Dehydration
  - Reduced fibre in diet
  - Inconvenient or unfamiliar toilet arrangements
  - Depression
  - Confusion
- Cancer
  - Colonic malignancy
  - Extrinsic compression
    - advanced pelvic tumour
    - peritoneal carcinomatosis
  - Hypercalcaemia
  - Spinal cord compression
    - including cauda equina compression
  - Paraneoplastic visceral neuropathy
- Anorectal pathology
  - Haemorrhoids
  - Anal fissure

Clinical features

Symptoms

- Infrequent stool
- Hard/uncomfortable stool
- Distension
- Abdominal pain
  - colicky
- Nausea and vomiting
- Flatulence
- Urinary retention
- left iliac fossa
- Diarrhoea +/- faecal incontinence if there is faecal impaction

Signs
- Abdominal distension
- Lower abdominal tenderness
- Bowel sounds may be quiet or scant
- Palpable colon
  - faecal mass
    - indentable — mobile
- Rectal examination (or digital examination of colostomy)
  - faecal impaction   • anal fissure
  - tumour mass   • haemorrhoids
  - empty rectum
    - bowel obstruction — high faecal impaction
  - loss of perianal sensation and loss of tone of anal sphincter
    - spinal cord/cauda equina compression
- Non-functioning ileostomy
  - suspect small bowel obstruction
- Check for signs of bowel obstruction (see Gastrointestinal obstruction 📖 p238)
- Check for signs of spinal cord/cauda equina compression (see Malignant extradural spinal cord compression 📖 p194)

Investigations
Investigations are only necessary if constipation is persistent or the cause is not obvious.

Bloods
- U&E
  - dehydration
    - cause or effect
- Ca^{2+}
  - hypercalcaemia

Imaging
- AXR
  - faecal loading   • bowel obstruction

Management
Pre-emptive
- Anticipate and monitor bowel function
- Advise adequate intake of fluid and dietary fibre
- Prescribe laxatives to all patients on strong opioids unless they have diarrhoea
  - Senna 15–30 mg *nocte*
  - Co-danthrusate 1–3 capsules *nocte*

Management of established constipation
- Correct dehydration and increase fluid intake
- Treat hypercalcaemia if present (see Hypercalcaemia 📖 p164)
- Increase dietary fibre if the patient is able to tolerate it
- Consider stopping or changing drugs that may slow bowel transit

- Laxatives
  - For regular hard stool, prescribe a softening laxative
  - For infrequent soft stool, prescribe a stimulant laxative
  - For infrequent hard stool prescribe a stimulant plus a softening laxative or a combination laxative
  - Titrate up the dose until it is effective
  - Reduce dose or change laxative if poorly tolerated
  - Consider adding in rectal laxatives if oral laxatives are ineffective
  - Rectal laxatives should not be used without adequate oral laxatives to maintain bowel movements once the rectal laxatives have initiated bowel movements
- If constipation due to morphine persists in spite of adequate doses of laxatives, consider switching morphine to fentanyl (there is some evidence that it is less constipating)

Management of faecal impaction

- It may respond over a few days to oral polyethylene glycol (movicol) 4–8 sachets/day if the patient can tolerate this volume (each sachet 125 ml fluid)
- For soft stool give bisacodyl suppositories PR 10 mg od
- For hard stool
  - low in the rectum give sodium citrate or phosphate enemas
  - high in the rectum give an arachis oil enema overnight
- For difficult low stool consider disruption and removal of stool with a gloved finger
  - the patient may need sedation with midazolam IV
- Prescribe oral laxatives to prevent recurrence

Laxatives

Stimulant laxatives

- Stimulate peristalsis and reduce transit time
  - therefore also soften by reducing reabsorption of water
- Relieve the hypersegmentation of the bowel caused by opioids
- May cause abdominal colic
- Examples
  - Senna 15 mg *nocte*
  - Bisacodyl 5–10 mg *nocte*
  - Dantron
    - only available in combination laxatives

Softening laxatives

- Osmotic laxatives
  - draw water into the bowel increasing stool water content
  - lactulose
    - 15 ml bd and then adjusted to patients' needs
    - may cause flatulence, bloating and colic
  - magnesium hydroxide mixture
    - 25–50 ml PRN
    - may increase Mg^{2+} levels with persistent use
- Iso-osmotic laxatives
  - taken in larger volume and retain water during transit, therefore useful in dehydration

- effective with faecal impaction
- polyethylene glycol (movicol)
  — 1–2 sachets od-bd, up to 8 sachets/day in faecal impaction
- Surface-wetting agents
  - gentle, lubricating action makes them suitable for use in functional bowel obstruction
  - prescribe with a stimulant in established constipation
  - Docusate sodium
    — 100–200 mg bd
- Bulk-forming agents
  - useful in elderly patients where inadequate dietary fibre is the principal cause of constipation
  - may exacerbate opioid induced constipation
  - fybogel
    — 1 sachet bd

Combination laxatives

- Contain a stimulant and a softener
- Co-danthrusate
  - Dantron 50 mg/docusate sodium 60 mg
  - 2 capsules *nocte*, titrate up to 1–3 capsules at night
  - 5–15 ml suspension *nocte*
- Co-danthramer
  - Dantron 25 mg/poloxamer 200 mg
  - 2 capsules *nocte*
  - 5–10 ml suspension *nocte*
- Dantron is carcinogenic in animal studies
  - these laxatives are only licensed for use in 'terminal illness'.
  - avoid in curable or early stage malignancy
- Warn patients that dantron discolours urine red/orange
- It may cause a painful perineal rash
  - avoid if there is faecal incontinence or damaged perineal skin

Rectal laxatives

- Usually given od
- Sodium citrate compound (micolette/micralax enema)
  - osmotic softening enema for low rectal stool
- Sodium phosphate enema
  - osmotic softening
- Arachis oil enema
  - softening for high rectal stool
  - can be administered via a Foley catheter for high impaction
- Glycerol suppositories
  - mildly stimulant
- Bisacodyl suppositories
  - stimulant

⑦ **Abdominal distension**

Abdominal distension is a common symptom in cancer patients, particularly those with advanced disease.

Causes

- Generalized abdominal distension
  - Ascites
  - Constipation
  - Bowel obstruction
    — subacute
    — small bowel
    — large bowel

- Localized abdominal distension
  - Primary tumour mass
  - Tumour infiltration
    — Hepatomegaly
    — Isolated deposits
      – subcutaneous
    — Lymphadenopathy
      – peritoneal

Clinical features

Symptoms

- Increasing girth/weight
  - usually despite anorexia
- Increasing abdominal discomfort or pain
- Early satiety and anorexia
  - reduced space for gastric expansion
- Oesophageal reflux
  - increased intra-abdominal pressure
- Increasing breathlessness
  - diaphragmatic splinting
  - reactive pleural effusion
- Altered bowel habit
  - constipation
  - overflow diarrhoea
- Inability to wear normal clothes
- Nausea and vomiting

Signs

- Abdominal distension
- Shifting dullness, fluid thrill
  - ascites
- Palpable masses
  - organomegaly
  - tumour
- Jaundice
  - liver disease
    — malignant involvement
    — cirrhosis
- Scars
  - laparotomy
  - breast
- Colostomy, ileostomy, ileal conduit
  - are they working normally?
- Tympanic abdomen
  - bowel obstruction
  - viscus perforation
  - check for rebound tenderness which would indicate peritonism
- Everted umbilicus
- Previous ascitic drain sites

- Abdominal tenderness
  - malignant infiltration or deposit
  - if accompanied by fever may be abscess or collection
    - post-surgery
- Suprapubic dullness
  - distended bladder (urinary retention)
- Digital rectal examination
  - hard faeces or faecal loading in rectum of a constipated patient

Investigations

Bloods
- FBC
  - infection
- U&E
  - vomiting
  - fluid shifts
    - ascites   - bowel obstruction
- LFTs
  - hepatic metastases
  - tumour deposits at the porta hepatis causing obstruction
- Coagulation screen
  - liver infiltration can affect its synthetic function and the production of clotting factors
  - any abnormality should be corrected if necessary e.g. bleeding
  - important prior to consideration of invasive procedures
- Blood cultures
  - if fever is present
- Tumour markers
  - to monitor recurrent malignancy
    - CEA   - CA125

Urine
- MSU
  - urinary tract infection can predispose to retention

Imaging
- AXR
  - dilated loops of bowel in bowel obstruction ± fluid levels
  - faecal loading of the caecum/transverse colon
- Erect CXR
  - free air under the diaphragm if perforated viscus
- Abdominal USS
  - free fluid   - tumour masses
  - abscesses and collections within the abdomen
- CT scan
  - can more accurately determine level of obstruction in small bowel obstruction

Biopsy
- Ascitic fluid sampling
  - diagnostic
  - sample sent for MC&S if fever present
- Biopsy of solid masses
  - diagnostic
  - USS or CT-guided

Management
- Nil by mouth if bowel obstruction or perforation is suspected.
- Symptomatic management of pain (see Pain 📖 p2).
  - consider the patient's current analgesic regimen.
  - morphine PO/SC may be required.
  - consider SC syringe driver if requiring multiple injections of analgesia and anti-emetic.
  - hyoscine butylbromide may relieve colicky pain
    — 20–40 mg SC qds.
    — 20–60 mg/24 hours SC infusion via syringe driver.
- Management of nausea and vomiting (see Nausea and vomiting 📖 p38).
  - anti-emetics
    — cyclizine IM/IV 150 mg/24 hours
  - dexamethasone
    — may reduce oedema around tumour and relieve subacute bowel obstruction.
    — acts as an anti-emetic.
    — 8–12 mg SC od.
  - NG tube if bowel obstruction.
- Assessment of fluid status.
  - Replace fluid ± electrolytes as necessary.
  - Insert urinary catheter
    — urinary retention   — poor urine output
- Antibiotics for patients with fever or suspected perforation.
  - Cefuroxime IV 1.5 g tds + metronidazole IV 500 mg tds.
  - In neutropenic patients
    — Piperacillin-tazobactam IV 4.5 g qds + gentamicin IV 5–7 mg/kg od
  - Consult local microbiology guidelines.
- Laxatives for patients with constipation (see Constipation 📖 p54).
- Ascitic drainage (see Paracentesis 📖 p250).
- Consider surgical or endoscopic intervention for obstructed patients.
  - Stenting or laser procedures.
  - Seek expert advice.
- Consider surgical intervention for abdominal masses.
  - Debulking or excision.
- Consider radiotherapy if appropriate.
- Intravenous or intraperitoneal chemotherapy may be an option.
  - Ovarian carcinoma
    — can increase interval between ascitic drainage procedures.

⑦ Jaundice

Jaundice is the yellow discolouration of the skin and sclera owing to the accumulation of bilirubin. The minimum bilirubin level in the blood for clinically apparent jaundice is 35 μmol/l, but usually it will be higher by the time of presentation.

Jaundice in the cancer patient is usually caused by impaired biliary flow owing to locally advanced or metastatic disease and therefore is a poor prognostic sign. Jaundice can also have implications for further treatment as many cytotoxic chemotherapy drugs are metabolized in the liver and cannot be used in the presence of deranged LFTs. However, it is important not to overlook other possible causes for jaundice, and therefore a systematic approach is useful.

Causes

See Fig. 1.3.

Unconjugated jaundice
- ↑ Bilirubin production
  - haemolysis
- ↓ Hepatocellular uptake and conjugation
  - Gilbert's syndrome

Conjugated jaundice
- Hepatocellular damage
  - acute viral hepatitis
  - alcoholic hepatitis
  - drugs
    - prescription
    - over-the-counter
    - complementary
    - alternative
  - sepsis
  - Budd–Chiari syndrome
  - right heart failure
  - cirrhosis
    - alcohol
    - viruses
    - autoimmune
    - drugs
    - haemochromatosis
    - α_1-antitrypsin deficiency
    - Wilson's disease
- Impaired bile flow
  - Intrahepatic cholestasis
    - primary biliary cirrhosis
    - primary sclerosing cholangitis
    - massive liver metastases
    - hepatocellular carcinoma
  - Extrahepatic cholestasis
    - gallstones
    - malignancy
      - carcinoma of the head of pancreas
      - cholangiocarcinoma
      - porta hepatis lymphadenopathy due to metastatic carcinoma
      - ampullary carcinoma
    - biliary stricture

Investigations

See Fig. 1.4

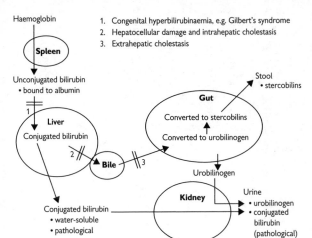

Fig. 1.3 Jaundice.

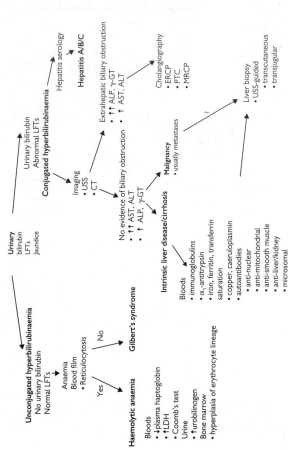

Fig. 1.4 Investigation of the jaundiced cancer patient.

Conjugated jaundice

This is caused by failure of excretion of bile from the hepatocytes into the biliary system. This may be due to:
- Hepatocellular damage
- Intrahepatic biliary obstruction
- Extrahepatic biliary obstruction

Clinical features
Symptoms
- Infective symptoms
  - acute viral hepatitis
  - cholangitis
  - liver abscess
- Pale stools and dark urine
  - particularly with extrahepatic cholestasis
- Anorexia
- Pruritus
- RUQ pain
- Abdominal distension due to ascites

Signs
- Signs of chronic liver disease
- Hepatomegaly
  - metastases
  - hepatitis
- Splenomegaly
  - secondary to cirrhosis and portal hypertension
- Ascites
  - malignancy
  - cirrhosis

Management
- Cessation of any putative causative drugs.
- Correct coagulopathy prior to any invasive investigations or if there is bleeding.
  - vitamin K 5–10 mg slow IV infusion.
  - FFP if immediate investigation is required or vitamin K is not effective.
- For those patients with non-malignant causes discuss with the appropriate specialty team
  - gastroenterologist
  - haematologist
  - hepatobiliary surgeon
- Few patients with malignant causes for their jaundice are suitable for radical treatment. All patients with hepatobiliary malignancies must be referred to the hepatobiliary multidisciplinary team (MDT) meeting to discuss suitability for radical surgery.
- For those patients with malignant obstruction not suitable for radical surgery, consider referral for palliation with endoscopic stenting.
  - ensure coagulation is corrected.
  - prophylactic antibiotics
    — ciprofloxacin

- For some patients alternative procedures may be more appropriate.
  - palliative surgical bypass procedures
    - often occur at the time of attempted radical surgery if, at the operation, a radical approach is no longer deemed appropriate.
  - percutaneous transhepatic stent insertion.
- Recurrent jaundice due to stent occlusion as a result of tumour regrowth is unfortunately common; however, this may be amenable to re-stenting.
- Patients with chemosensitive disease may be suitable for palliative chemotherapy, although care needs to be taken, particularly with cytotoxic drugs that require hepatic metabolism (see Chemotherapy-related hepatotoxicity 🔲 p358).
  - anthracyclines
  - vinca alkaloids
  - taxanes
  - etoposide
  - irinotecan

Management of cholestatic itch

Itch can be a distressing and intractable symptom of cholestasis although there is no clear relationship between the level of jaundice and the degree of itch. Cholestatic itch is thought to have peripheral and central components. Endogenous opioids rather than histamine may be the main chemical mediators and antihistamines do not appear to give effective relief other than through night sedation.

- Relief of cholestasis
  - Stenting of common bile duct can relieve extrahepatic cholestasis.
  - Dexamethasone 6–8 mg PO od may help to relieve intrahepatic cholestasis associated with malignancy.
- Symptomatic management
  - Skin care
    - Moisturizers should be used first and may give adequate relief.
      - Aqueous cream
      - E45
    - Topical calamine lotion or aqueous cream with 2% menthol may be helpful.
  - Drugs
    - Consider night sedation
      - Temazepam
      - Sedative antihistamine
    - If cholestasis cannot be relieved consider specialist palliative care input
      - Rifampicin
        - start at 75 mg od; titrate to 150 mg bd if tolerated.
        - it may increase hepatic dysfunction, therefore use lowest effective dose.
        - it is a hepatic enzyme inducer; therefore check for its many interactions with other drugs.
        - it turns urine orange and may discolour contact lenses.
      - An oral opioid antagonist
        - in patients not taking opioids for pain relief.
      - Androgen stanozol
        - 5–10 mg od.
        - in patients with a limited prognosis.

Unconjugated jaundice

Haemolysis

Intravascular breakdown of red blood cells releases haemoglobin into the bloodstream. A small proportion of this is bound to plasma haptoglobins, which become saturated and rapidly depleted. Free plasma haemoglobin is filtered by the kidney and can appear in urine as haemoglobinuria. Unconjugated bilirubin swamps the capacity of the liver to form water-soluble conjugated bilirubin. If liver function is normal, haemolysis usually produces mild elevation in serum bilirubin (68–102 µmol/l). Clinically patients may present with anaemia and splenomegaly.

In cancer patients haemolysis may occur because of:
- Autoimmune haemolysis
  - particularly in lymphoma and CLL.
- Drug-induced immune haemolysis
  - fludarabine
- Haemolytic transfusion reaction
- Microangiopathic haemolytic anaemia
  - haemolytic uraemic syndrome has been reported following mitomycin C.

Gilbert's syndrome

This is present in 2–7% of the population; 5–15% of patients will have a family history of jaundice. This is most often caused by reduced glucuronidation of bilirubin by a mutated UDP-glucuronosyl transferase gene product. The patient remains asymptomatic and there is usually only a mild elevation of total bilirubin on routine testing (17–102 µmol/l). Bilirubin levels may rise during fasting or illness. No treatment is required.

Hepatorenal syndrome

Hepatorenal syndrome is an acute oliguric renal failure occurring without intrinsic renal disease in the presence of advanced liver disease. The pathogenesis is thought to be due to peripheral vasodilatation (due to release of nitric oxide) causing hypotension and subsequent release of renal vasoconstrictors which restrict renal blood flow, resulting in a reduction in GFR and avid sodium and water retention.

There are four major criteria that must be present for the diagnosis:
- Low GFR
  - serum creatinine ≥133 µmol/l or 24-hour creatinine clearance ≤40 ml/minute.
- Absence of:
  - shock
  - fluid loss
  - infection
  - nephrotoxic drug treatment
- No sustained improvement in renal function despite cessation of nephrotoxic drugs and volume expansion with 1.5 litres of plasma expander.
- Proteinuria < 50 mg/day and no USS evidence of obstruction or renal disease.

Additional criteria provide supportive evidence but are not required for the diagnosis.

- Urine volume <500 ml/day
- Urine $[Na^+]$ <10mmol/l
- Urine osmolality > plasma osmolality
- Urinary red blood cells <50/high powered field
- Serum $[Na^+]$ <130 mmol/l

There are two recognized types of hepatorenal syndrome:

- Type 1
  - serum creatinine increases to ≥221 µmol/l or creatinine clearance falls to ≤20 ml/min in less than 2 weeks.
  - high mortality (<10% survival).
- Type 2
  - more indolent increase in creatinine.
  - mortality ~50%.

Management

- Stop nephrotoxic drugs and diuretics.
- Treat any infection.
- Ensure adequate volume expansion.
- Seek expert help.
- Some patients may benefit from use of vasopressin analogues
  - terlipressin 1 mg IV bd.
- Transjugular intrahepatic portosystemic shunting (TIPS) may be appropriate in certain patients once stabilized with medical therapy.
- The best treatment option is orthotopic liver transplantation; however, this is highly unlikely to be appropriate in the majority of cancer patients.

Further reading

Arroyo, V., Ginès, P., Gerbes, A.L., Dudley, F.J., Gentilini, P., Laffi, G., Reynolds, T.B., Ring-Larsen, H. and Schölmerich, J. (1996). Definition and diagnostic criteria of refractory ascites and hepatorenal syndrome in cirrhosis. *Hepatology* **23**(1): 164–176.

O'Beirne, J.P. and Heneghan, M.A. (2005). Current management of the hepatorenal syndrome. *Hepatology Research* **32**(4): 243–249.

Twycross, R., Greaves, M.W., Handwerker, H., Jones, E.A., Libretto, S.E., Szepietowski, J.C. and Zylicz, Z. (2003). Itch: scratching more than the surface. *Q. J. M.* **96**: 7–26.

:☼: **Drowsiness and decreased Glasgow Coma Scale**

Drowsiness, decreased Glasgow Coma Scale (GCS), and ultimately true coma (GCS<8) can occur in the cancer patient for a number of reasons. The degree of urgency in the management of such situations can vary widely according to the clinical context. The key to managing these patients lies in stabilizing the patient and quickly establishing a likely list of differential diagnoses, such that specific treatment may commence as rapidly as possible, if appropriate.

Common causes of decreased GCS in cancer patients
- Toxic
  - Opioid overdose
  - Radiation injury
    - somnolence syndrome
  - Chemotherapy-induced encephalopathy
    - ifosfamide
    - cytarabine
    - high dose methotrexate
- Metabolic
  - Hypercalcaemia
  - Hyponatraemia
  - Hypoglycaemia
- Systemic infection
  - Generalized sepsis
    - neutropenic sepsis
- Structural lesions causing raised intracranial pressure
  - Primary CNS tumours
  - Cerebral metastases
  - Cerebral haemorrhage
    - into a cerebral metastasis
    - secondary to thrombocytopenia
- Meningeal irritation
  - Infective meningitis
  - Subarachnoid haemorrhage
  - Carcinomatous meningitis
    - leptomeningeal metastases

Immediate management
- Stabilize the patient
  - Open the airway, technique depends on level of coma
    - lay the patient semi-prone
    - insert oropharyngeal airway
    - intubate and ventilate
  - Give oxygen
  - Support the circulation
    - correct hypotension with fluids
  - Treat seizures if present
- Rapid assessment
  - Is an obvious cause immediately apparent?
  - History from witness/family

- Immediate specific treatment if indicated
  - 50 ml 50% dextrose IV for hypoglycaemia
    — if patient is at risk of Wernicke's encephalopathy give thiamine 250 mg IV (one pair of IVHP ampoules).
  - naloxone for opioid overdose
    — dilute a 400 µg ampoule of naloxone to 10 ml with 0.9% saline.
    — give naloxone 40 µg (1 ml) increments every 2 minutes until the patient is rousable

Assessment

- Glasgow Coma Scale (3–15), sum of:

Eye opening

Spontaneously	4
To speech	3
To painful stimuli	2
No response	1

Best verbal response

Orientated	5
Disorientated	4
Inappropriate words	3
Incomprehensible sounds	2
No response	1

Best motor response

Obeys verbal commands	6
Localizes painful stimuli	5
Withdrawal to pain	4
Flexion to pain	3
Extension to pain	2
No response	1

- General examination
  - Core temperature
    — fever   — hypothermia
  - Cardiovascular status
    — poor cerebral perfusion
  - Respiratory status
    — hypoxia
    — slow shallow breathing
      - opioid intoxication
    — Kussmaul breathing
      - acidosis
    — abnormal respiratory patterns
      - brainstem compromise
  - Abdominal examination
    — acute intra-abdominal event
  - Skin
    — rash   — signs of trauma

- General neurological examination
  - Papilloedema
    - raised intracranial pressure
  - Meningism
    - meningitis   — haemorrhage
    - encephalitis
  - Lateralizing signs
    - suggests a focal or structural lesion
- Assess brainstem function (if deeply comatose)
  - Pupillary response
    - size   — reaction to light
  - Corneal reflex
  - Resting position of eyes
  - Eye movements
    - spontaneous
    - oculocephalic (Doll's head manoeuvre)
  - Respiratory pattern

Initial investigations

Bloods

- Glucose
  - BM stick   • venous
- FBC and coagulation screen
- U&Es
- LFTs
- Ca^{2+}, Mg^{2+} and phosphate
- Toxicology
  - including urgent paracetamol and salicylate levels if overdose is suspected or possible
- Blood cultures
  - peripheral   • central venous lines

Urine

- MSU
- Urinary osmolality and electrolytes if hyponatraemic
- Urine for toxicology if suspected

ECG

- Arrhythmia or myocardial infarction may result in cerebral hypoperfusion and drowsiness

Imaging

- CXR
  - infection or another cause for hypoxia leading to drowsiness
- CT brain
  - focal lesions   • haemorrhage
- MRI brain
  - meningeal disease   • brainstem pathology

Lumbar puncture

- If no evidence of toxic, metabolic or systemic infection to cause decreased GCS.
- CT brain is normal and no sign of raised intracranial pressure.
- Send CSF for
  - MC&S
  - protein levels
  - glucose
  - cytology

Further management

Subsequent management should be directed at the specific cause.
- Infection should be treated with appropriate antibiotics.
- Metabolic abnormalities should be corrected.
  - Hypercalcaemia (see Hypercalcaemia 📖 p164)
  - Hyponatraemia (see Hyponatraemia 📖 p176)
  - Hypoglycaemia (see Hypoglycaemia 📖 p172)
- Raised intracranial pressure (see Raised intracranial pressure 📖 p206)
  - Dexamethasone 10 mg IV initially, then 4 mg IM every 6 hours as required for 2–4 days then gradually reduced and stopped over 5–7 days
    — acts within hours and effect lasts for several days.
    — useful for cerebral oedema associated with intracerebral malignancy.
  - Mannitol
    — 1 g/kg as a 20% solution given by rapid IV.
    — acts within minutes and effect lasts for several hours.
    — may be repeated.
  - Intubation and hyperventilation
    — requires admission to ICU.
    — acts within minutes and effect lasts for a few hours.
  - Occasionally, neurosurgical intervention may be indicated in the case of intracranial mass lesions.
- Somnolence syndrome (see Radiotherapy-related neurotoxicity 📖 p386)
  - occurs 1–6 months after whole brain radiotherapy.
  - improvement may occur over weeks to months.
  - dexamethasone may reduce the duration of somnolence syndrome.
- Ifosfamide encephalopathy (see Chemotherapy-related neurotoxicity 📖 p352)
  - Methylene blue 1% 50 mg tds/qds IV
    — treatment.
    — primary prophylaxis if encephalopathy risk is high.
    — secondary prophylaxis on subsequent cycles.
- Leptomeningeal metastases (see Leptomeningeal metastases 📖 p214)
  - Whole brain +/– neuroaxis radiotherapy.
  - Intrathecal chemotherapy.

Further reading

Plum, F., Posner, J.B., Saper, C.B. and Schiff, N. (2007). *The Diagnosis of Stupor and Coma*, 4th edn. Oxford: Oxford University Press.

Ramrakha, P.S. and Moore, K.P. (2004). *Oxford Handbook of Acute Medicine*, 2nd edn. Oxford: Oxford University Press.

ⓘ **Collapse, weakness, 'off-legs'**

Collapse, weakness, 'off-legs' is a common acute presentation in cancer patients. Often it is due to progression of the underlying cancer; however, it is important to perform a thorough assessment of patients and not to assume the deterioration is due to progressive disease. There may be a tendency to under-investigate some patients with metastatic cancer, when they may have conditions that could respond well to active management, improving their quality of life.

The common causes in cancer patients are similar to the causes found in non-cancer patients, although there are some causes that must always be remembered and excluded in patients with a known malignancy.

Common causes in oncology patients

- Neurological
  - Cerebral metastases
    - UMN weakness, seizures or stroke
    - new diagnosis
    - progression/complication of existing disease
  - Spinal cord compression and cauda equina syndrome
    - can present gradually or suddenly with cord infarction
  - Proximal myopathy
    - steroid use
  - Paraneoplastic neurological syndromes
    - cerebellar degeneration
    - peripheral neuropathies
    - polymyositis/dermatomyositis
- Cardiovascular
  - Pulmonary embolism
  - Myocardial infarction
  - Arrhythmias
  - Malignant pericardial effusion
- Metabolic
  - Hypercalcaemia
    - bone metastases
    - PTH-rp secretion
  - Hyponatraemia
  - Hypokalaemia
- Infection
  - Local infection may cause general deterioration in debilitated patients
    - UTI
    - pneumonia
  - Generalized sepsis (especially when patient is neutropenic) can present with a lack of focal symptoms, leading to a generalized 'collapse'
- Other important causes in cancer patients
  - Pain
  - Pathological fracture
  - General debility/cachexia

Clinical features

Symptoms

A thorough history, including a full oncological/general past medical history, drug history and detailed history of the presenting episode, can give vital clues as to the correct differential diagnosis and appropriate investigations.

It is important to recognize common symptom complexes in oncology patients as they require urgent management. These are:

- Spinal cord compression/cauda equina syndrome
  - back pain
  - leg weakness
  - sensory loss
  - sphincter dysfunction
- Hypercalcaemia
  - weakness
  - drowsiness
  - confusion
  - nausea
  - polyuria
  - bone and abdominal pains
  - constipation
  - depression
- Neutropenic sepsis
  - sepsis in neutropenic patients can cause a generalized collapse, sometimes in the absence of fever or other obvious signs of infection

Signs

A full systemic examination is vital upon admission for patients presenting with collapse/weakness/'off-legs', and a thorough neurological examination is vital.

Specific signs to seek actively in cancer patients include:

- Spinal cord compression
  - sensory and UMN motor loss at and below the level of the lesion
  - a band of hyperaesthesia at the level of the lesion
  - tenderness on palpation/percussion over the vertebrae involved
- Cauda equina syndrome
  - flaccid, areflexic, LMN motor loss in the lower limbs (often asymmetrical)
  - saddle anaesthesia
  - loss of anal tone on rectal examination

Investigations

Bloods

- FBC
- U&Es
- LFTs
- Ca^{2+}
- Blood cultures
- Magnesium and phosphate
- Glucose

  - always exclude hypercalcaemia in acutely unwell cancer patients
- Further bloods as indicated by clinical differential diagnosis
  - cardiac enzymes if cardiac ischaemia possible
- Specialist tests may be indicated in certain circumstances
  - immunological tests for auto-antibodies in paraneoplastic neurological conditions (anti-Hu, anti-Yo)

Urine
- MSU

ECG
- Arrhythmia
- Ischaemia

Imaging
- As directed by history and examination
- CXR
  - infection
  - pericardial effusion
- Plain X-rays of any areas of bone pain
  - pathological fracture
  - painful metastasis
- MRI whole spine
  - if spinal cord or cauda equina compression needs to be excluded
- CT brain
  - if new or progressive intracranial disease needs to be confirmed
- MRI brain
  - more sensitive than CT for detection of leptomeningeal disease
- V/Q scan or CTPA
  - PE

Neurophysiology
- Nerve conduction studies
  - neuropathy

Management
The management is directed at the underlying cause or causes. Often the cause of reduced mobility in cancer patients is multifactorial and a multidisciplinary approach with physiotherapy and occupational therapy is essential. In complex cases the advice of a specialist in elderly care medicine may also be useful as they are experts in assessing complex and interacting medical problems and may have access to specialist rehabilitation services. Ultimately, the aim must be to try and correct the under lying causes and return the patient to their previous mobility. However, in patients with a limited prognosis, some longer courses of rehabilitation may not be fruitful. The emphasis in these cases should be on optimizing their quality of life by ensuring that the appropriate care and appliances are in place for their current needs and not on working towards unobtainable goals. The loss of mobility may sometimes herald the final stages of a malignant illness and it is important that aims are realistic and that palliative care needs are addressed appropriately.

For the management of specific causes important in cancer patients see:
- Spinal cord compression/cauda equina syndrome (see Malignant extradural spinal cord compression 📖 p194)
- Hypercalcaemia (see Hypercalcaemia 📖 p164)
- Hypokalaemia (see Hypokalaemia 📖 p180)
- Hyponatraemia (see Hyponatraemia 📖 p176)
- Pain (see Pain 📖 p2)
- Pathological fracture (see Bone pain and pathological fracture 📖 p220)
- Neutropenic sepsis (see Infections in the neutropenic patient 📖 p326)
- Raised intracranial pressure (see Raised intracranial pressure 📖 p206)
- Leptomeningeal metastases (see Leptomeningeal metastases 📖 p214)
- Pulmonary embolus (see Venous thromboembolism 📖 p98)

:☼: Seizures

Seizures are relatively common in cancer patients, mainly owing to the incidence of cerebral metastases (which is increasing with improved systemic therapies) and primary CNS malignancy (2% of cancers in the UK). Other causes of seizures also occur in patients with cancer, either because of co-morbidity or treatment-related toxicities. It is therefore important to be aware of the differential causes and management of single seizures, status epilepticus and chronic intermittent seizures. It is also important to remember the practical limitations that the occurrence of seizures may place on a patient (e.g. driving restrictions) who may have to make many hospital visits for management of their malignancy.

Common causes of seizures in cancer patients

- Cerebral tumours
  - primary or metastatic
  - seizures may by precipitated by radiotherapy or chemotherapy treatment
- Electrolyte disturbance
  - hyponatraemia
  - hypocalcaemia
  - hypomagnesaemia
  - common in cancer patients and may be precipitated or exacerbated by treatments
    — cisplatin chemotherapy   — bisphosphonates
- Drug overdose or toxicity
  - alcohol
  - tricyclic antidepressants
  - cytotoxic chemotherapy agents (uncommon)
    — ifosfamide   — dacarbazine
    — paclitaxel
- Drug withdrawal
  - dacarbazine
  - anti-epileptic drugs
- Intracranial infection
- Stroke
- Hypoglycaemia
- Head injury
- Hypoxia

Differential diagnosis of seizures

- Rigors due to sepsis
- Myoclonic jerks
  - opioid toxicity
- Generalized dystonia
  - metoclopramide-induced
- 'Pseudo-seizures'

☺: Status epilepticus

Status epilepticus occurs when there is:
- a single continuous seizure lasting >30 minutes.
- intermittent seizure activity lasting >30 minutes without recovery of full consciousness between seizures

It is a true medical emergency, with 10–15% mortality from cardiorespiratory failure, and all doctors should be aware of its immediate management.

Management
- Secure airway
  - semi-prone position with head slightly lower to avoid aspiration
  - insert oral airway if possible between seizures
- High flow O_2
- Obtain IV access if possible between seizures and take blood for investigations
- Monitor
  - ECG
  - BP
- Termination of seizures with benzodiazepines
  - lorazepam IV
    - 4 mg at <2 mg/minute
    - can be repeated once after 10 minutes
  - diazepam PR
    - 0.5 mg/kg to max of 30 mg
- Check blood glucose and correct hypoglycaemia if present
  - 50 ml of 50% glucose
    - if alcohol excess suspected give concomitant thiamine 250 mg IV (one pair of IVHP ampoules) to prevent the increased risk of Wernicke's encephalopathy
- Correct hypotension with fluid resuscitation to maintain cerebral perfusion pressure
- If seizures resolve maintain recovery position as conscious level recovers
- Administer second line therapy if seizures are not terminated within 20 minutes or recur before conscious level improves for longer than 10 minutes
  - phenytoin infusion
    - 15–18 mg/kg diluted to 10 mg/ml in 0.9% saline at <50 mg/minute
    - care in patients with known cardiac conduction abnormalities
- In refractory status, >60 minutes after initial therapy, call for specialist help to consider
  - general anaesthesia, intubation, and ventilation
  - management in ICU
  - further drug therapies
    - propofol
    - thiopental
    - midazolam
  - specialist monitoring and management of complications

Investigations

Bloods
- Glucose
- Ca^{2+} and Mg^{2+}
- U&Es
- FBC
- Toxicology
  - serum (5 ml) and urine (50 ml) samples
- LFTs
- Coagulation screen
- Anticonvulsant levels
- ABGs

Imaging
- CXR
  - aspiration
  - primary lung cancer
- CT brain
  - cerebral metastases
  - stroke
  - head injury
- MRI brain
  - cerebral metastases
  - leptomeningeal metastases

Invasive
- Lumbar puncture
  - Send for
    — MC&S
    — protein levels
    — glucose
    — cytology
  - infectious meningitis
  - carcinomatous meningitis

Single seizures

Single tonic–clonic seizures can in most cases be managed with simple first aid alone.
- Stay calm and note the time of onset.
- Protect the patient, e.g. cushion the head, but only attempt to move them if they are in danger. Do NOT attempt to restrain them.
- Wait for the seizure to run its course, although benzodiazepines (e.g. diazepam 0.5 mg/kg to max of 30 mg PR) may be used to terminate the seizure if readily available.
- Following the seizure, place the patient in the recovery position.
- Open and protect the airway and give oxygen if available.
- Investigate as for status epilepticus.

Chronic intermittent seizures

Cancer patients with seizures often have either a limited life expectancy (e.g. cerebral metastases) or have a transient precipitating cause for their seizures (e.g. treatment toxicity) such that the long-term management of their seizures may not be a major issue. There is a subset of oncology patients, e.g. those with low-grade glioma, who will require chronic treatment with anticonvulsant drugs to control an underlying tendency for seizures.

Principles of management
- Joint management by oncologist, neurologist, general practitioner, and nurse specialists.
- Education of the patient, their family and/or carers about their condition, its management, its side effects, and the management of individual seizures.
- Anticonvulsant drugs should be considered after a first unprovoked seizure if brain imaging reveals a structural abnormality.
- Drug treatment should be individualized according to the seizure type, co-medications, co-morbidity, and tolerability by the patient.
- Monotherapy should be used initially and the dose increased until seizure control is achieved or tolerance is exceeded.
- If control is not achieved with monotherapy a second drug is added.
- Routine blood monitoring of anticonvulsant drug levels is not necessary; however, it can be useful for phenytoin as the therapeutic level is well defined. Serum drug levels are also useful when compliance or toxicity are issues.

Driving advice

In the UK, patients should be advised that they are legally obliged to inform the DVLA of the occurrence of a seizure. Driving licences are revoked until the patient has been free from seizures, treated or untreated, for 1 year. If the patient continues to have nocturnal seizures, they must be free from daytime seizures for 3 years. Drivers of large goods or passenger vehicles ('group 2' licence holders) have their licence revoked until they are seizure-free off medication for at least 10 years, i.e. often permanently in practice.

Further reading

The epilepsies: The diagnosis and management of the epilepsies in adults and children in primary and secondary care. NICE Clinical Guideline 20. 2004. www.nice.org.uk
DVLA website www.dvla.gov.uk

⑦ **Fever**

A temperature of >38°C in a cancer patient is generally considered as significant.

There is a fairly wide differential diagnosis which depends on individual patient factors.

Differential diagnosis

- Infection
  - Particularly important in a neutropenic patient (see Infections in the neutropenic patient 📖 p326), but patients may be profoundly immunosuppressed with a normal neutrophil count, e.g. after a stem cell transplant, with underlying myeloma or chronic lymphocytic leukaemia
- Malignancy
  - The malignant process itself may produce fevers
  - This is particularly prominent with:
    — lymphoma
    — renal cell carcinoma
- Drug fever
  - Some chemotherapy drugs are associated with fever, e.g. cytarabine, cladribine
  - However, many other drugs may cause a fever, e.g. antibiotics
- Transfusion reaction
  - Acute haemolytic transfusion reaction (AHTR)
  - Non-haemolytic febrile transfusion reaction
  - Bacterial contamination of the unit of red cells or platelets
- PE
- Connective tissue diseases

Investigations

- Fever owing to underlying malignancy is a diagnosis of exclusion
- No specific test is available to determine whether a fever is drug-induced. In some instances, the only test is to stop a drug and assess for resolution of the fever

Bloods

- FBC
- U&Es
- LFTs
- CRP
- Blood cultures
  - from indwelling catheter and peripheral blood
  - repeat whenever patient spikes a temperature, even after commencing antibiotics
- ABG
  - hypoxia due to infection or PE
- In a patient receiving a blood transfusion with symptoms and signs suggestive of an AHTR
  - Coagulation screen to assess for DIC
  - U&E to assess for renal failure
  - Repeat blood group and antibody screen from the patient

- Send the unit of red cells to be re-grouped and to assess for bacterial contamination
- Assess for haemolysis
  - direct antiglobulin test
  - bilirubin
  - LDH
  - serum haptoglobins
- Blood film for spherocytes

Urine/sputum/stool
- MSU for MC&S
- Sputum cultures
- Stool cultures if diarrhoea present

Imaging
- CXR
- TOE
  - If signs of infective endocarditis
    - new murmur
    - splinter haemorrhages
    - septic emboli
    - microscopic haematuria
- CT abdomen and pelvis
  - To look for occult source of sepsis
    - paracolic abscess
    - subphrenic abscess
    - prostatitis
- V/Q scan or CTPA
  - PE

Immunosuppressed patient
- In a patient who is immunosuppressed, e.g. post-stem cell transplant, opportunistic infections should also be borne in mind
  - Nasopharyngeal aspirate with immunofluorescence for respiratory viruses, e.g. RSV, adenovirus, influenza, and parainfluenza
  - PCR on a peripheral blood sample for reactivation of CMV infection
  - CT chest to look for signs of fungal infection or PCP
  - Bronchoscopy with washings
    - MC&S with silver staining for PCP
    - MC&S for fungal infection

Management
- Treatment should be directed at the underlying cause.
- In a neutropenic patient with a fever, empirical antibiotics should be administered as a matter of urgency (see Infections in the neutropenic patient p326).
- If fevers continue despite an adequate course of antibiotics to cover the diagnosed infection, consider stopping all antibiotics and perform further blood cultures if the patient spikes a temperature to obtain a microbiological diagnosis

⑦ **Bleeding**

Bleeding is a common occurrence in cancer patients. One of the commonest causes is erosion of the malignancy into a blood vessel (see Eroded artery 📖 p124). In the absence of such an anatomical cause, however, haematological disorders should be considered.

There are two main patterns of bleeding related to underlying haematological problems.

Platelet-type
- Low numbers of circulating platelets
- Dysfunctional platelets
- Abnormalities of von Willebrand's factor (which mediates platelet adhesion to the vessel wall)

The following clinical features are seen:
- Purpura (frequently around the ankles)
- Mucosal haemorrhage
  - nose bleeds
  - gum bleeds
  - GI bleeds
- Menorrhagia
- Superficial bruising
- Excessive bleeding after minor procedures

Coagulation-type
- Deficit in one or more clotting factors

The following clinical features are seen:
- Intramuscular haematomas
- Intra-articular bleeding with haemarthrosis
- Superficial bruising
- Excessive bleeding after minor procedures

Causes

In cancer patients, the following causes are the most common.

Platelet-type
- Low number of platelets (see Thrombocytopenia 📖 p288)
  - Chemotherapy-induced marrow suppression
  - Radiotherapy-induced marrow suppression
  - Metastatic malignancy involving the bone marrow
  - Sequestration of platelets in the periphery
    - splenomegaly
  - Consumption of platelets in the periphery
    - sepsis
    - DIC
    - ITP
- Dysfunctional platelets
  - Anti-platelet medication, e.g. aspirin, dipyridamole, clopidogrel
  - Renal failure

- Abnormalities of von Willebrand's factor
  - Acquired von Willebrand's disease
    - a rare condition usually associated with a paraprotein (due to myeloma, Waldenström's syndrome or monoclonal gammopathy of undetermined significance (MGUS)) resulting in reduced circulating von Willebrand's factor.

Coagulation-type

- Multiple clotting factor deficiency
  - DIC (note: also a cause of low platelets) (see Disseminated intravascular coagulation 🕮 p278).
  - Warfarin therapy
  - Secondary to massive transfusion
- Single clotting factor deficiency
  - Acquired haemophilia
    - a rare but very serious condition characterized by an immune response targeting factor VIII. Can be associated with underlying malignancy.

Investigations

A bone marrow aspirate and trephine is helpful in diagnosing metastatic involvement of the marrow. In a patient with DIC, a septic screen is required to rule out infection as a precipitating cause.

Table 1.6 Haematological test results in various conditions associated with malignancy

Condition	PT	APTT	Platelet count	Bleeding time	Blood film
Therapy-related marrow suppression	N	N	↓	↑	Pancytopenia
Metastatic marrow involvement	N	N	↓	↑	Pancytopenia Leukoerythroblastic Tear drop red cells
DIC	↑	↑	↓	↑	Occasional fragments
ITP	N	N	↓	↑	N
Acquired haemophilia	N	↑	N	N	N
Acquired von Willebrand's disease	N	↑	N	↑	N

Management

Treat the underlying cause

- Therapy-related thrombocytopenia or marrow infiltration
  - Platelet transfusion
    — aiming for count of $>50\times10^9$/l in a patient actively bleeding
- DIC
  - If APTT and/or PT prolonged give FFP 12–15 ml/kg
  - If platelets low give a platelet transfusion aiming for count of $>50\times10^9$/l
  - If fibrinogen low after FFP consider 10 units cryoprecipitate aiming for level of >1 g/l
- ITP
  - Prednisolone 1 mg/kg PO or methylprednisolone 1 g IV with Ivlg 0.4 g/kg/day for 5 days
  - If life-threatening bleed, may give platelets after Ivlg
- Acquired haemophilia
  - For acute bleed, give recombinant factor VIIa or FEIBA after liaison with haematologist
  - Commence prednisolone 1 mg/kg PO (or methylprednisolone 1 g IV)
- Acquired von Willebrand's disease
  - Multiple doses of intermediate purity factor VIII will normally neutralize the pathogenic antibody temporarily as it is normally of low titre
  - Ivlg may be used in an attempt to eradicate the inhibitor

Further reading

Delgado, J., Jimenez-Yuste, V., Hernandez-Navarro, F. and Villar, A. (2003). Acquired haemophilia: review and meta-analysis focused on therapy and prognostic factors. *Br. J. Haematol.* **121**: 21–35.

⑦ Haematuria

Haematuria is the presence of blood in the urine.

Microscopic haematuria is >3 RBC per high power field in urinary sediment.

Macroscopic haematuria is the presence of blood in the urine visible to the naked eye.

Any haematuria should never be ignored. In adults haematuria should be regarded as a symptom of urological malignancy until proven otherwise. Patients under 40 years of age with microscopic haematuria should be referred to the renal physician for investigation for glomerulonephritis.

Causes

Upper tract (kidney and ureter)

- Malignant renal tumours:
  - Renal cell carcinoma
  - Renal/ureteric transitional cell carcinoma
- Benign renal tumours:
  - Renal cyst
  - Angiomyolipoma
- Renal or ureteric calculi
- Glomerulonephritis
- Pyelonephritis
- Papillary necrosis
- Trauma

Lower tract (bladder, urethra, and prostate)

- Bladder tumours
  - Transitional cell carcinoma — common
  - Adenocarcinoma — rare
  - Squamous cell carcinoma — rare
- Urinary tract infection
- Cystitis
  - Drug-related (e.g. ifosfamide, cyclophosphamide)
  - Radiation
  - Interstitial cystitis
  - Schistosomiasis
- Prostate tumours
  - Benign prostatic hyperplasia
  - Adenocarcinoma of the prostate
- Trauma

Rare causes of haematuria

- Arteriovenous malformation
- TB
- Arteritis

The most common cause (20–25%) of macroscopic haematuria in a patient >50 years of age is carcinoma of the bladder.

Investigations
Bloods
- FBC
- Coagulation screen
  - Patients with an INR in the therapeutic range must be fully investigated, as haematuria is not a normal consequence of anticoagulation
- U&Es

Urine
- Urine dipstick
  - If protein detected → 24-hour protein collection, and consider referral to renal physician
- Urine sample
  - MC&S
  - Cytology

Microscopic haematuria

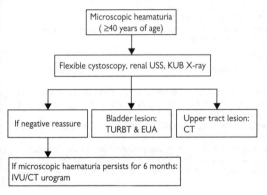

Fig. 1.5 Investigation of microscopic haematuria.

NB. All cases of bladder carcinoma should have an IVU or CT urogram at diagnosis to exclude a concomitant upper tract lesion.

Macroscopic haematuria

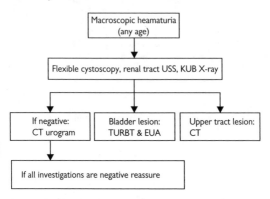

Fig. 1.6 Investigation of macroscopic haematuria.

NB. In suspected ureteric lesions further information can be obtained from a retrograde study or by direct inspection using the ureteroscope.

Management

- Most cases of haematuria settle by increasing the patient's oral fluid intake.
- If the haematuria becomes severe and the patient develops clot retention, urethral catheterization with a three-way irrigating catheter is required (usually a 22-F catheter).
- Initially bladder washouts are required to remove any clot from the bladder.
- Bladder irrigation is then set up using either saline or sterile water.
- If bladder washouts and bladder irrigation do not clear the clots a formal bladder washout +/− TURBT under anaesthesia is generally required.

Further reading

American Urological Association Microscopic Hematuria guidelines (2001). www.auanet.org/guidelines

Cardiovascular emergencies

① **Superior vena cava obstruction**

Superior vena cava obstruction (SVCO) is a commonly encountered problem in certain subgroups of cancer patients.

The SVC is formed by the fusion of the left and right brachiocephalic veins. It extends caudally for 5–8 cm and drains into the right atrium. The azygos vein also arches over the right main bronchus to fuse posteriorly with the SVC. The SVC is contained within a confined anatomical space with the mediastinal parietal pleura laterally and the mediastinal lymph nodes medially. As the vein is thin-walled and only filled at relatively low pressure, any significant compression within this space can result in obstruction to blood flow. External compression (by tumour, lymphadenopathy or some other process) is often complicated by internal thrombosis within the blood vessel. The severity of the resulting syndrome depends on the rapidity of onset and the level of the obstruction. Secondary thrombosis often results in a more rapid onset and more severe symptoms. A more gradual onset allows the establishment of collateral blood flow and limits the severity. If the obstruction is above the level of the azygos vein, this system can readily dilate and shunt blood, thus limiting the severity of symptoms.

Clinical features

Symptoms
- Fullness of face, neck, and arms
- Dyspnoea
- Cough
- Dysphagia
- Headache
- Visual disturbance
- Hoarseness
- Syncopal episodes
- Symptoms of underlying malignancy
  - haemoptysis
  - weight loss
  - night sweats
- Symptoms worse first thing in the morning and exacerbated by bending or lying down

Signs
- Facial suffusion and oedema
- Chemosis
- Arm oedema
- Fixed engorgement of veins with downward flow in distribution of SVC
  - head
  - neck
  - arms
  - upper thorax
- Papilloedema
  - uncommon and late sign
- Signs of underlying malignancy
  - lymphadenopathy
  - pleural effusion
    — especially right-sided
  - hepatomegaly
- See Fig. 2.1

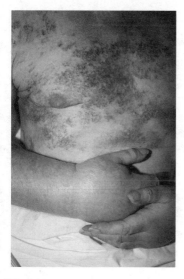

Fig. 2.1 Dilated chest wall collateral veins and bilateral arm oedema in a patient presenting with SVCO.

Causes

Malignant causes (85–95%)
- Small cell lung carcinoma (SCLC)
- Non-small cell lung carcinoma (NSCLC)
  - Squamous cell carcinoma of the lung
  - Adenocarcinoma of the lung
  - Large cell carcinoma of the lung
- Non-Hodgkin's lymphoma
- Rarely
  - germ cell neoplasms
  - metastatic breast cancer
  - metastatic colon cancer
  - Kaposi's sarcoma
  - oesophageal carcinoma
  - mesothelioma
  - Hodgkin's disease

Non-malignant causes
- Mediastinal fibrosis
- SVC thrombosis
  - indwelling central lines
  - pacemaker wires
- Rarely
  - Behçet's disease
  - sarcoidosis
  - retrosternal goitre
  - tuberculosis

Differential diagnosis
- Heart failure
- Cardiac tamponade
- External jugular vein compression

Investigation

The diagnosis of SVCO is often clinically obvious and much of the investigation is aimed at establishing the underlying cause. Unless the condition is complicated by another life-threatening condition (e.g. tracheal obstruction), then definitive treatment can, and should, await the histological diagnosis.

Imaging
- CXR
  - mediastinal widening (60%)
  - mass
    — right upper lobe
    — mediastinal
  - pleural effusion (25%)
  - lobar collapse
  - normal CXR is unusual (<20%)
- CT of thorax with contrast
  - anatomy of disease
    — may guide choice of biopsy technique
  - venous patency and associated thrombus
  - establishment of collateral flow
  - See Figs 2.2 and 2.3
- MRI, USS, and venography may also be useful

Tissue diagnosis
- Sputum cytology
- FNA or biopsy
  - Bronchoscopy
  - Transcutaneous
    - CT or USS-guided
  - Mediastinoscopy
    - very high diagnostic accuracy
  - From site of other disease
    - if technically and clinically more appropriate
    - lymphadenopathy
      - supraclavicular   – cervical
    - liver metastases
  - Occasionally, open biopsy may be necessary
    - thoracotomy   — mediastinotomy

Management
The primary treatment depends on:
- Urgency of relief required
- Underlying histological diagnosis

The most appropriate treatment is usually to treat the underlying cause. This, therefore, requires previous knowledge of the presence of malignancy; otherwise, treatment should be delayed to obtain a tissue diagnosis. In the presence of cerebral oedema or disabling symptoms, stent placement provides the most rapid relief and provides time for definitive tissue diagnosis. Chemotherapy and radiotherapy should be withheld until the cause of the obstruction is known, as in a minority of cases the cause is non-malignant.

Immediate management
- Nurse with the head of the bed elevated
- Corticosteroids
  - Dexamethasone 8 mg PO bd with proton pump inhibitor cover
  - May reduce diagnostic accuracy of lymphoma
    - if commenced before biopsy
- Diuretics

Chemotherapy
- The treatment of choice in chemosensitive disease
  - SCLC   • germ cell tumours
  - lymphoma
- Response rates are not affected by the presence of SVCO and mirror those of the underlying disease

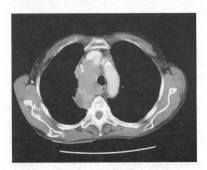

Fig. 2.2 CT scan (with IV contrast) shows a right mediastinal lymph node mass compressing the SVC.

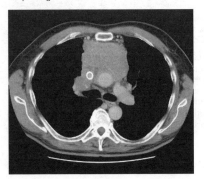

Fig. 2.3 CT scan post-stent insertion for SVCO caused by a large mediastinal mass in a patient with small cell lung cancer.

Radiotherapy

- For non-chemosensitive disease
- Usually treated with a parallel pair covering the disease compressing the SVC
- A variety of schedules have been used, from 8 Gy/1# to 50 Gy/25#.
- Response rates vary according to underlying disease, with symptomatic relief in:
  - 60–80% of patients with SCLC
  - 40–50% of patients with NSCLC

Radiological stent placement

- Radiologically placed intravascular expandable stent gives rapid and reliable symptomatic relief in 90–95% of patients.
- The need for anticoagulation following stent placement has yet to be confirmed.
- Stent insertion is the treatment of choice for recurrent chemoresistant and radioresistant disease.
- This requires the expertise of an interventional radiologist confident in SVC stent insertion; this may not therefore be available in all centres.

Thrombolysis

- Patients with documented thrombus in association with partial SVCO may benefit from thrombectomy (rarely) and/or thrombolysis.
- For most cancer patients simple anticoagulation with LMWH and subsequent warfarin may be more appropriate.

Surgery

- The use of surgical bypass is possibly best restricted to benign conditions but this approach has also been used in malignant disease.

Prognosis

- Rather than being dependent on the diagnosis of SVCO itself, the prognosis with this condition is entirely dependent on the histology and stage of the underlying disease and the patient's general condition.
- SVCO commonly relapses, with symptoms recurring in 15–20% of those cases caused by lung cancer.

Further reading

Ostier, P.J., Clarke, D.P., Watkinson, A.F. and Gaze, M.N. (1997). Superior vena cava obstruction: A modern management strategy. *Clin. Oncol.* **9**: 83–89.

Rowell, N.P. and Gleeson, F.V. (2002). Steroids, radiotherapy, chemotherapy and stents for superior vena cava obstruction in carcinoma of the bronchus: A systematic review. *Clin. Oncol.* **14**(5): 338–351.

⑦ **Venous thromboembolism**

Venous thromboembolism (VTE) comprises:
- Deep venous thrombosis (DVT)
- Inferior vena cava thrombosis
- Pulmonary embolus (PE)

VTE is relatively common in cancer patients. Cancer is a major risk factor for development of VTE and this is thought to be due to a number of factors, including a hypercoagulable state that develops with the presence of cancer.

There is an increased risk of cancer being detected within 6–12 months of a first episode of VTE, particularly in those with no other risk factors and/or recurrent episodes. VTE may be the presenting symptom of occult malignancy, present in 7–12% of those with VTE and no other risk factors.

Pulmonary embolism has an untreated mortality rate of 30% and a treated mortality rate of 12% at 1 month. The occurrence of VTE in patients already known to have cancer is a poor prognostic factor. Non-fatal recurrence, particularly in the first year, is common in those with disabling neurological disease and cancer, and least likely in those with temporary risk factors.

Virchow's triad of features that promote thrombus formation:
- Abnormal blood constituents
  - cancer may produce thrombophilic substances
- Abnormal vessel wall
  - cancer may compress or invade into vessel
- Abnormal flow
  - cancer may compress vessel

Risk factors for VTE
- Major risk factors (relative risk 5–20)
  - Malignancy
    - abdominal/pelvic
    - advanced/metastatic
  - Surgery
    - major abdominal/pelvic
    - postoperative ICU
    - lower limb
  - Lower limb trauma/fracture
  - Obstetrics
    - late pregnancy
    - puerperium
    - caesarean section
  - Previous thromboembolism
  - Immobility

- Minor risk factors (relative risk 2–4)
  - Cardiovascular
    - — CCF — hypertension
    - — indwelling central venous catheter
      - – PICC line – Groshong line
      - – Hickman line
  - Oestrogens
    - — tamoxifen — HRT
    - — combined oral contraceptive pill
  - Obesity
  - Other
    - — myeloproliferative disorders — nephrotic syndrome
    - — COPD — chronic dialysis
    - — neurological disability — IBD
    - — thrombophilia — Behçet's disease
    - — paroxysmal nocturnal haemoglobinuria

⑦ Deep vein thrombosis (DVT)

- Typically presents as unilateral swelling of a lower limb.
  - Bilateral DVT is unusual and bilateral lower limb swelling raises the possibility of:
    - — IVC obstruction
    - — hypoalbuminaemia
    - — CCF
    - — lymphoedema secondary to malignant involvement of draining pelvic lymph nodes
- May involve:
  - Only veins distal to the knee
  - Veins proximal to the knee
  - Proximal large veins within the pelvis
    - — common iliac — external iliac
- May occur in the upper limb, especially in association with an indwelling central venous catheter (PICC, Hickman line, Groshong line).
- Can also occur as a complication of tumour growth and direct compression of a vein.

Clinical features

- Swollen oedematous limb
- Pain and tenderness
- Erythema or discoloration
- Increased warmth
- Collateral circulation
  - distended superficial veins, especially in the upper limb

Investigations

- Patients must be stratified by determining their pre-test probability for the presence of DVT.
- All patients with a previously objectively diagnosed DVT/PE are regarded as high risk.

- All other patients are assessed according to the following criteria:
  - Active cancer   1
  - Paralysis, plaster   1
  - Bed >3 days or surgery within 4 weeks   1
  - Tenderness along veins   1
  - Entire leg swollen   1
  - Calf swollen >3 cm   1
  - Pitting oedema   1
  - Collateral superficial veins   1
  - Alternative diagnosis likely   −2
    — ruptured Baker's cyst
    — superficial thrombophlebitis
    — cellulitis
      Low probability   ≤0
      Moderate probability   1–2
      High probability   ≥3
- Low probability patients
  - If D-dimer is negative (<500 µg/l) DVT is reliably excluded and no further investigation is required.
  - If D-dimer is positive (>500 µg/l) proceed to compression USS.
- Moderate and high probability patients
  - Proceed directly to compression USS.
    — If this is negative, a DVT proximal to the knee has been excluded.
      – If D-dimer is then found to be negative no further investigation is required.
      – If D-dimer is found to be positive, a further compression USS is required after 1 week to exclude the presence of a distal DVT that has progressed to become a proximal DVT.

Bloods
- D-dimer levels are non-specific, being elevated during infection, inflammation, postoperatively, and even by the presence of malignancy alone. False negative results can occur.
- Prior to commencing anticoagulation, a patient's baseline coagulation screen (PT, APTT) must be measured. Other blood tests are also required to assess the risks from anticoagulation.
  - FBC
    — evidence of occult bleeding   — platelet count
  - LFTs
  - U&Es
    — LMWH should not be used in patients with severe renal impairment.

Imaging
- Contrast venography remains the gold standard investigation for DVT; however, it is an invasive investigation.
- Compression USS is highly sensitive for detecting proximal DVT; however, it is less accurate for isolated distal below-knee DVT. The risk of PE is low from isolated below-knee DVT and there is no evidence to support the need for anticoagulation in these patients.

⑦ IVC thrombosis

This represents a subset of DVT; however, some specific situations only relate to IVC thrombosis.
- Renal cell cancer
  - intravascular tumour propagating into the IVC
- Direct compression of the IVC
  - retroperitoneal lymphadenopathy
    — germ cell tumours   — prostate cancer
  - retroperitoneal leiomyosarcoma
  - adrenal cortical carcinoma
  - retroperitoneal fibrosis

Clinical features
- Classically bilateral lower limb oedema with dilated superficial veins.
- If the thrombosis occurs above the level of the renal veins, renal function may deteriorate owing to reduction in renal perfusion.

Investigations
Imaging
- USS
  - less sensitive in the abdomen than in the legs
    — presence of bowel gas
    — difficulty in assessing venous compressibility
- Contrast-enhanced CT

☼ Pulmonary embolism (PE)

Obstruction of part of the pulmonary vascular tree by a thrombus that has travelled from a distant site. Other rare causes include tumour embolism, air embolism, and fat embolism.

Typically occurs in the presence of DVT (70%, but only clinically apparent in 25%) but occasionally no source of embolus is found.

Clinical features

No symptoms or signs are diagnostic.
- Dyspnoea and tachypnoea (>20 breaths/minute)
  - if absent, pleuritic pain/haemoptysis usually reflect other pathology
  - acute onset for acute PE
  - insidious onset for chronic PE, owing to recurrent small volume clots
- Pleuritic chest pain
- Cough
  - may be productive of blood-stained sputum (haemoptysis)
- Tachycardia
  - loud P_2 • split S_2
- Hypotension
  - suggests massive PE causing right heart failure
- Palpitations
- Hypoxia
- Pleural rub
- Raised JVP

Investigations
- Patients must be stratified by determining their pre-test probability for the presence of PE.
- In all patients presenting with features compatible with PE
  - Dyspnoea and tachypnoea +/− pleuritic chest pain +/− haemoptysis
  - Two other factors are sought
    — the absence of another reasonable clinical explanation
    — the presence of a major risk factor (see p98)
  - Where both factors are true the pre-test probability is high
  - If only one is true the pre-test probability is intermediate
  - If neither is true the pre-test probability is low
- In cancer patients, therefore, any patient presenting with features compatible with PE will be high probability unless there is a reasonable alternative clinical explanation for their symptoms, when they will be intermediate probability.
- Low and intermediate probability patients
  - If D-dimer is negative (<500 µg/l) PE is reliably excluded and no further investigation is required.
  - If D-dimer is positive (>500 µg/l) proceed to imaging investigations.
- High probability patients
  - Proceed directly to imaging investigations (ideally within 24 hours).

Bloods
- D-dimer levels are non-specific, being elevated during infection, inflammation, postoperatively, and by the presence of malignancy alone. False negative results may occur in patients with subsegmental PE.
- ABG
  - Hypoxia is common; however, oxygen saturation may be normal.
- Alveolar–arterial O_2 gradient (A–a gradient)
  - Estimate of alveolar–arterial O_2 gradient
    — A–a = $[(FiO_2) - (PaO_2 + PaCO_2/0.8)]$
      - FiO_2 in % (room air 21%)
      - PaO_2 and $PaCO_2$ in kPa (from ABG).
  - Normal A–a gradient ~2 kPa
    — at sea level with normal humidity
    — increases with increasing age.
  - An elevated A–a gradient with a normal CXR is highly suggestive for PE.
- Troponin elevation is certainly common in PE. In a patient with chest pain, dyspnoea, T wave inversion and a raised troponin, the differential diagnosis includes MI and PE.
  - Distinguishing between these two diagnoses relies on:
    — the characteristics of the chest pain
      - pleuritic in PE
      - chest tightness radiating to the neck and arms in MI
    — an echo may be required.

- Prior to commencing anticoagulation, a patient's baseline coagulation screen (PT, APTT) must be measured. Other blood tests are also required to assess the risks from anticoagulation.
  - FBC
    - evidence of occult bleeding — platelet count
  - LFTs
  - U&Es
    - LMWH should not be used in patients with severe renal impairment.

ECG
- Non-specific changes are commonest
  - sinus tachycardia
  - atrial fibrillation
  - right bundle branch block
  - anterior T wave inversion
- Uncommonly
  - $S_IQ_{III}T_{III}$
    - S wave in lead I
    - Q wave in lead III
    - T wave inversion in lead III
- See Fig. 2.4

Imaging
- CXR
  - No specific features are characteristic
  - Small effusions are present in 40% of patients with PE
- V/Q scan
  - Can only be used in patients with:
    - a normal CXR
    - no concurrent cardiopulmonary disease
  - A normal/low probability result reliably excludes PE
  - A high probability result is not diagnostic of PE
    - false positives are possible in those with previous rather than current PE
  - Further imaging (e.g. CTPA) is mandatory in all those patients with:
    - an indeterminate result
    - discordant clinical assessment and V/Q scan
- CTPA
  - The investigation of choice for PE
    - more specific than V/Q scanning
    - may provide the correct diagnosis when PE has been excluded
  - See Figs 2.5 and 2.6
- Echo
  - Echo is very non-specific for the diagnosis of PE; it may show evidence of right heart dilatation and raised pulmonary pressures
  - Its main uses are:
    - in the emergency setting in the absence of imaging with a CTPA
    - exclusion of an MI
      - evidenced by regional wall motion abnormalities

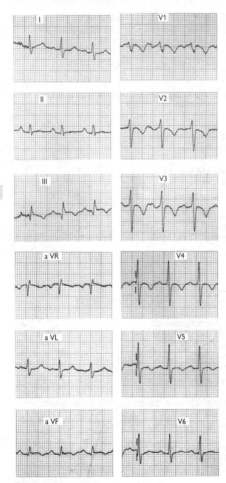

Fig. 2.4 12-lead ECG in acute massive PE.
- Sinus tachycardia.
- Incomplete right bundle branch block.
- T wave inversion in the right precordial leads.
- Right atrial dilatation
  - tall peaked T waves in lead II.
- $S_IQ_{III}T_{III}$
  - S wave in lead I
  - Q wave in lead III
  - T wave inversion in lead III.

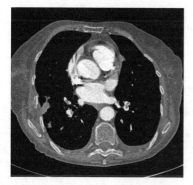

Fig. 2.5 CTPA shows extensive pulmonary embolic disease.
- Thrombus within the lobar and segmental branches of both pulmonary arteries.
- There is also a right-sided rib metastasis, confirming the diagnosis of metastatic cancer. For this patient the PE was the presenting symptom of occult metastatic malignancy.

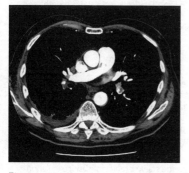

Fig. 2.6 CTPA shows extensive pulmonary embolic disease.
- There is also a small right pleural effusion.

Management of VTE

- Remove any precipitating indwelling venous catheter
- Oxygen as required
- Adequate analgesia

Anticoagulation

- Formal anticoagulation should commence as soon as the diagnosis is confirmed. If PE is considered LMWH should be started in patients with a high or intermediate pre-test probability before imaging.
- Anticoagulation will reduce the risk of recurrent embolism.
- Length of anticoagulation:
  - 6 weeks in the presence of an identifiable temporary risk factor (e.g. indwelling venous catheter).
  - 3–6 months for first episode of idiopathic VTE.
  - Indefinite anticoagulation in those with persisting risk factors (e.g. cancer)
    - although evidence suggests that this results in an increased risk of bleeding with no evidence for a reduction in mortality.
- Bleeding on treatment is common.
  - The risk of bleeding is related both to the intensity and duration of anticoagulation.
  - The rate of major bleeding in all patients is <3% at 3 months and mortality is <0.5%.
  - The risk of bleeding is six times higher in cancer patients than non-cancer patients:
    - haemoptysis   — thrombocytopenia
    - GI bleed   — NSAIDs
    - haemorrhage into brain metastases
  - The risk of significant bleeding must be weighed against the risk to the patient of not being anticoagulated.
  - If bleeding risk is high, consider the use of long term LMWH in place of warfarin, because the anticoagulating effect of LMWH:
    - is more predictable than trying to control the INR.
    - only lasts for 24 hours after each SC injection.

LMWH

- Once daily SC injections provide stable predictable anticoagulation.
- Lee *et al.* (2003) report that in cancer patients LMWH is more effective than oral anticoagulation in reducing the risk of recurrent thromboembolism without increasing the risk of bleeding.
- LMWH is becoming increasingly popular as the first choice for anticoagulation in certain groups of cancer patients
  - CNS primary   - Hepatic metastases
  - Brain metastases   - Deranged liver function
  - Those on capecitabine chemotherapy
  - Those at high risk of recurrent thromboembolism

Warfarin
- Target INR
  - 2.5 for VTE
  - 3.5 for recurrent VTE in patients on warfarin with an INR >2.0
  - An INR within 0.5 of the target value is generally satisfactory
- Commence LMWH at therapeutic dose and continue until INR is therapeutic (INR >2.0)
- Commence warfarin
  - Many trusts now have outpatient anticoagulation clinics who will oversee warfarin anticoagulation and monitoring
  - Dosing regimes vary, therefore follow local policy
    — An example
      - Day 1 and 2
        5 mg each evening if INR<1.4 (PT<16 seconds)
      - Day 3

<1.5	10 mg	2.6–3.0	1 mg
1.5–2.0	5 mg	>3.0	0 mg
2.1–2.5	3 mg		

      - Day 4

<1.6	10 mg	2.8–3.0	3 mg
1.6–1.7	7 mg	3.1–3.5	2 mg
1.8–1.9	6 mg	3.6–4.0	1 mg
2.0–2.3	5 mg	>4.0	0 mg
2.4–2.7	4 mg		

Fondaparinux
- A synthetic pentasaccharide that binds antithrombin and enhances its activity towards factor Xa, but has no activity against thrombin.
- There is no risk of heparin-induced thrombocytopenia (unlike LMWH).
- Once daily SC injection.
- Licensed for the prophylaxis and treatment of VTE.

Recurrent thromboembolism
- Cancer patients have three times the risk of recurrent thromboembolism than patients without cancer.
- Options for treatment are:
  - Aim for an INR of 3.5
  - Change to LMWH
  - Addition of LMWH to warfarin therapy (increased risk of bleeding)
  - Consider insertion of an IVC umbrella filter

IVC filter
- An IVC filter can be used where anticoagulation
  - is contraindicated
  - is unsuccessful in preventing recurrence of PE from continuing DVT.
- It is inserted under image guidance by an interventional radiologist.
- It can be temporary or permanent.
- It is designed to filter out clots as they travel upwards from the pelvic veins through the IVC.
- Good evidence that filters improve long term recurrence rates or mortality is, however, lacking.

Management of acute massive PE

- 10–15% of patients with PE present with circulatory collapse owing to acute massive PE resulting in right heart failure.
- The diagnosis of acute massive PE is suggested by severe hypoxia and hypotension.
- Give high flow oxygen.
- Investigations are driven by the clinical situation
  - Balancing the need to confirm the diagnosis and the patient's suitability for investigation and treatment.
    - Is the patient stable enough to move to radiology department?
      - Consider unfractionated heparin IV 80 units/kg prior to imaging.
    - If acute massive PE is confirmed, is the patient suitable for thrombolysis?
  - Consider
    - ECG   — ECHO
    - CXR   — CTPA
- If the patient is not suitable for thrombolysis, owing to significant risk of bleeding, then treat as for standard PE.
- If the patient is suitable for invasive treatment and PE is confirmed, then commence thrombolysis as early as possible.
  - Alteplase 10 mg by IV injection over 1–2 minute, followed by IV infusion of 90 mg over 2 hours, max 1.5 mg/kg in patients less than 65 kg
  - Streptokinase IV 250 000 U over 30 minutes, then 100 000 U per hour for up to 12–72 hours according to condition.
- If a diagnosis of PE is likely and the patient is deteriorating and at risk of cardiac arrest, do not wait for CTPA/echo before considering thrombolysis.
- Cardiac arrest:
  - PE accounts for:
    - 10% of patients admitted with non-traumatic sudden death.
    - 50% of patients arriving with EMD or asystole on ECG.
  - In spite of aggressive treatment, very few survive to discharge.
  - However, should cardiac arrest occur while in hospital and massive PE is strongly suspected clinically, an immediate IV bolus of 50 mg alteplase administered during CPR may be life-saving.

Reference

Lee, A.Y.Y., Levine, M.N., Baker, R.I., Bowden, C., Kakkar, A.K., Prins, M., Rickles, F.R., Julian, J., Haley, S., Kovacs, M. and Gent, M. (2003). Low-molecular-weight heparin versus a coumarin for the prevention of recurrent venous thromboembolism in patients with cancer. *N. Engl. J. Med.* **349**: 146–153.

Further reading

Blann, A.D. and Lip, G.Y.H. (2006). Venous thromboembolism. *BMJ* **332**: 215–219.

Campbell, I.A., Fennerty, A. and Miller, A.C. (2003). British Thoracic Society guidelines for the management of suspected acute pulmonary embolism. *Thorax* **58**: 470–483.

Capstick, T. and Henry, M.T. (2005). Efficacy of thrombolytic agents in the treatment of pulmonary embolism. *Eur. Respir. J.* **26**: 864–874.

Ho, W.K., Hankey, G.J., Lee, C.H. and Eikelboom, J.W. (2005). Venous thromboembolism: diagnosis and management of deep vein thrombosis. *Med. J. Aust.* **182**: 476–481.

Robinson, G.V. (2006). Pulmonary embolism in hospital practice. *BMJ* **332**: 156–160.

① Pericardial effusion and tamponade

Pericardial effusion denotes the presence of excess fluid in the pericardial space and is not uncommon in patients with advanced malignancy. Cardiac tamponade occurs when a pericardial effusion causes haemodynamically significant cardiac compression. Tamponade is a clinical diagnosis, supported by echocardiographic findings, and exhibits a spectrum of severity. The haemodynamic consequences of fluid in the pericardial space depend on the volume of fluid and principally how quickly it has accumulated. In malignant effusions there has generally been time for the stiff pericardium to distend and so large volumes (~2 litres) may often be accommodated without symptoms.

Immediate drainage is only indicated in the case of overt tamponade, which is very uncommon in patients with malignancy.

Causes of pericardial effusion

- Malignancy
  - Lung
  - Breast
  - Leukaemia
  - Lymphoma
  - Melanoma
- Infection
  - TB
  - Viral, e.g. coxsackie
  - Bacterial, e.g. septicaemia
  - Fungal
- Radiotherapy
- Uraemia
- Collagen vascular disease
  - SLE
  - PAN
- Hypothyroidism
- Trauma/iatrogenic

Clinical features

Symptoms

- Asymptomatic
- Dyspnoea
- Positional chest pain
- Cough
- Light-headed/dizzy

Signs

- Beck's triad
  - Hypotension
  - Muffled heart sounds
  - Raised JVP
- Pulsus paradoxus (an exaggeration of the physiological drop in blood pressure on inspiration)
- Kussmaul's sign (a rise in the JVP with inspiration)
- Sinus tachycardia
- Pericardial rub (in the early stages)
- Signs of right and, eventually, left heart failure

Investigations

Bloods
- FBC
  - infection
  - leukaemia
  - lymphoma
- U&Es
  - uraemia
- TFTs
  - hypothyroidism
- Autoimmune screen
  - collagen vascular disease

ECG
- Reduced QRS voltages
- Electrical alternans
- 'Saddle-shaped' ST elevation
- Sinus tachycardia

Imaging
- CXR
  - cardiomegaly
  - lung cancer
  - pneumonia
  - TB
- ECHO (investigation of choice)
  - small effusions are <1 cm thick and often localized posteriorly
  - large effusions are >1 cm thick and surround the heart
  - early signs suggestive of incipient tamponade are right atrial collapse and, later, right ventricular diastolic collapse
- TOE/CT/MRI
  - not usually required unless effusion is small or loculated

Management of pericardial effusion and tamponade

- The management is dependent on:
  - haemodynamic status of the patient
  - whether diagnostic aspiration is required
- The size of an effusion is not necessarily a good guide to the presence or absence of tamponade.
- In asymptomatic patients with large effusions, serial echo and observation is prudent whilst a definitive treatment strategy is decided.
- Routine pericardial drainage is rarely justified owing to the inherent risks of the procedure and the likelihood of fluid reaccumulation unless the underlying cause has been addressed.
- When to drain an effusion
  - Tamponade
  - Tamponade prophylaxis
  - Aid to diagnosis (typically only 7% diagnostic yield)
    - Samples should be sent for:
      - culture
      - Gram stain and ZN stain
      - cytology

- Pericardiocentesis is a potentially hazardous procedure and should be undertaken under echo guidance or with the aid of fluoroscopy, by experienced practitioners.
- Patients requiring pericardiocentesis should be closely monitored and their circulation should be supported with IV fluids.

Definitive management of malignant pericardial effusion

Malignancy is the most common cause of reaccumulation of pericardial effusion. Definitive treatment requires the creation of a pericardial window or instillation of sclerosant.

- Pleuropericardial window
- Pericardiectomy
- Percutaneous balloon pericardiotomy
- Intrapericardial sclerosants

Further reading

Soler-Soler, J., Sagristà-Sauleda, J. and Permanyer-Miralda, G. (2001). Management of pericardial effusion. *Heart* **86**: 235–240.

Vaitkus, P.T., Herrmann, H. and LeWinter, M.M. (1994). Management of malignant pericardial effusion. *JAMA* **272**: 59–64.

Zipes, D.P., Libby, P., Bonow, R.O. and Braunwald, E. (eds) (2004). *Braunwald's Heart Disease*, 7th edn. Philadelphia W.B. Saunders.

⑦ **Cardiac masses**

Metastatic involvement of the heart is 20 times more common than primary cardiac tumours. The clinical presentation of cardiac tumours is more closely related to their size, location, and effect on surrounding cardiac structures than on their histological type.

The common clinical presentations include:
- Heart failure
- Peripheral embolism
- Arrhythmia

Left atrial tumours

- 90% of primary cardiac left atrial tumours are myxomas.
- Signs and symptoms mimic those of mitral valve disease, particularly mitral stenosis. Atrial fibrillation is less common as the tumour is intracavitary and does not lead to left atrial dilatation.
- Physical examination reveals a pansystolic murmur, resembling mitral regurgitation, and a diastolic murmur secondary to obstruction of the mitral valve by the tumour. In addition, a loud S_1, S_4 and early diastolic sound (tumour plop) may also be heard.

Right atrial tumours

- 50% of primary cardiac right atrial tumours are sarcomas.
- Frequently present with symptoms of right heart failure.

Ventricular tumours

- Intracavitary ventricular tumours may present with either left- or right- sided heart failure dependent on their location.
- Intramural tumours may be asymptomatic or may mimic restrictive or dilated cardiomyopathies.

Clinical features

Symptoms

Left ventricular failure
- Reduced exercise tolerance
- Cough (pink frothy sputum)
- Dyspnoea
  - Exertional
  - Paroxysmal nocturnal dyspnoea
  - Orthopnoea
- Fatigue

Right ventricular failure
- Peripheral oedema
- Abdominal distension
- Malaise
- Nausea/anorexia

Arrhythmia
- Palpitations
- Syncope

Embolism
- Commonly neurological symptoms, although symptoms dependent on site of embolism

Signs
Left ventricular failure
- Tachypnoea
- Tachycardia
- Fine lung crackles or wheeze (cardiac asthma)
- Anxious, sweaty
- Raised JVP
- S_3/gallop rhythm

Right ventricular failure
- Raised JVP
- Hepatomegaly
- Abdominal distension
- Pitting oedema

Investigations
Bloods
- FBC, U&Es, cardiac enzymes, ABG
  - to assess the severity of heart failure

ECG
- 24-hour tape/telemetry
  - arrhythmia

Imaging
- CXR
  - pulmonary oedema
- Echo (investigation of choice)
  - cardiac structure and function
- TOE/CT/MRI
  - cardiac structure and function

Management
Pulmonary oedema
- Treatment of acute pulmonary oedema
  - Sit the patient upright
  - 100% oxygen (provided no history of CO_2 retention)
  - IV access and cardiac monitor
  - 2.5–5 mg diamorphine IV
  - 40–120 mg furosemide IV
  - Start nitrates IV (e.g. GTN 2–10 mg/h)
    - titrate to keep SBP >90 mmHg (caution if moderate to severe aortic stenosis)
- Further treatment is dependent on the underlying cause of the pulmonary oedema. If there is any uncertainty arrange urgent echo and discuss with cardiologist
- Consider
  - Urgent surgical referral if LVF secondary to severe valvular dysfunction or structural defects
  - Rate control of acute tachycardia
  - Dobutamine/dopamine and central line if refractory pulmonary oedema secondary to severe left ventricular impairment

Embolism

- Discuss with cardiology/surgical cardiothoracic team, as prompt surgery may be required.
- Anticoagulation may be needed (See Venous thromboembolism 📖 p98).

☼ Arrhythmias

- Any patient with a rhythm disturbance must be assessed for cardiovascular compromise.
- Diagnosis and immediate management should follow the Resuscitation council arrhythmia guidelines (see Appendix 📖 p409).
  - Tachycardia algorithm (with pulse)
  - Bradycardia algorithm
- If the patient is not immediately at risk then an attempt should be made to establish the:
  - Source of the abnormal rhythm
    — sinoatrial node   — atria
    — atrioventricular node   — ventricle
  - Integrity of the conducting system
    — heart block   — accessory pathway
    — bundle branch block
- Outlined below are some general management principles for acute rhythm disturbances. However, the Resuscitation council arrhythmia guidelines are recommended both for diagnostic and therapeutic interventions. Longer term management should be discussed with a cardiologist.

Tachycardia

- Important questions include:
  - broad or narrow complex tachycardia?
  - regular or irregular rhythm?
- Narrow complex tachycardia
  - In general, supraventricular arrhythmias with rates <200 bpm rarely cause immediate haemodynamic compromise unless there is pre-existing cardiac disease or other significant co-morbidity. Nevertheless, there are always exceptions, and uncontrolled supraventricular tachycardia will eventually lead to tachycardia-mediated cardiomyopathy if not treated promptly.
  - The priority initially is correct identification of the rhythm disturbance.
    — Irregular narrow complex tachycardia
      - most likely to be atrial fibrillation
      - rarely
        • atrial flutter with variable conduction
        • multifocal atrial tachycardia
        • other supraventricular rhythms

- Rate control of atrial fibrillation can be obtained with a number of agents, all of which have limitations and contraindications.
  - digoxin
  - amiodarone
  - beta blockers
  - verapamil
- Acute rate control (1–2 hours)
  - amiodarone IV
    - if patient is compromised by the atrial fibrillation
    - 5 mg/kg over 20–120 minutes, up to max 1.2 g in 24 hours
    - has the potential to cause cardioversion to sinus rhythm with the associated thromboembolic risk
  - metoprolol IV
    - if patient has:
      - good blood pressure (SBP >120 mmHg)
      - no asthma
      - no prior structural heart disease
    - up to 5 mg bolus at rate 1–2 mg/minute, repeated after 5 minutes if necessary, total dose 10–15 mg
    - with no potential to cause cardioversion
    - beware:
      - hypotension
      - heart failure
      - asthma
      - heart block
- Subacute rate control (12–24 hours)
  - digoxin PO/IV
    - 1–1.5 µg in divided doses over 24 hours. Less urgent digitalis 250–500 µg daily
    - digoxin IV 0.75–1 mg over 2 hours
      - may result in faster loading; however, if acute rate control is needed use amiodarone or metoprolol
    - doses may need to be reduced in elderly patients and those with renal impairment
  - digoxin alone may not be sufficient to control rate so have a low threshold for adding:
    - beta blockers
      - atenolol 25–100 mg PO od
      - bisoprolol 2.5–10 mg PO od
    - calcium antagonists
      - diltiazem MR 120–360 mg PO od
      - verapamil MR 120–480 mg PO od
    - never combine verapamil/diltiazem with a beta blocker owing to the combined negative ionotropic effect
- Consideration should also be given to the patient's thromboembolic risk and aspirin 300 mg od or LMWH can be used as an interim measure depending on the risk-benefit ratio.
- New onset atrial fibrillation always requires investigation for potential triggers
  - MI
  - hyperthyroidism
  - sepsis
  - PE
- Treatment of the precipitant may ultimately be the most effective way to treat the atrial fibrillation

- Regular narrow complex tachycardia
  - should be investigated as per Resuscitation Council guidelines
    - vagal manoeuvres
    - adenosine
      - contraindications
        - active wheeze
        - known Wolff–Parkinson–White syndrome
  - treatment initiated as per Resuscitation Council guidelines
- Broad complex tachycardia
  - Broad complex tachycardia should always be assumed to be VT until proven otherwise as VT is by far the commonest broad complex tachycardia and inappropriate administration of drugs designed to treat supraventricular tachycardia (e.g. verapamil) can be fatal in the event of misdiagnosis
  - For further details see Resuscitation Council tachycardia algorithm 📖 p412

Bradycardia
- Important questions include:
  - Is the patient currently on any negatively chronotropic medications?
    - beta blockers   — diltiazem
    - verapamil
  - Is there an extrinsic cause?
    - electrolyte disturbance   — hypothyroidism
    - raised intracranial pressure
  - In the event of symptomatic bradycardia a temporary pacing wire can be considered if there are:
    - prolonged symptomatic pauses
    - clinical evidence of compromise
    - bradycardia-mediated VT
  - If a patient is tolerating a significant bradycardia without deleterious effect on their blood pressure or overt symptoms, then the associated risks of temporary pacing by unskilled operators may outweigh the associated benefits. If temporary pacing is required the most experienced operator available should be involved, ideally a cardiologist.

Further reading
Resuscitation guidelines (2005). www.resus.org.uk

Cardiomyopathy

⑦ **Cardiomyopathy**

Cancer and cardiovascular disease are both common and share some mutual risk factors such as smoking and obesity. Consequently, it is not uncommon to encounter oncology patients with restrictive or dilated cardiomyopathy secondary to neoplasia, as a complication of treatment or as coexistent conditions.

Malignancies associated with cardiac involvement include:

- Malignant melanoma
- Lung cancer
- Breast cancer
- Renal carcinoma
- Soft tissue sarcomas
- Leukaemia and lymphoma
- Oesophageal cancer
- Hepatocellular carcinoma
- Thyroid cancer

Dilated cardiomyopathy

Dilated cardiomyopathy is characterized by dilatation and impaired contraction of one or both ventricles. This leads to impaired systolic function and patients can be asymptomatic or may present with heart failure, atrial and ventricular arrhythmias or, more rarely, sudden cardiac death.

There are a large number of causes of dilated cardiomyopathy, the most common being ischaemic heart disease and hypertension. Cancer-related dilated cardiomyopathy is most likely to be caused by the treatment of the cancer (chemotherapy, radiotherapy) rather than the cancer itself. Metastatic cardiac involvement is a rare cause and care should be taken to ensure other common treatable aetiologies have been excluded. Phaeochromocytoma can cause catecholamine-induced dilated cardiomyopathy.

Clinical features
Symptoms
- Asymptomatic
- Heart failure
- Palpitations/syncope

Signs
- Signs of CCF
- Displaced apex
- S_3 and S_4

Investigations
ECG
- Sinus tachycardia
- Arrhythmias
- ST and T wave abnormalities
- Intraventricular conduction defect
- 24-hour tape/telemetry if there is a suspicion of malignant arrhythmias

Imaging
- CXR
  - Cardiomegaly
  - Pulmonary venous hypertension
- Echo (investigation of choice)
  - LV dilatation, dysfunction, and abnormal diastolic mitral valve motion

Management of dilated cardiomyopathy

- Treatment of acute pulmonary oedema and arrhythmias (see Cardiac masses 📖 p114).
- Management of dilated cardiomyopathy is similar to that of chronic heart failure with:
  - ACE inhibitors/angiotensin II receptor antagonists being the mainstay of therapy.
  - Diuretics to maintain euvolaemia.
  - The addition of beta blockers and spironolactone if symptomatic.

Restrictive cardiomyopathy

Impaired ventricular relaxation leading to diastolic dysfunction is the hallmark of restrictive cardiomyopathy. The ventricles are excessively stiff and rigid. The LV is neither dilated nor hypertrophied, and systolic function is preserved.

Causes

Restrictive cardiomyopathy is relatively rare in Western countries but has a number of causes other than malignancy and treatment-related complications, including endomyocardial fibrosis, storage disorders, and amyloid deposition (can be secondary to multiple myeloma or Hodgkin's disease).

Clinical features

Symptoms
- Dyspnoea
- Malaise/fatigue
- Right sided heart failure

Signs
- Signs of right heart failure
- S_3 or S_4
- Inspiratory increase in venous pressure (Kussmaul's sign)

Investigations

ECG
- P mitrale or P pulmonale
- AF
- Reduced QRS voltages
- Poor R wave progression

Imaging
- CXR
  - Pulmonary venous hypertension
  - Mild cardiac enlargement
- Echo
  - Normal LV size and function
  - Restrictive E:A mitral inflow pattern
  - Increased LV wall thickness
  - Bi-atrial enlargement
  - Pericardial effusion

Management of restrictive cardiomyopathy

Therapy is directed at symptoms, as no specific treatment exists, other than that of the underlying condition. The prognosis is variable, but patients are usually increasingly symptomatic and there is a high mortality rate.

Distinguishing restrictive cardiomyopathy from constrictive pericarditis
The clinical and haemodynamic features of constrictive pericarditis are very similar to those of restrictive cardiomyopathy. Constrictive pericarditis can be seen in any condition causing chronic pericarditis and in particular can be secondary to neoplasia, radiation exposure, and chemotherapeutic agents. The distinction from restrictive cardiomyopathy is important as constriction can be successfully treated surgically, whereas no definitive therapy short of cardiac transplantation exists for restrictive cardiomyopathy. A large number of clinical and haemodynamic parameters are available to help in the distinction but CT, endomyocardial biopsy, and radionuclide angiography are all increasingly utilized. It is now extremely rare for an exploratory thoracotomy to be needed.

Further reading

Hancock, E. (2001). Cardiomyopathy: differential diagnosis of restrictive cardiomyopathy and constrictive pericarditis. *Heart* **86**: 343–349.

☠ **Eroded artery**

The erosion of a major artery by a malignant process can cause sudden and torrential haemorrhage, resulting in death from exsanguination in a matter of minutes. If witnessed, it can be incredibly distressing to both staff and relatives alike.

It is an important occurrence in some subgroups of cancer patients. 'Carotid blow-out' has been estimated to be the cause of 10–20% of deaths in advanced and recurrent head and neck cancer. It also occurs in 3–4% of patients undergoing head and neck surgery.

The most important decision regarding the management of erosion of a major artery is between active and palliative management. This decision is best made in advance when the risk of arterial erosion is identified. For the majority of patients palliative management will be entirely appropriate. Whether the patient should be informed of the risk and involved in the decision-making process raises important ethical issues.

Anticipation

Risk factors

- Previous radiotherapy
  - increases risk 7-fold
  - especially if administered within 2 months of surgery
- Surgery
  - radical neck dissection
- Postoperative healing problems
  - flap necrosis
- Neck wound infection
- Pharyngocutaneous fistula
- Fungating tumour
- Tumour invading artery
- Systemic factors
  - age
  - poor nutrition/weight loss
  - diabetes mellitus
  - atherosclerosis

'Warning signs'

- 'Sentinel' or 'herald' bleeds
  - minor bleeding locally
- Pulsation or 'ballooning' of the artery
- Sternal or high epigastric pain
- Surgical or radiological identification of arterial erosion

Patients with the above risk factors or warning signs should be discussed at the appropriate multidisciplinary team meetings and their management plans decided. Following this, discussion with the patient and relatives may be considered appropriate and any 'Do Not Attempt Resuscitation' decisions formalized.

Active resuscitation and treatment

- Resuscitation
  - high flow O_2
  - large bore IV access and aggressive fluid resuscitation
- Specific surgical measures aimed at stopping the bleeding
  - immediate attendance by a vascular or head and neck surgeon

Palliative management

If it has been decided that the occurrence of carotid artery rupture will represent a life-ending event then the goals of management must be to minimize anxiety, ease suffering, and ensure death with dignity in a calm, reassuring, and caring atmosphere. The key to achieving this is in the preparation of staff and equipment.

Patients should be nursed in a side room if at all possible.

The following items should be kept discreetly but readily available:

- Call bell
- Suction equipment
- Bowl
- Syringes (10 ml) for cuff inflation on tracheostomy tube (if applicable)
- Gloves, plastic aprons, and eye protectors/face shields
- Dark coloured towels (to camouflage the presence of blood)
- Clinical waste bags
- Equipment to obtain IV access
- Appropriate sedation
  - Midazolam 5–10 mg IV stat and then titrated to response
  - Diazepam 5–10 mg PR is an alternative
- Diamorphine (5–10 mg IV stat) should be used only if the patient is suffering pain and/or breathlessness

What to do

- Avoid panic, stay with the patient and calmly call for assistance
- Be aware of relatives, visitors, and other patients, provide privacy and support as needed
- Apply towels to the bleeding site to absorb as much bleeding as possible
- Inflate cuff of tracheostomy tube to prevent choking (if applicable)
- Apply gentle suction
- Administer sedation

Further reading

Potter, E. (2005). The management of carotid artery rupture, related to the terminal care of the head and neck cancer patient – Information and Guidelines. *British Association of Head and Neck Oncology Nurses*. www.bahnon.org.uk

Respiratory emergencies

⑦ **Malignant pleural effusion**

Excess pleural fluid accumulates in the pleural space when there is disruption of the parietal pleural lymphatic drainage. VEGF may also play a role in the pathophysiology of malignant pleural effusions.

Malignant effusions are classically 'exudative' as predicted by one or more of Light's criteria being present.

- Pleural fluid protein:serum protein >0.5
- Pleural fluid pH:serum pH >0.6
- Pleural fluid LDH >2/3 of serum 'upper limit of normal'

The most common cause of an exudative effusion in the over 60s is malignancy; however, a transudative effusion is also common in this age group.

The diagnosis of a malignant pleural effusion renders non-small cell lung cancer T4 (at least Stage IIIB) and all other malignancies metastatic (Stage IV). However, not all effusions in oncology patients are malignant in nature, and in patients with otherwise curable disease, the exact nature of the effusion should be established. Confirmation of an effusion being 'malignant' conventionally demands the presence of malignant cells in pleural fluid cytology or a diagnostic pleural biopsy (CT-guided or by thoracoscopy).

Malignant pleural effusions can occur in almost any malignancy; however, they are most common in lung and breast carcinomas.

- Lung   37.5%
- Breast   16.8%
- Lymphoma   11.5%
- GU tract   9.4%
- GI tract   6.9%
- Other   7.3%
- Unknown primary   10.7%

Median survival from diagnosis of a malignant pleural effusion is 6 months, although this does depend critically on the primary tumour site, with the shortest survival time in patients with lung carcinoma and the longest survival time in patients with ovarian carcinoma.

Differential diagnosis of pleural effusion in the oncology patient

Transudate

- Raised venous pressure
    - Cardiac failure
    - Constrictive pericarditis
    - SVCO
- Hypoproteinaemia
    - Nephrotic syndrome
    - Cirrhosis with ascites
    - Protein-losing enteropathy
- Hypothyroidism
- Meigs' syndrome
    - Benign ovarian tumour producing a right-sided pleural effusion

Exudate

- Malignancy
  - Including mesothelioma
- Parapneumonic effusion
- Empyema
- Pulmonary infarction
- Benign asbestos effusion
- Drugs
  - Oncology-related
    - methotrexate
    - G-CSF
    - cyclophosphamide
  - General
    - amiodarone
    - phenytoin
    - carbamazepine
    - nitrofurantoin
    - propylthiouracil
    - bromocriptine
- Connective tissue disorder
- TB
- Pancreatitis

Clinical features

Symptoms

- Small effusions may be asymptomatic
  - incidental finding on CXR
  - malignant effusions are typically large volume
- Dyspnoea
- Pain
  - pleural thickening on imaging and history of asbestos exposure is highly suggestive of mesothelioma
- Cough/haemoptysis
  - suggests large airway involvement
- Systemic
  - weight loss
  - paraneoplastic phenomena
  - anorexia

Signs

- Trachea may be pushed away from the affected side
- Reduced expansion on affected side
- Stoney dullness to percussion
- Reduced air entry
  - may have bronchial breathing at fluid level

Differential diagnosis from signs
  - pleural thickening
  - lobar/lung collapse
    - trachea may be pulled towards affected side
  - raised hemidiaphragm
- May have other features of malignancy
  - clubbing
  - enlarged cervical/axillary lymph nodes
  - SVCO

Investigations

Bloods

- FBC
  - infection

- Coagulation screen
  - prior to drain insertion
- LDH/albumin/protein
  - diagnosis of exudate/transudate on Light's criteria
- TFTs

Imaging
- CXR
  - is usually diagnostic of effusion (see Fig. 3.1)
  - USS/CT can reveal smaller volumes of fluid and guide drain insertion
- CT
  - with contrast can delineate pleural appearance
    — thickening   — nodularity
  - may reveal
    — a primary lesion
    — distant disease/lymph nodes
    — pulmonary vascular status (PE)

Interventional
- Diagnostic aspiration
  - Cytology
    — sensitivity approx. 60%
    — a second cytological sample/analysis may improve sensitivity by a further 10%
  - Protein/pH/LDH
    — diagnosis of exudate/transudate on Light's criteria
  - MC&S
    — empyema
      - pH<7.2
      - may relate to a recent pleural procedure
  - Staining and culture for TB
- Pleural biopsy
  - Guided biopsy (USS needle/CT-guided cutting biopsy) in presence of visible pleural thickening
  - Abrams' biopsy
    — rarely used
    — poor sensitivity (40–50%) for diagnosis of malignant disease
    — sensitivity higher for *Mycobacterium tuberculosis* detection if suspected
- Thoracoscopy
  - allows direct visualization of pleura+/− biopsy
  - performed under GA or LA/sedation
  - perform when diagnosis of malignant effusion needs ruling out in the presence of negative cytology samples (usually two) and low likelihood of guided biopsy success as judged by imaging
  - sensitivity >90%
  - often preferred earlier in diagnostic pathway if high probability of mesothelioma, as simultaneous talc pleurodesis can be performed whilst minimizing pleural access

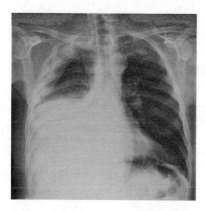

Fig. 3.1 A large right pleural effusion in a patient with recurrent non-small cell lung cancer.

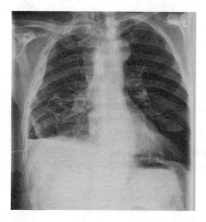

Fig. 3.2 There remains a small residual right hydropneumothorax, but the effusion has reduced significantly in size since the insertion of the drain.

Management

The decision to intervene for a malignant effusion depends on:

- patient wishes
- severity of symptoms
- response to previous intervention
- prognosis
- primary tumour

Following diagnosis, observation is an option for small or minimally symptomatic effusions.

For larger effusions, removal of pleural fluid often improves dyspnoea; however, pleural encasement by disease can result in 'trapped lung' which does not expand following fluid removal. This typically gives a poor symptomatic result. Do not keep removing fluid if the patient is having little discernible benefit. Consider other causes of dyspnoea if good lung re-expansion appears to have been achieved with little symptom improvement. Following removal, fluid reaccumulation should be expected without further treatment.

Common approaches

- Thoracocentesis
  - palliation of effusion
  - no need for admission
  - see Thoracocentesis and talc pleurodesis 📖 p134
  - do not remove more than 1–1.5 l per aspiration
    — avoids re-expansion pulmonary oedema
  - high recurrence rate in the absence of systemic treatment for the malignancy, so if appreciable life expectancy proceed to formal drainage and pleurodesis
- Cytotoxic chemotherapy
  - after thoracocentesis, cytotoxic chemotherapy may prevent reaccumulation of pleural fluid in some chemosensitive tumours
    — lymphoma
    — germ cell tumour
    — SCLC
    — breast carcinoma
    — ovarian carcinoma
- Intercostal drain insertion and talc pleurodesis
  - this is the treatment of choice for recurrent, symptomatic malignant effusions.
  - see Fig. 3.2
  - see Thoracocentesis and talc pleurodesis 📖 p134
  - small-bore (10–14 F) drains are usually satisfactory even in quite heavily blood-stained effusions
  - fibrinolytics are sometimes used (e.g. 250 000 U streptokinase) to aid drainage of loculated effusions
    — seek advice from respiratory physician
  - the most common choice of sclerosant for pleurodesis is talc slurry
  - corticosteroids (and possibly NSAIDs) may reduce the success rate for talc pleurodesis (anti-inflammatory action)
  - pleurodesis can be repeated if initially unsuccessful and conditions are otherwise favourable

More specialized approaches

- Thoracoscopy with talc pleurodesis
  - Can also allow interruption of pleural septation to improve drainage
  - 90% success rate
- Indwelling pleural catheter
  - patients can manage effusion drainage independently
  - familiarization with insertion procedure and post-procedure drain care needed
  - can result in spontaneous pleurodesis
  - complications
    - localized infection
    - cutaneous tumour seeding
- Pleuroperitoneal shunt
  - rarely used
  - complications
    - shunt occlusion
    - infection
    - tumour seeding into the peritoneal cavity
- Surgical pleurectomy
  - can be performed in conjunction with a VATS procedure
  - good performance status and appreciable life expectancy needed

Further reading

Antunes, G., Neville, E., Duffy, J. and Ali, N. (2003). BTS guidelines for the management of malignant pleural effusions. *Thorax* **58** (Suppl. II): ii29–ii38.

Maskell, N.A. and Butland, R.J.A. (2003). BTS guidelines for the investigation of a unilateral pleural effusion in adults. *Thorax* **58** (Suppl. II): ii8–ii17.

⑦ Thoracocentesis and talc pleurodesis

Intercostal drain insertion

Preparation
- Check indication and need for procedure
  - Pneumothorax
    — in any ventilated patient
    — tension pneumothorax after initial needle relief
    — persistent or recurrent pneumothorax after simple aspiration
    — large secondary spontaneous pneumothorax in patients
       >50 years
  - Malignant pleural effusion
  - Empyema and complicated parapneumonic pleural effusion
  - Traumatic haemopneumothorax
  - Postoperative
    — thoracotomy
    — oesophagectomy
    — cardiac surgery
- Check FBC and coagulation screen
  - Known liver disease/abnormal LFTs
  - Anticoagulated
  - Possibility of neutropenia/bone marrow failure
  - Consider delaying procedure if patient neutropenic
  - Consider vitamin K if INR >1.5
  - Consider platelet transfusion if platelet count <50 ×10^9/l
- Consider USS guidance for drain insertion for:
  - Selected cases post-pneumonectomy
  - Loculated effusions
  - Abnormal anatomy
  - Bulky intrathoracic soft tissue disease
  - Failed insertion
- Explain procedure and possible complications
  - Complications
    — pain
    — bleeding
    — poor therapeutic outcome
    — pneumothorax
    — empyema (1%)
    — misplacement
      - intrapulmonary (5–6%)
    — re-expansion pulmonary oedema
    — surgical emphysema
- Obtain consent for procedure
- Insertion of IV cannula useful
  - Cautious use of sedation (midazolam 1–5 mg IV titrated for effect)
- Ensure all equipment, connectors, and underwater seal prepared

Procedure
- Position patient
  - sitting forward over a table with extended arms
  - lying with insertion side rotated 45–90° with arm on the side of the pneumothorax behind the patient's head to expose the axillary area
  - if the patient has had a site marked by USS for drain insertion, ensure that he or she is positioned in exactly the same posture as when the USS took place
- Strict aseptic technique should be maintained at all times; use an assistant if available
- Select site for drainage
  - safest position is within 'triangle of safety'
    - anteriorly   pectoralis major
    - posteriorly   latissimus dorsi
    - inferiorly   5th intercostal space
  - more posterolateral insertion is common but less comfortable for the patient to lie on
- Infiltrate with 5–10 ml of 1% lignocaine above the lower rib of the chosen intercostal space
  - so avoiding the intercostal neurovascular bundle
  - insert until the parietal pleura is reached (usually experienced as sharp pain) and infiltrate at least a further 10 ml 1% lignocaine at this depth
- Confirm aspiration of fluid (effusion) or air (pneumothorax) at this point with a green needle on the syringe used for infiltrating local anaesthetic
  - a green needle usually reaches the required depth
- Seldinger type drains (12–14 F) are increasingly used
  - these are inserted via an introducer needle and guidewire
  - the position of the introducer needle in the pleural space can be confirmed by further aspiration of fluid (or air)
  - leave the needle in position, remove syringe (the open end of the needle can be temporarily covered with a finger) and insert guidewire through needle; it should pass easily into the pleural space
  - remove introducer needle over the wire, keeping hold of the guidewire at all times
  - slide dilator over the wire, again keeping hold of the wire, and dilate down through the subcutaneous tissue
    - a skin incision with a scalpel may be required
  - remove the dilator, and slide the drain over the wire (again, never let go of the guidewire!)
  - when the drain has passed into the pleural space, remove guidewire and connect drain to the tubing and underwater seal, ideally with a three-way tap in series
  - fix the drain to the chest wall
    - place a suture to the chest wall then tie the ends round the drain

   — special dressings are sometimes available for fixing smaller
      drain types
   — cover the insertion site with a single, breathable, secure
      dressing, which can be easily removed if needed
- Seek senior advice before insertion of a 'Trochar' type drain
- Obtain a CXR to confirm drain is in the thoracic cavity

Further considerations
- Drain management
  - flush small drains with 10–20 mls of saline tds
  - prescribe prophylactic heparin (e.g. 5000 U heparin SC bd) unless
    contraindicated
  - ensure patient has adequate analgesia prescribed in the event of
    pain
  - warn patient not to lift drain above level of insertion when
    mobilizing
  - record drain output/flushes in the observation notes
  - a 'swinging' drain refers to movement of a fluid column in the drain
    tubing with respiration; it implies continuity with the pleural space
    and a patent drain
  - when draining large effusions to dryness, output can be controlled
    by tap closure (or clamping) after each litre
    — never tap/clamp off for more than 1 hour and immediately
       resume free drainage if patient experiences increasing dyspnoea
       whilst the drain is closed (and consider obtaining urgent CXR)
  - high volume-low pressure suction can be attempted to assist lung
    expansion, but should only be initiated after discussion with a
    respiratory physician/thoracic surgeon
- Drain removal
  - remove drain by releasing any anchoring suture and withdrawing
    during a single expiratory manoeuvre or Valsalva manoeuvre. Cover
    drain site with a simple dressing
  - record CXR appearance post-withdrawal
- Mesothelioma
  - seeding along the drain insertion tract is much more common than
    with other tumours
  - prophylactic radiotherapy is routinely given at the port site
    following drain removal (usually 21 Gy in 3# with electrons)
  - smaller drain sites may need to be marked with Indian ink

Pleurodesis
Sterile talc is currently the most commonly used sclerosant in the UK.

Preparation
- Explain procedure and possible complications
  - Complications
    — pain   — fever
    — failure (10–20% with talc)
    — risk of ARDS with talc (<1%)
- Obtain consent for procedure

- Ensure analgesia prescribed
  - NSAIDs may reduce success rate
- Small bore (10–14 F) drains are usually satisfactory for drainage of effusion and pleurodesis
- A good result usually demands that the visceral and parietal pleura are in apposition
  - the effusion has been drained to dryness and the lungs well expanded (80% success rate)
  - failure of pleurodesis is predominantly caused by incomplete lung expansion
- Incomplete lung re-expansion may be due to:
  - 'trapped lung'
  - pleural loculations
  - proximal large airway obstruction
  - persistent air leak
- Where complete lung re-expansion or pleural apposition is not achieved and the patient is unsuitable for surgical intervention, pleurodesis should still be attempted
- The amount of pleural fluid drained per day before the instillation of a sclerosant (<150 ml/day) is less relevant for successful pleurodesis than radiographic confirmation of fluid evacuation and lung re-expansion
- Once effusion drainage and lung re-expansion have been radiographically confirmed, pleurodesis should not be delayed while the cessation of pleural fluid drainage is awaited

Procedure

- Consider pre-medication
  - 5–10 mg morphine PO
  - 1 mg lorazepam PO
  - relative caution in elderly and those with chronic respiratory disease
- Instil 3 mg/kg of 1% lignocaine (max. 250 mg) into the pleural cavity via drain, using a sterile syringe. Flush drain with 20 ml normal saline to ensure dose enters the chest. This is easy via a three-way tap. Close tap (or clamp drain)
- Make up talc slurry in a sterile syringe
  - 4 mg sterile talc + 30 ml 0.9% saline
  - do not use >5 mg of talc as this increases the risk of ARDS
- Instil talc slurry via drain, flush again with saline and close off tap/clamp
- Resume free drainage after 1 hour
- Monitor observations closely (half-hourly for at least 2 hours)
  - transient pyrexia is not unusual
  - paracetamol can be given if needed
  - pyrexia beyond 48–72 hours is unusual and pleural infection should be considered
- ARDS usually becomes evident within 48 hours
  - increasing dyspnoea   • hypoxia
  - diffuse pulmonary infiltrate on CXR

- Suction may be required for incomplete lung expansion and to aid pleurodesis
  - when suction is applied, the use of high volume-low pressure systems is recommended with a gradual increment in pressure from 5 to 20 cmH$_2$O
  - full lung expansion is not achievable in all patients (due to trapped lung)
- Remove drain when fluid satisfactorily drained and lung expanded on CXR
  - most patients manage to have their drain removed with 72 hours

Further reading

Antunes, G., Neville, E., Duffy, J. and Ali, N. (2003). BTS guidelines for the management of malignant pleural effusions. *Thorax* **58**(Suppl. II): ii29–ii38.

Laws, D., Neville, E. and Duffy, J. (2003). BTS guidelines for the insertion of a chest drain *Thorax* **58**(Suppl. II): ii53–ii59.

① Airway obstruction

Airway obstruction in the cancer patient can occur anywhere from the base of the tongue to the terminal bronchioles. The most common site for obstruction is the larger intrathoracic airways (trachea to lobar bronchi). Obstructing lesions may occur higher in the respiratory tract from pharyngeal or laryngeal disease.

Obstructive complications may be the first presentation of bronchial carcinoma, e.g. dyspnoea with lobar collapse found on the CXR.

Proximal disease, rapid onset, and poor underlying respiratory reserve usually give rise to more severe symptoms.

Causes
- Intraluminal tumour mass
  - bronchial carcinoma
    - NSCLC   — SCLC
  - bronchial carcinoid
  - laryngeal carcinoma
  - tracheal carcinoma
  - pulmonary metastases
    - usually parenchymal, rarely endobronchial
- Extrinsic compression
  - tumour
    - oesophageal carcinoma   — thymic tumour
    - thyroid carcinoma
  - lymphadenopathy
    - bronchial carcinoma
      - NSCLC   - SCLC
    - non-Hodgkin's lymphoma
    - oesophageal carcinoma
    - thyroid carcinoma
- Intraluminal tumour mass and extrinsic compression

Clinical features
Symptoms
- Dyspnoea
  - almost always present to some degree
- Cough
- Cough, sputum, fever (non-resolving pneumonia)
  - poor antibiotic response
  - slow (>6 weeks) resolution of consolidation
  - recurrent episodes
  - may herald lobar obstruction
- Voice change
  - mediastinal invasion of recurrent laryngeal nerves
- Haemoptysis
  - new bleeding and clot formation on a partially obstructing lesion can cause a rapid increase in dyspnoea

Signs
- Stridor
  - more prominent inspiratory than expiratory phase
  - extrathoracic obstruction
- Tachypnoea
- Cyanosed if severe obstruction
- Lobar collapse or consolidation
  - trachea may be pulled towards affected side
  - dullness to percussion
  - ↓ breath sounds with collapse
  - ↑ breath sounds with consolidation
- Assess for SVCO (see Superior vena cava obstruction 📖 p92)
  - large volume mediastinal disease
  - right upper lobe primary

Investigations

Bloods
- FBC
  - anaemia may exacerbate symptoms of hypoxia
- ABGs
  - assess severity of hypoxia
  - to guide O_2 therapy

Spirometry
- Usually not indicated in the acute setting
- Flow-volume loops may have characteristic appearance

Imaging
- CXR
  - Mass
  - Mediastinal lymphadenopathy
  - Lobar collapse
  - Consolidation
    — air space opacification   — air bronchogram
  - Other malignancy-related source of dyspnoea
    — pleural effusion   — lymphangitis carcinomatosis
- Chest CT
  - Better delineates extent of disease than CXR
  - Helps planning of elective bronchoscopic procedures
  - Aids palliative radiotherapy planning
  - Diagnosis of pulmonary vascular obstruction (PE)

Fibreoptic bronchoscopy
- Obtain tissue diagnosis
  - biopsy
    — endobronchial lesion
    — transbronchial for extrinsic lesion
  - bronchial–alveolar lavage
  - endobronchial brushings
- Therapeutic applications

Management

Malignant airways obstruction does not usually present with acute respiratory failure, allowing diagnostic and therapeutic procedures to proceed in a timely fashion.

Rapid onset or severe dyspnoea demands prompt symptomatic relief and discussion with a thoracic physician/surgeon as to whether early bronchoscopy (flexible or rigid) is appropriate.

- Assess oxygenation status
- High flow O_2 therapy
  - use arterial PaO_2 to guide delivery
- Nebulized salbutamol may relieve added bronchospasm
- Consider trial of helium–oxygen (Heliox 79%/21%) mixture if severe dyspnoea
  - may need to entrain additional oxygen
  - maintains laminar airflow distal to stenosis
  - reduces work of ventilation
- Assist removal of expectorated/pooled secretions from oropharynx
- If interventional treatment is inappropriate and patient is distressed give opioids and/or benzodiazepines
  - morphine 5–10 mg PO
  - diamorphine 1.25–2.5 mg IV
  - diazepam 5–10 mg PO
  - midazolam 1.25–2.5 mg IV
- Treat haemoptysis if contributing to symptoms (See Haemoptysis 📖 p146)
- Consider commencing trial of steroid
  - dexamethasone 4–8 mg bd IV
    — may reduce vasogenic oedema associated with a tumour mass
    — no acute benefit
    — little evidence
    — is there active respiratory infection?
- All newly diagnosed cancer patients should have appropriate staging investigations to assess the potential for radical surgical clearance. In those patients presenting with airway obstruction, the proximity of local disease to the carina often means surgery is not an option. Palliation of symptoms is the primary aim in most cases.
- External beam radiotherapy (radical or palliative) can relieve symptoms of airway obstruction over a period of days
- Chemotherapy can relieve symptoms of airway obstruction over a period of days if the obstruction is caused by a chemotherapy-sensitive tumour
  - SCLC
  - lymphoma
- Discuss interventional bronchoscopic approaches with a respiratory specialist
  - a clear plan should be made early as to the timing and extent of all investigations/treatment
  - some modalities can be used to complement conventional systemic chemotherapy or external beam radiotherapy

- utilization of the different interventional bronchoscopy techniques is governed by:
  - local expertise and availability
  - patient presentation
    - performance status and life expectancy
    - site of obstruction
- availability is generally limited to tertiary centres

Acute upper airway obstruction

Extrathoracic upper airways obstruction, e.g. owing to an advanced laryngeal carcinoma, may present with acute stridor and impending respiratory obstruction. These patients require urgent review by the ENT team for assessment and to protect the airway.

- Emergency tracheostomy
- Mechanical or laser debulking
- Emergency laryngectomy

Acute large airway obstruction

External compression of airway

- Stent placement
  - a stent can be deployed using a flexible or rigid bronchoscope
  - multiple stents can be deployed in an individual patient
  - stents are available for bifurcation of the airway
  - stents are used in patients with good performance state and appreciable life expectancy (>1 month)
  - removal and reinsertion may be performed
  - complications
    - cough
    - haemoptysis
    - pain
    - re-stenosis
      - tumour overgrowth
    - halitosis
    - stent migration

      - granulation tissue

Tracheal or proximal bronchial tumour ± acute dyspnoea and/or urgent coagulation needed for bleeding

- Rigid bronchoscopy and debulking
  - needs general anaesthetic
  - only for lesions in the trachea or proximal bronchi
  - can combine with other techniques
  - contraindications
    - obstructing laryngeal disease
    - unstable cervical spine
- Nd:YAG laser
  - usually used via rigid bronchoscope
  - sessions can be repeated as, and when, symptoms recur
  - small risk of bleeding or perforation
  - risk of fire means inspired oxygen concentration must be <40%
- Electrocautery (diathermy)

Subacute airway obstruction
- External beam radiotherapy
  - palliative treatment
  - dose options 8–10 Gy/1#, 17 Gy/2#, 20 Gy/5#
- Systemic chemotherapy for chemosensitive tumours
- Cryotherapy
  - localized disease
  - multiple sessions usually needed
  - may be performed using a flexible bronchoscope
  - when the maximum dose of external beam radiotherapy has been reached
- Endobronchial brachytherapy
  - single high dose of radiation (10–20 Gy at 1 cm)
  - can be used to give localized radiotherapy when the maximum dose of external beam radiotherapy has been reached
  - risk of significant haemoptysis
- Photodynamic therapy (PDT)
  - photosensitizing agent given intravenously is activated to generate a cytotoxic effect when exposed to light of the appropriate wavelength delivered by the bronchoscope
  - risk of haemoptysis and skin photosensitivity

Further reading

Bolliger, C.T., Sutedja, T.G., Strausz, J. and Freitag, L. (2006). Therapeutic bronchoscopy with immediate effect: laser, electrocautery, argon plasma coagulation and stents. *Eur. Respir. J.* **27**: 1258–1271.

Vergnon, J-M., Huber, R.M. and Moghissi, K. (2006). Place of cryotherapy, brachytherapy and photodynamic therapy in therapeutic bronchoscopy of lung cancers. *Eur. Respir. J.* **28**: 200–218.

⃠ **Haemoptysis**

Haemoptysis is a common feature in cancer patients, either as the presenting feature of malignancy (lung cancer or lung metastases) or as a complication of the underlying malignancy or its treatment.

About 60% of cancer patients with haemoptysis have a primary lung cancer; the other 40% have disease metastatic to the lung (particularly breast, colorectal, lymphoma, laryngeal). Around 50% of lung cancer patients will experience haemoptysis at some stage in their illness. Massive haemoptysis only accounts for 10% of haemoptysis.

Haemoptysis in the cancer patient usually results from direct malignant invasion of blood vessels within the lung, or breakdown of friable endo-bronchial disease; however, non-malignant causes must also be considered, especially if the extent of known malignant disease does not suggest involvement of the larger airways. Atypical infections should be considered in the presence of prolonged immunosuppression.

Causes
- Bleeding endobronchial mass
- Malignant invasion into pulmonary vasculature
- Lower respiratory tract infection
  - pneumonia
  - lung abscess
  - fungal
  - TB
    — invasive bronchopulmonary aspergillosis
    — aspergilloma
- Pulmonary embolism
- Spurious haemoptysis
  - bleeding from mouth or nasopharynx
- Iatrogenic
  - post-biopsy
- Other
  - bronchiectasis
  - Wegener's granulomatosis
  - AVM
  - SLE
  - mitral stenosis
  - Goodpasture's syndrome
  - pulmonary hypertension

Clinical features
History
- Known history of lung cancer or other malignancy
- Recent bronchial intervention or lung biopsy
- Coagulopathy
  - patient on warfarin
  - acute promyelocytic leukaemia
  - known extensive malignant liver involvement
- Features of infection
  - fever
  - purulent sputum
- Previous TB

- History of immunosuppression
  - intensive chemotherapy
  - HIV infection
- Clinical suspicion of PE
  - disproportionate dyspnoea compared to CXR appearance
  - new calf swelling or pain
  - previous thromboembolism

Examination

- Examination may be normal
- Bleeding points in the gums or nasopharynx
- Petechial rash, excessive bruising
- Tachypnoea
- Hypotension
  - blood pressure likely to be normal even in massive haemoptysis
- Clinical features of pneumonia
  - area of dullness on percussion
  - bronchial breath sounds
- Lower limb thromboembolism
  - >2 cm difference between legs
  - distended superficial veins
  - tenderness along deep leg veins
- Other causes of dyspnoea in the chest
  - lobar collapse
  - pleural effusion

Investigations

Bloods

- FBC
  - thrombocytopenia
- LFTs
- Coagulation screen
  - if PT, APTT, and platelets abnormal request thrombin time and fibrin degradation products to confirm DIC
- Crossmatch
  - only for massive haemoptysis
- ABGs
  - rarely needed unless indeterminate reading of peripheral SaO_2 or increasing respiratory distress/compromise
- Autoantibodies
  - ANA
  - ANCA
  - Anti-GBM
- Aspergillus precipitins

Sputum

- Sputum cytology
  - usually redundant if lung cancer previously diagnosed
- Sputum
  - MC&S
    — useful for diagnosing infections
  - state clearly on the microbiology request if TB or fungal infections considered
  - ≥3 samples should be sent for acid-fast bacilli

Imaging
- CXR
  - malignant disease
  - infective consolidation
  - collapsed lobe
  - bronchiectasis
  - large volumes of blood cause opacification on the CXR
- CT chest
  - parenchymal or mediastinal disease
  - involvement of major thoracic vessels
  - characteristic appearances of aspergilloma
  - nodular disease suggestive of TB
  - compare with previous scans if available
- CT pulmonary angiogram (CTPA)
  - first choice investigation for suspected pulmonary embolic disease in the cancer patient with an abnormal CXR or prior history of lung disease
- Echo
  - right ventricular strain in large PE
  - mitral stenosis
  - pulmonary hypertension
- Fibreoptic bronchoscopy
  - can anatomically locate bleeding points under direct vision in the major airways or subdivisions
  - microbiological material can be obtained
  - in patients with known endobronchial malignant disease, broncho-scopy provides little additional information unless a prelude to more formal intervention
- Bronchial angiography
  - rarely indicated unless:
    — arterial embolization of the bleeding site is considered
    — the site of bleeding remains unknown after other investigations
  - embolization is a highly specialized intervention and unusual for malignant haemoptysis
- ENT review +/− flexible nasendoscopy
  - if bleeding suspected from the nasopharynx

Management

① *Mild to moderate haemoptysis (<100 ml/24 hours)*
- Reverse coagulopathy
  - re-establish therapeutic INR if raised
  - the decision to continue anticoagulation if haemoptysis is encountered within the therapeutic INR range needs individual risk-benefit analysis
- Platelet transfusion
  - aim for platelets >50x10^9/l in the presence of haemoptysis
- Anticoagulation
  - will usually reduce haemoptysis caused by acute PE
  - if bleeding endobronchial disease coexists, a period of monitored heparin/LMWH treatment is a practical way to proceed
- Treat bronchitis/pneumonia with usual empirical antibiotics unless microbiology or allergy directs otherwise
  - amoxicillin 500 mg tds PO/IV +/− clarithromycin 500 mg bd PO

- Oral tranexamic acid (500 mg tds PO) can reduce symptoms of small infrequent haemoptysis. Possible small increased risk of thromboembolism
- Bronchoscopic treatment depends on centre, physician/surgeon preference, and availability of a rigid bronchoscopy service
  - discuss options with thoracic physicians/surgeons
    — cryotherapy   — electrocautery
- Systemic chemotherapy, if indicated by diagnosis and performance status, may reduce the degree of haemoptysis, although this will have an appreciable time lag to effect
- Palliative external beam radiotherapy can reduce symptomatic haemoptysis in patients of all performance states if endoscopic therapy is not appropriate or available
  - 10 Gy/1# to tumour mass
- Surgery
  - once patient has been investigated and found to be operable

:Ö: *Massive haemoptysis*

Massive haemoptysis refers to blood loss sufficient to obstruct the airway and threaten life, usually >500 ml/24 hours. Quantification of blood loss is difficult as expectoration of blood may vary as much of the blood may be swallowed.

Massive haemoptysis is usually preceded by small volume haemoptysis. In lung cancer massive haemoptysis conveys a high mortality (80–100%). Its occurrence should prompt appropriate discussion with the family. Given its distressing nature, it is fortunately an unusual cause of death.

- 3% lung cancer deaths
  - 7% squamous cell carcinoma
  - 2% large cell carcinoma
  - <1% adenocarcinoma
  - <1% small cell carcinoma
- If intervention and further investigation is not indicated, good symptom control of distress and dyspnoea should be the priority
  - Appropriate sedation
    — midazolam 5 mg IV stat and then titrated to response.
    — diazepam 5–10 mg PR is an alternative
  - Diamorphine 5 mg IV stat
- Patients can compromise their airway and effectively drown in blood, long before circulatory volume is compromised
  - Basic airway manoeuvres if upper airway obstructed
  - Assist removal of secretions/blood with suction
  - Secure airway with endotracheal intubation if indicated
    — this may need careful consideration depending on prognosis
    — consult a senior physician and/or liaise with ICU urgently
    — consider double lumen endotracheal tubes or selective intubation of one lung to protect the uninvolved lung from aspirated blood
    — do not delay treatment if in doubt

- Give oxygen
  - 40–60% FiO_2
  - 4 l/minute via nasal route may have to suffice for practical reasons if rapid, repeated expectoration
- Obtain IV access and fluid resuscitate
  - if a central line is indicated, use the high internal jugular approach to minimize the risk of pneumothorax
- Arrange urgent portable CXR
- If the side of bleeding (right or left) can be inferred from known disease or CXR shadowing, lay patient on the affected side
  - reduces aspiration into the unaffected lung
  - patients often position themselves as such spontaneously
- Nebulized adrenaline 0.5–1 mg (5–10 ml of 1:10 000 solution)
  - to reduce secondary bronchospasm and/or bleeding
- Reverse coagulopathy
  - vitamin K (5–10 mg IV stat)
    — may take several hours to take effect.
    — lower doses (1mg IV) if prosthetic heart valves
  - FFP (12–15 ml/kg, usually 4 units for an average adult)
    — rapid effect but short-lived
- Transexamic acid 1 g PO/IV stat
- Vasopressin
  - 20 units IV over 15 minutes
  - relative contraindication in coronary artery disease
- Flexible bronchoscopy can be attempted once the airway is stabilized
  - localization of bleeding source often obscured by blood/clot
  - therapeutic
    — iced saline lavage
    — topical adrenaline (1:20 000 solution)
    — balloon catheter tamponade
      - specialized balloon catheters can be left in place for up to 24 hours and removed later under direct vision
- Rigid bronchoscopy
  - offers superior suction and electrocautery
- Bronchial artery embolization
  - has shown promise in massive haemoptysis from benign aetiologies, but limited usefulness in malignant disease
- Emergency surgery
  - often inappropriate in cancer patients

Further reading

Bolliger, C.T., Sutedja, T.G., Strausz, J. and Freitag, L. (2006). Therapeutic bronchoscopy with immediate effect: laser, electrocautery, argon plasma coagulation and stents. *Eur. Respir. J.* **27**: 1258–1271.

Vergnon, J-M., Huber, R.M. and Moghissi, K. (2006). Place of cryotherapy, brachytherapy and photodynamic therapy in therapeutic bronchoscopy of lung cancers. *Eur. Respir. J.* **28**: 200–218.

⑦ **Lymphangitis carcinomatosis**

The lungs are a common site for metastatic disease. This is commonly nodular, but occasionally (6–8% of lung metastases) can present as lymphangitis carcinomatosis. Lymphangitis carcinomatosis is often unilateral when associated with bronchial carcinoma, whilst bilateral lymphangitis carcinomatosis is more often due to metastatic spread. Lymphangitis carcinomatosis refers to the diffuse infiltration of lymphatic channels by tumour, resulting in obstruction and interstitial oedema. The patient's symptoms of dyspnoea often appear out of proportion to the physical signs or X-ray findings.

Clinical features
Symptoms
- Dyspnoea
- Dry cough
- Fever
- Night sweats
- Chest pain
- Haemoptysis

Signs
- Increased pulse and respiratory rate
- Fine crepitations

Common causative tumours
- Adenocarcinoma (80%)
  - breast (35%)
  - stomach (20%)
  - lung (20%)
- Other cell types
  - Squamous carcinoma
    - lung
    - cervix

Differential diagnosis
- Pulmonary oedema
- Interstitial pneumonitis
- Pulmonary lymphoma
- Pulmonary Kaposi's sarcoma
- Pulmonary sarcoidosis

Investigations
The CXR and HRCT are usually diagnostic and no further investigations are usually required. Occasionally other conditions may mimic classical lymphangitis carcinomatosis. If this is suspected then other investigations may be required to obtain a correct diagnosis and give the appropriate management. This is particularly important if it is thought to be a first presentation of cancer or a first presentation with suspected metastatic relapse.

Bloods
- FBC
  - anaemia increasing dyspnoea
  - infection

- Cardiac enzymes
  - if cardiac cause of dyspnoea suspected
- LDH
  - lymphoma
- Immunology
  - chronic interstitial lung disease

ECG
- Pulmonary oedema secondary to CCF is highly unlikely in the presence of a normal ECG

Imaging
- CXR
  - reticular or reticulonodular shadowing
  - septal lines (Kerley A and B lines)
  - peribronchial cuffing
  - associated features
    — mediastinal lymphadenopathy
    — pleural effusion
  - normal in 50% of patients with histologically proven disease.
  - sensitivity only 25%
- HRCT scan
  - interlobular septal thickening
  - thickening of the fissures
  - peribronchovascular thickening
  - pattern may be:
    — unilateral or bilateral
    — focal or diffuse
    — symmetrical or asymmetrical
  - associated features
    — mediastinal lymphadenopathy
    — pleural effusion
  - highly suggestive in a suspicious clinical context

Biopsy
If lymphangitis carcinomatosis is the presenting feature of a malignancy then confirmation of the histological diagnosis may be appropriate.
- Biopsy of obvious primary
- Biopsy of other metastatic disease
- Bronchoscopy
  - transbronchial biopsy
  - bronchial brushings
  - bronchoalveolar lavage
- Open lung biopsy

Management of lymphangitis carcinomatosis

- Symptomatic treatment of dyspnoea and cough
- Corticosteroids may provide some relief
  - Prednisolone 100 mg PO od or dexamethasone 8 mg PO bd with PPI cover
  - Try for 1 week
    - if response, then titrate steroids down to lowest effective dose
    - if no symptomatic improvement then stop
- Specific systemic treatment of the underlying malignancy may have a good effect if the disease remains responsive to treatment
  - Chemotherapy
  - Hormone therapy

Prognosis

The prognosis of lymphangitis carcinomatosis is poor and patients generally only survive weeks or months. The prognosis is, however, dependent on the underlying disease and its response to specific treatment. Approximately 50% of patients die within 3 months of symptomatic presentation.

Further reading

Bruce, D.M., Heys, S.D. and Eremin, O. (1996). Lymphangitis carcinomatosa: a literature review. *J. R. Coll. Surg. Edin.* **41**(1): 7–13.

⚠ **Pneumothorax**

Pneumothorax is defined as the abnormal presence of air in the pleural space.

Pneumothorax is conventionally classified as:
- Primary
  - no underlying lung disease
- Secondary
  - related to underlying lung disease
    - COPD
    - asthma
    - cystic fibrosis
    - lung abscess
    - carcinoma
      - primary
      - metastatic

Primary pneumothorax is thought to result from the rupture of occult pleural 'blebs' or bullae. Active smoking greatly increases the chance of pneumothorax and its recurrence.

Pneumothorax associated with malignancy is typically considered secondary; however, malignant pleural involvement is not always demonstrable or responsible.

Causes of pneumothorax in the cancer patient
- Spontaneous
- Iatrogenic
  - Central venous line
    - Hickman line
    - Groshong line
  - Radiologically guided lung biopsy
  - Post-thoracocentesis
    - inadvertent access of air during procedure
    - 'trapped lung'
      - the inability of underlying lung to re-expand following drainage of pleural effusion due to malignant disease coating the visceral pleura
- Malignant invasion of pleura
  - Sometimes results in formation of bronchopleural fistula. This can also occur after-lung surgery, e.g. following lobectomy
- Treatment effect (following chemotherapy or radiotherapy)
  - Tumour cavitation and/or necrosis
- Mechanical effect from bronchial/airway obstruction

Clinical features
History
- Dyspnoea
- Pleuritic chest pain
- Cough
- Awareness of 'bubbling' or noises in chest
- Soft tissue swelling around neck or chest wall
  - surgical emphysema

Examination
- Mediastinal shift (away from pneumothorax)
  - tracheal deviation
  - displacement of apex beat
- Reduced expansion on affected side
- Hyper-resonant percussion note
- Reduced air entry on auscultation
- Reduced vocal resonance

Investigations

Bloods
- ABGs
  - may be necessary if there is obvious respiratory compromise
    — SaO_2 <90–92%
- Coagulation screen
  - before insertion of chest drain
    — especially if known/suspected
      – malignant liver disease
      – bone marrow infiltration

Imaging
- CXR
  - usually diagnostic
  - visible lung edge and absence of lung markings peripheral to the edge
  - a small amount of pleural fluid is common
    — ipsilateral blunting of the costophrenic angle
  - anterior pneumothorax may be better visualized on a lateral CXR
  - The British Thoracic Society guidelines:
    — <2 cm rim of air
      – small pneumothorax
    — ≥2 cm rim of air
      – large pneumothorax
    — 1 cm rim of air ≈25% pneumothorax
    — 2 cm rim of air ≈50% pneumothorax
- Chest CT scan
  - malignant pleural disease
  - differentiate large bullae from pneumothorax
  - pneumothorax in patients with significant surgical emphysema

Management

The treatment of pneumothorax depends on:
- The severity of symptoms
- The size of pneumothorax
- Whether the pneumothorax is primary or secondary

Where a background of malignancy involving the chest exists, treatment should proceed as for secondary pneumothorax.

- See Fig. 3.3
- All patients with a secondary pneumothorax should be admitted
- All patients should receive high flow O_2 (10 l/min) where feasible (not with CO_2 retaining patients) to increase the reabsorption of the pneumothorax
  - The rate of reabsorption of air in a pneumothorax is 1.25–1.8% of the volume of hemithorax every 24 hours
- Observation is only an option if the patient is asymptomatic and
  - <1 cm rim of air
  - isolated apical pneumothorax
- Many patients with secondary pneumothorax will require intervention
  - Aspiration should only be attempted in patients with:
    - <2 cm rim of air
    - <50 years of age
    - minimally breathless
    — If simple aspiration is successful (lung re-expansion on CXR) the patient should be admitted for 24 hours with a further CXR at 24 hours
    — Repeat aspiration for failure of initial aspiration is not indicated in secondary pneumothorax
  - Owing to the high failure rate of simple aspiration in secondary pneumothorax, intercostal drain insertion should be carried out in all other patients
    — Consider USS guidance for drain insertion if the patient is clinically stable and has abnormal anatomy or bulky intrathoracic soft tissue disease
    — Complications
      - visceral trauma is now very rare with the Seldinger technique
      - pleural infection/empyema 1–6%
      - misplacement 4%
      - surgical emphysema
    — Small bore chest drains (10–14 F) are sufficient to drain most pneumothoraces and pleural fluid
    — Larger drains (20–24 F) may need to be inserted if there is:
      - gross surgical emphysema
        - especially if involving the neck
      - failure to achieve lung expansion with small bore drains, because of the presence of a large air leak which exceeds the capacity of the smaller tubes
    — Failure of lung expansion may also be due to 'lung trapping' from soft tissue pleural disease
    — Chest drains should never be clamped unless under the supervision of a respiratory specialist with appropriately trained nursing staff to look after the patient. If the patient is to be moved, keep the drain bottle below chest height
    — Refer to a respiratory physician after 48 hours if there is:
      - failure of lung expansion
      - persistent air leak ('bubbling' at the underwater seal) despite lung expansion on the CXR

- check drain is still 'swinging' (this implies continuity with the pleural space) and that air is not entering between tube connectors
— High volume-low pressure suction can be attempted to assist lung expansion
  - it should not be applied within 48 hours of insertion of the chest drain and should be initiated only after discussion with a respiratory physician/thoracic surgeon

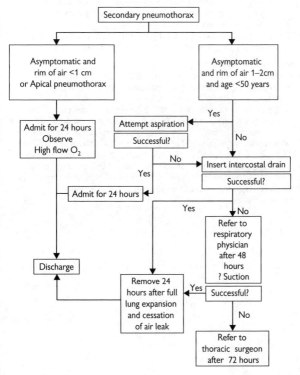

Fig. 3.3 Management of pneumothorax.

- — Refer to a thoracic surgeon after 3–5 days if there is:
  - – failure of lung expansion
  - – persistent air leak
- — Surgical options
  - – open thoracotomy and pleurectomy
    - • lowest recurrence rate
  - – minimally invasive procedures
    - • thoracoscopy (VATS)
    - • pleural abrasion
    - • surgical talc pleurodesis
- — Most cancer patients are not suitable candidates for invasive surgical procedures. Recurrent pneumothoraces in cancer patients may be managed more appropriately with medical talc pleurodesis (via an intercostal drain)
- Commercial airlines advise that there should be a 6-week interval between having a pneumothorax and travelling by air

Iatrogenic pneumothorax

- Many patients with an iatrogenic pneumothorax may not have underlying lung disease or chest malignancy and can therefore be managed as a primary pneumothorax
  - If patient is asymptomatic with <2 cm rim of air, patient can be discharged with a repeat CXR at 2 weeks. Patient should be advised to return to hospital if they experience worsening breathlessness
  - If patient is symptomatic or >2 cm rim of air attempt aspiration of air; if this fails consider a further attempt at aspiration. After two attempts at aspiration consider insertion of an intercostal drain
- Patients with an iatrogenic pneumothorax and underlying lung disease or chest malignancy should be managed as for a secondary pneumothorax.

:☠: **Tension pneumothorax**

Tension pneumothorax is a respiratory emergency.

It describes a clinical syndrome, which is not necessarily proportionate to the size of the pneumothorax or the degree of mediastinal shift.

Urgent evacuation of intrapleural air is necessary.

Clinical features

- Clinical examination findings consistent with pneumothorax
    AND
- Extreme respiratory distress
    - may be cyanosed
- Raised JVP
- Tachycardia
- Hypotension

Differential diagnosis

- PE
- Pericardial effusion/cardiac tamponade

Management of tension pneumothorax

- The diagnosis is clinical: do not wait for a CXR
- Give high flow oxygen to correct hypoxia
- Insert the largest available venous cannula into the thorax
    - perpendicular to the chest wall
    - via the second intercostal space, midclavicular line
- Immediate escape of air ('hissing') should be evident
- If this does not occur diagnosis is likely to be incorrect and cannula should be removed
- Leave cannula in place until hissing stops
- Temporarily occlude cannula whilst preparation for formal chest drainage is made

Further reading

Chapman, S., Robinson, G., Stradling, J. and West, S. (2005). *Oxford Handbook of Respiratory Medicine.*, Oxford: Oxford University Press.

Henry, M., Arnold, T. and Harvey, J. (2003). BTS guidelines for the management of spontaneous pneumothorax. *Thorax* 58(Suppl. II): ii39–ii52.

Metabolic emergencies

! Hypercalcaemia

Corrected serum $[Ca^{2+}]$ >3.0 mmol/l.
Corrected $[Ca^{2+}]$ = measured $[Ca^{2+}]$ + 0.02(40 − [albumin]).
Occurs in up to 20% of all malignancies, especially
- Breast cancer
- Lung cancer
- Myeloma
- Lymphoma
- Prostate cancer
- Renal cell carcinoma

Causes of malignant hypercalcaemia
- Lytic bone metastases
  - osteoclast stimulation
  - cytokine release
- Secretion of PTH-related peptide (PTHrP)
  - especially squamous cell carcinoma of the lung
- Renal impairment
  - in myeloma, deposition of Bence Jones proteins in the renal tubules results in renal impairment and reduced Ca^{2+} excretion resulting in hypercalcaemia
  - hypercalcaemia itself causes renal dysfunction and diuresis, resulting in dehydration. Hypovolaemia stimulates Na^+ reabsorption in the kidney with concomitant Ca^{2+} reabsorption
- Excess vitamin D activity
  - some lymphomas produce active metabolites of vitamin D, resulting in increased intestinal absorption of Ca^{2+}

Clinical features
- Fatigue
- Drowsiness
- Nausea and vomiting
- Polyuria
- Bone pain
- Dehydration
  - dry mouth
- Abdominal pain
  - constipation
  - renal colic
- Anorexia
- Depression
- Confusion
- Seizures
- Weakness

  - postural hypotension

  - peptic ulceration

Investigations
Bloods
- Serum Ca^{2+}
- Phosphate
- Mg^{2+}
- Serum PTH
  - should be undetectable in malignant hypercalcaemia
  - if present consider primary (or tertiary) hyperparathyroidism
- LFTs
- U&Es
- Serum electrophoresis

ECG
- Long PR interval
- Widened QRS complexes
- Short QT interval
- Hypercalcaemia causes increased sensitivity to digoxin

Imaging

- X-ray painful area of bone
- Consider a bone scan for full staging of bone metastases
  - myeloma deposits generally do not show up on a bone scan

Management

- $[Ca^{2+}] \geq 3.0$ mmol/l should be treated
- Patients with $[Ca^{2+}] <3.0$ mmol/l but above the normal range should only be treated if symptomatic
- Rehydration is essential
  - patients are dehydrated
  - renal impairment exacerbates hypercalcaemia
- Rehydrate with 0.9% saline
  - Na^+ required for Ca^{2+} excretion by the renal tubules
  - aim for 3–6 l over first 24 hours if cardiac function and urinary output permits
  - continue rehydration over subsequent days (≥ 3 l/day), with careful assessment of fluid status
- Monitor U&Es, Ca^{2+}, phosphate, Mg^{2+} and albumin daily
  - replace electrolytes as appropriate
- Bisphosphonate infusion
  - Pamidronate IV 90 mg in 500 ml 0.9% saline over 90 minutes
  - Zoledronic acid IV 4 mg over 15 minutes
  - Onset of action within 48 hours
  - Patient is usually normocalcaemic within 3–7 days
  - Bisphosphonate dose cannot be repeated within 7 days, therefore the mainstay of ongoing management while bisphosphonate acts is to maintain adequate hydration
  - Bisphosphonate infusion can be given regularly, ≥ 3 weeks apart
  - If renal function is compromised, reducing the dose and prolonging the infusion time is suggested (although this is not evidence-based)
  - Side effects
    - acute phase reaction, especially with the first dose
      - fever, malaise, bone pain
    - bisphosphonates are associated with acute tubular necrosis of the kidney in about 10% of patients, therefore renal function must be monitored over time, and bisphosphonates must be discontinued if renal function deteriorates
    - osteonecrosis of the jaw has been reported in patients who have received many repeated monthly doses of bisphosphonate, and who have also had dental work carried out, e.g. tooth extraction
- Corticosteroids and calcitonin no longer have any useful role in hypercalcaemia of malignancy
- Hypercalcaemia usually occurs in the presence of widespread metastatic disease. Treatment of the underlying malignancy, where possible, may result in symptomatic improvement and potentially increase life expectancy
  - palliative systemic chemotherapy
  - palliative radiotherapy to painful bone lesions

☉ **Tumour lysis syndrome**

Tumour lysis syndrome (TLS) is a group of metabolic complications arising from treatment of a rapidly proliferating neoplasm. Rapid cell lysis results in the acute release of intracellular products into the circulation. Occasionally the syndrome can occur prior to the initiation of treatment, presumably as a result of tissue ischaemia causing tumour cell death.

Pathophysiology

Rapid tumour cell death results in the following metabolic abnormalities
- Hyperuricaemia
  - Rapid cell death leads to a massive release and catabolism of nucleic acids. Purine nucleic acid breakdown leads to formation of hypoxanthine and xanthine. Xanthine oxidase catalyses the final step in the pathway with formation of uric acid. Uric acid is excreted mainly by the kidneys but is poorly soluble in water and can precipitate in the tubules, leading to urate nephropathy with associated ARF.
- Hyperphosphataemia
  - Tumour cell death releases large amounts of phosphate into the circulation. The kidney can respond by increasing clearance but this mechanism can become saturated (particularly if there is coexisting renal impairment owing to urate nephropathy). Calcium phosphate precipitation within the renal tubules can lead to (or exacerbate) ARF.
- Hyperkalaemia
  - Lysed tumour cells can release massive amounts of K^+ which the kidneys may have difficulty clearing, especially if their function is already compromised by the above mechanisms. Rapid rises in serum $[K^+]$ can result in potentially fatal arrhythmias.
- Hypocalcaemia
  - This is usually the result of a high phosphate level leading to precipitation of calcium phosphate in the renal tubules (resulting in renal failure) and other tissues (skin deposition results in pruritus and gangrene).
- Uraemia
  - This is commonly caused by one of the above metabolic abnormalities. However, there may be other contributory factors:
    — obstructive uropathy due to a tumour mass
    — sepsis-related ATN
    — tumour cell infiltration

Risk factors

The most important consideration in the management of TLS is the identification of patients at high risk with institution of appropriate preventative measures. The following risk factors have been identified:
- Patient-related factors
  - decreased urine output
  - pre-existing renal impairment
  - pre-existing hyperuricaemia
  - dehydration
  - acidic urine
- Tumour-related factors
  - high tumour cell proliferative rate
  - high tumour burden
  - high sensitivity to cytotoxic agents

The tumours most commonly associated with TLS are:
- Acute lymphoblastic leukaemia
  - especially with a high peripheral blast count
- High grade non-Hodgkin's lymphoma
  - especially Burkitt's lymphoma and lymphoblastic lymphoma

Less commonly
- Acute myeloid leukaemia
  - usually with high peripheral blast count
- Chronic lymphocytic leukaemia
- Myeloma
- Certain solid tumours
  - testicular cancer
  - breast cancer
  - SCLC

Clinical features

The clinical features are caused by the underlying metabolic disturbances (see Table 4.1).

Table 4.1 Clinical features of tumour lysis syndrome

Metabolic disturbance	Symptom
Hyperuricaemia	Haematuria, flank pain, acute obstructive nephropathy (anuria/oliguria)
Hyperphosphataemia	Nausea, vomiting, diarrhoea, seizures, hypocalcaemia, acute obstructive uropathy
Hyperkalaemia	Nausea, vomiting, diarrhoea, cramps, weakness, paraesthesiae, arrhythmias, sudden death
Hypocalcaemia	Muscle cramps, spasms, tetany, arrhythmias, confusion, hallucinations, seizures
Uraemia	Lethargy, anorexia, nausea, vomiting, confusion, encephalopathy, pericarditis, acidosis, oedema, hypertension

'Clinical tumour lysis syndrome' can be defined as:
- Creatinine ≥1.5× upper limit of normal
- Cardiac arrhythmia/sudden death and/or seizure
- Having ruled out an alternative cause for the clinical features

Investigations

The following tests need to be performed at baseline and at regular intervals (at least tds for at least 72 hours) after the initiation of treatment in high risk patients.
- Twice daily weight
- Fluid balance
- Bloods
  - Urea and creatinine
  - Serum K^+
  - Serum phosphate
  - Serum Ca^{2+}
  - Serum urate
- ECG
  - hyperkalaemia
    — peaked T waves
    — broad QRS complexes

'Laboratory tumour lysis syndrome' is the presence of abnormal laboratory results, as outlined in Table 4.2.
Additional tests which may be helpful include:
- Bloods
  - FBC
    — high blast count in acute leukaemias increases risk of TLS
  - LDH
    — in lymphoid neoplasms a high level indicates high tumour burden
  - CRP and blood cultures
    — coexisting sepsis increases the risk of complications in TLS
  - ABG
    — metabolic acidosis may indicate underlying renal impairment or tissue ischaemia, both increasing the risk of TLS
- Urine
  - MC&S
    — haematuria may indicate renal damage
    — white cells and nitrites may indicate urinary sepsis
- Imaging
  - CXR
    — as part of a septic screen

Prevention

Prevention requires the identification of patients at high risk of TLS with the institution of appropriate preventative measures. These measures include:
- Vigorous hydration, aiming for twice the daily fluid requirement (approximately 3 l/m^2/d) with a urine output of >100 ml/m^2/h.

- Low risk cases
  - allopurinol 300 mg daily increasing to 600–900 mg (10 mg/kg daily) in 2–3 divided doses. Start allopurinol 24 hours before the first chemotherapy treatment. Dose should be reduced in renal impairment or if concomitant azathioprine, mercaptopurine or 6-thioguanine treatment.
- High risk cases
  - rasburicase 200 mcg/kg once daily for up to 7 days according to plasma uric acid concentration. To measure uric acid levels in a patient on rasburicase, the sample needs to be taken to the laboratory immediately and on ice.
  Note: rarely causes bronchospasm and should avoid in G6PD-deficient patients.
- Urinary alkalinization is controversial. Although this may reduce uric acid precipitation, it increases the risk of xanthine crystal formation. Local protocols should be followed.

Treatment

Treatment is aimed at correcting the electrolyte imbalances and optimizing renal function (see Table 4.3).
Haemodialysis may be needed for:
- Symptomatic uraemia (usually >45 mmol/l)
  - tremor
  - confusion
  - coma
  - seizures
  - pericarditis
- $[K^+]$ >7 mmol/l and refractory to other measures
- Metabolic acidosis (arterial pH <7.1, $[HCO_3]$ <12 mmol/l)
- Fluid overload unresponsive to diuretics

Table 4.2 Cairo–Bishop definition of laboratory tumour lysis syndrome

Chemical	Serum level
Uric acid	≥476 μmol/l or 25% increase from baseline
K^+	≥6.0 mmol/l or 25% increase from baseline
Phosphate	Children: ≥2.1 mmol/l or 25% increase from baseline
	Adults: ≥1.45 mmol/l or 25% increase from baseline
Ca^{2+}	≤1.75 mmol/l or 25% decrease from baseline

Table 4.3 Treatment of electrolyte imbalances in tumour lysis syndrome

Electrolyte imbalance	Treatment
Hyperuricaemia ≥476 µmol/l	Intravenous fluids
	Loop diuretics increase excretion of uric acid
	Rasburicase (recombinant urate oxidase)
Hyperkalaemia	Calcium gluconate (10 ml of 10% IV over 2 minutes) as a cardioprotectant, repeat until ECG normalizes
[K⁺] ≥6.0 mmol/l Calcium resonium	Actrapid insulin 10 units plus 50 ml of 50% dextrose as an infusion over 30 minutes to drive K⁺ into the intracellular compartment.
[K⁺] ≥6.5 mmol/l Insulin and dextrose	Monitor blood glucose and K⁺ regularly
	Correct acidosis where possible (50–100 ml 8.4% $NaHCO_3$ via central line)
ECG changes Calcium gluconate, insulin and dextrose	Calcium resonium 15 g PO three-four times daily (not with fruit squash) (with laxative) or 30 g PR followed 3–6 hours later by an enema
	Avoid IV or PO K⁺ supplements and stop ACE inhibitors/K⁺-sparing diuretics
	Consider dialysis if [K⁺] >7 mmol/l and refractory to other measures
Hyperphosphataemia Children: ≥2.1 mmol/l	Avoid IV phosphate infusion
	Aluminium hydroxide 15 ml 6-hourly PO
Adults: ≥1.45 mmol/l	If severe, consider dialysis
Hypocalcaemia ≤1.75 mmol/l	If asymptomatic, no therapy indicated
	If symptomatic, calcium gluconate 2.25 mmol (10 ml) to correct symptoms. Can repeat or give a continuous IV infusion of 9 mmol (40 ml of 10%) daily

Further reading

Cairo, M.S. Bishop, M. (2004). Tumour lysis syndrome: new therapeutic strategies and classification. *Br. J. Haematol.* **127**: 3–11.

Flombaum, C.D. (2000). Metabolic emergencies in the cancer patient. *Semin. Oncol.* **3**: 322–334.

☼ Hypoglycaemia

Blood glucose <2.5 mmol/l with symptoms of neuroglycopenia.

Hypoglycaemia can be caused by a number of neoplasms, both pancreatic and non-pancreatic. Tumours other than insulinomas are thought to cause hypoglycaemia through unregulated production of insulin-like growth factors.

Causes
- Drugs
  - Insulin
  - Oral hypoglycaemic agents
  - Ethanol
  - Salicylates
  - Quinine
  - Pentamidine
- Tumours
  - Insulinoma
  - Carcinoid
  - Sarcoma
  - Lymphoma
  - Mesothelioma
  - Phaeochromocytoma
  - Haemangiopericytoma
  - Leiomyoma
  - Carcinoma
    — adrenal
    — breast
    — cervix
    — colon
    — prostate
    — stomach
    — pancreas
- Postoperative
  - Gastrectomy
  - Pancreatectomy
- Hepatic dysfunction
  - Cirrhosis
  - Paracetamol overdose
- Impaired oral intake
  - Dysphagia
  - Nausea
- Addison's disease
- Pituitary insufficiency
- Chronic renal failure

Clinical features
Due to sympathetic stimulation
- Tachycardia
- Palpitations
- Sweating
- Anxiety
- Tremor

Due to neuroglycopenia
- Confusion
- Slurred speech
- Blurred vision
- Focal neurological deficit
- Convulsions
- Coma

Investigations

Bloods
- Blood glucose monitor
- Laboratory glucose
- U&Es
- LFTs
- Ethanol
- Cortisol
- Insulin + C-peptide levels (before administering glucose)
  - High insulin, low C-peptide—exogenous insulin
  - High insulin, high C-peptide—insulinoma, 2° to sulphonylurea

Immediate management

- If history of malnourishment or chronic ethanol abuse, give thiamine 2–3 pairs every eight hours to avoid precipitating Wernicke's encephalopathy.
- In a conscious patient give 50 g oral glucose in warm water, lucozade or GlucoGel.
- In an unconscious patient give glucose IV (50 ml 50% dextrose); this is highly irritant to veins, therefore give 0.9% saline flush.
- Repeat if symptoms persist after 10 minutes.
- If intravenous access is impossible give 1 mg glucagon IM. This increases hepatic glucose efflux; therefore glucose must be given simultaneously to avoid later hypoglycaemia. Glucagon is not suitable for sulphonylurea overdose or liver failure. Glucagon should only be given once, and not for the treatment of recurrent hypoglycaemia.
- If hypoglycaemia is caused by a long-acting sulphonylurea or insulin, start a 10% dextrose infusion and monitor glucose hourly.

Further management

- Patient should regain consciousness within 10 minutes.
- Consider long-acting carbohydrate once patient conscious.
- Closely monitor blood sugars for 24 hours as risk of rebound hypo/hyperglycaemia.
- If not responding to treatment, consider other cause for depressed consciousness level (e.g. head injury while hypoglycaemic).
- Prolonged severe hypoglycaemia (>4 hours) can lead to cerebral oedema.
- Hypoglycaemic attacks in previously well controlled diabetics may suggest a new pathology, e.g. liver failure, diabetic nephropathy (reduced renal clearance of insulin).

Insulinoma

Insulinoma is a tumour of the insulin-secreting β-cells of the pancreatic islets. Annual incidence: 1–2 cases/million population/year. The majority (95%) are benign. Most are sporadic, but may be associated with multiple endocrine neoplasia (MEN).

Present with symptoms of hypoglycaemia, associated with fasting or exercise.

Investigations
- 15-hour fasting glucose test
  - Hypoglycaemia with raised insulin and raised C-peptide
- To localize the tumour
  - CT
  - MRI
  - EUS
  - Intraoperative USS

Treatment
- Surgical excision
- If surgery fails or patient is unfit for surgery, somatostatin analogues (e.g. octreotide, lanreotide) and diazoxide can help symptoms
- Chemotherapy (e.g. streptozocin)

Further reading

Beckers, M.M., Slee, P.H. and Van Doorn, J. (2003). Hypoglycaemia in a patient with a gastrointestinal stromal tumour. *Clin. Endocrinol. (Oxf).* **59**(3): 402–404.

Ford-Dunn, S., Smith, A. and Sykes, N. (2002). Tumour-induced hypoglycaemia. *Palliat. Med.* **16**(4): 357–358.

Hirshberg, B., Cochran, C., Skarulia, M.C., Libutti, S.K., Alexander, H.R., Wood, B.J., Chang, R., Kleiner, D.E. and Gorden, P. (2005). Malignant insulinoma: spectrum of unusual clinical features. *Cancer* **104**(2): 264–272.

ⓘ **Hyponatraemia**

Normal plasma [Na^+] 135–145 mmol/l.
Symptomatic hyponatraemia is usually associated with a plasma [Na^+] <125 mmol/l.
Symptoms are related to the severity and the rapidity of the fall in the plasma [Na^+]. Symptoms are caused by osmotic movement of water into brain cells resulting in cerebral oedema, and the effects of extracellular fluid volume imbalances

Clinical features

Neurological

- Malaise
- Nausea and vomiting
- Weakness
- Ataxia
- Headache
- Confusion
- Seizures
- Coma

Volume status

- Hypovolaemia
  - decreased skin turgor
  - oliguria (if extrarenal Na^+ loss)
  - tachycardia
  - postural hypotension
- Hypervolaemia
  - raised JVP
  - peripheral oedema
  - pulmonary oedema
  - ascites

Causes

Normal serum osmolality

Pseudohyponatraemia

- Hyperlipidaemia
- Hyperproteinaemia

Excess solute

- Glucose
- Ethanol

Decreased serum osmolality

Hypovolaemia

- Renal Na^+ losses (urinary [Na^+] >20 mmol/l)
  - diuretics
  - mineralocorticoid deficiency (Addison's disease)
  - salt-wasting nephropathy
    — cisplatin chemotherapy
  - cerebral salt wasting
    — post-intracranial surgery
    — subarachnoid haemorrhage
  - renal tubular acidosis
- Extrarenal Na^+ losses (urinary [Na^+] <20 mmol/l)
  - GI losses
    — vomiting
    — external biliary drainage
    — diarrhoea

- Dermal losses
  - burns
  - sweating
- Fluid sequestration
  - peritonitis
  - ileus
  - pancreatitis
- Recurrent drainage of ascites

Normovolaemia (urinary [Na$^+$] >20 mmol/l)
- SIADH
  - Tumours
    - majority of malignancies, especially SCLC
  - Drugs
    - cyclophosphamide
    - chlorpropamide
    - vinca alkaloids
    - opioids
    - carbamazepine
    - haloperidol
    - phenothiazines
    - SSRIs
  - Pulmonary
    - pneumonia
    - abscess
    - TB
    - asthma
    - positive pressure ventilation
    - vasculitis
  - CNS
    - meningitis
    - tumours
    - encephalitis
    - head injury
    - subdural haematoma
    - vasculitis
    - subarachnoid haemorrhage
    - cerebral abscess
- Metabolic
  - Hypothyroidism
  - Porphyria
  - Glucocorticoid deficiency
- Water intoxication
  - Primary polydipsia
  - Post-TURP
  - Excessive hypotonic intravenous fluids

Hypervolaemia
- Urinary [Na$^+$] <20 mmol/l
  - Congestive cardiac failure
  - Nephrotic syndrome
  - Cirrhosis with ascites
- Urinary [Na$^+$] >20 mmol/l
  - Chronic renal failure

Investigations

Bloods
- U&Es
- Glucose
- LFTs
- Total protein
- Amylase
- TFTs
- Cortisol +/− short synacthen test
- Plasma osmolality

Urine
- Urinary osmolality
- Urinary [Na$^+$]

CXR
- Pulmonary pathology responsible for SIADH

① Hypokalaemia

Normal plasma $[K^+]$ 3.5–5.0 mmol/l.
Symptomatic hypokalaemia is usually associated with a plasma $[K^+]$ <2.5 mmol/l.

Causes

Decreased intake
- Usually due to anorexia secondary to tumour, chemotherapy or radiotherapy
- Decreased intake rarely causes significant hypokalaemia unless associated with increased loss of K^+

Increased entry into cells
- Metabolic alkalosis (e.g. secondary to vomiting)
- Insulin (often used with TPN)
- β-adrenergic agonists
- Thyrotoxicosis
- Increased blood cell production (e.g. G-CSF to treat neutropenia)
- Hypothermia

Increased GI losses
- Vomiting
- Diarrhoea
- NG tube drainage
- Tumour-related
  - villous adenoma
  - VIPoma
  - carcinoid syndrome
  - medullary carcinoma of the thyroid
- Laxatives
- Ileostomy
- Ureterosigmoidostomy

Increased urinary losses
- Diuretics
- Hypomagnesaemia
  - secondary to cisplatin
- Drug-induced renal tubular damage
  - cytotoxic chemotherapy
    - cisplatin
    - ifosfamide
    - streptozocin
  - aminoglycosides
  - amphotericin B
- Tumours producing ectopic ACTH
  - SCLC and others
- Primary mineralocorticoid excess (Conn's syndrome)
- Secondary hyperaldosteronism
  - cirrhosis
  - nephrotic syndrome
  - CCF
- Exogenous steroids (e.g. dexamethasone)
- Post-obstructive diuresis
- Renal tubular acidosis

Clinical features
- Neuromuscular
  - Weakness
  - Hypotonia
  - Confusion
  - Ileus
- Cardiac
  - Palpitations
    — atrial and ventricular ectopic beats
  - Potentiates digoxin toxicity
- Renal
  - Polyuria
  - Polydipsia

Investigations
Bloods
- U&Es
- Ca^{2+} and Mg^{2+}
- Phosphate
- Glucose
- TSH, fT_4
- ABG for metabolic alkalosis
- Aldosterone:renin ratio for Conn's syndrome

ECG
- ST depression
- T wave inversion
- Prolonged PR interval
- Prominent U wave

Management
- Treat $[K^+]$3–3.5 mmol/l with oral replacement
  - K^+ rich foods, e.g. bananas, oranges
  - K^+ tablets, e.g. sando-K (1 tablet=12 mmol K^+)
- Diuretic-induced hypokalaemia
  - Add a K^+-sparing diuretic to limit further urinary loss of K^+
    — amiloride, spironolactone
- Treat symptomatic hypokalaemia with IV KCl replacement
  - Usually infuse 20–40 mmol KCl in 1 litre over 4–8 hours
  - Maximum infusion rate 20 mmol/h, which must occur via a central line with ECG monitoring
  - Higher rates of infusion may cause arrhythmias
  - [KCl] >60 mmol/l can cause painful sclerosis of peripheral veins
- Hypomagnesaemia is a common complication of chemotherapy; check Mg^{2+} levels in resistant hypokalaemia, and replace if necessary (see Hypomagnesaemia 📖 p182)

Further reading
Gennari, F.J. (1998). Hypokalaemia. *New Engl. J. Med.* **339**(7): 451–458.

Schaefer, T.J. and Wolford, R.W. (2005). Disorders of potassium. *Emerg. Med. Clin. N. Am.* **23**(3): 723–727.

Welfare, W., Sasi, P. and English, M. (2002). Challenges in managing profound hypokalaemia. *BMJ.* **324**: 269–270.

⑦ **Hypomagnesaemia**

Hypomagnesaemia $[Mg^{2+}]$ <0.75 mmol/l.

In oncology, it is most commonly caused by chemotherapy agents, particularly those that are platinum-based, e.g. cisplatin causes proximal tubular damage which results in hypomagnesaemia.

Clinical manifestations are mainly caused by increasing neuromuscular excitability, similar to those of hypocalcaemia.

Mg^{2+} deficiency may cause secondary hypocalcaemia because of defective PTH secretion and end organ insensitivity to PTH.

Hypomagnesaemia can also cause renal K^+ wasting and hypokalaemia.

The hypocalcaemia and hypokalaemia will not improve until the underlying hypomagnesaemia is corrected.

Clinical features

Neurological
- Tetany
- Tremor
- Myoclonus
- Ataxia
- Convulsions
- Coma

Cardiovascular
- Arrhythmias
  - Ventricular
  - Supraventricular
  - Torsade de pointes
- Coronary artery spasm
- Increased risk digoxin toxicity

Metabolic
- Hypokalaemia
- Hypocalcaemia
- Hypophosphataemia

Other
- Agitation
- Delirium
- Depression

Investigations

Bloods
- U&Es
- Mg^{2+}
- Ca^{2+}
- Glucose
- Amylase

Urine
- 24-hour urinary Mg^{2+} excretion
- Urinary excretion >30 mg/day in a hypomagnesaemic patient suggests renal wasting (e.g. cisplatin, aminoglycosides, diuretics)

ECG
- Prolonged PR interval
- Widened QRS
- Prolonged QT interval

Causes

Decreased intake
- Poor diet
- Chronic alcohol intake
- Parenteral nutrition with inadequate Mg^{2+}

GI losses
- Malabsorption
- Vomiting
- Diarrhoea
- Fistulae
- Short bowel syndrome
  - post-bowel resection
- Pancreatitis
  - saponification of Mg^{2+} and Ca^{2+} occurs in necrotic adipose tissue

Renal losses
- Nephrotoxins
  - Cisplatin
  - Amphotericin B
  - Cyclosporine
  - Pentamidine
  - Aminoglycosides
- Loop and thiazide diuretics
- Cetuximab
- Alcohol
- Hypercalcaemia
- Diuretic phase of ATN
- Hyperaldosteronism

Others
- Hungry bone syndrome
  - increased Mg^{2+} uptake by renewing bone after parathyroidectomy
- Diabetes with persistently raised glucose

Management

This depends on severity of clinical manifestations.
- In mild hypomagnesaemia ($[Mg^{2+}]$ >0.6 mmol/l) and in the absence of symptoms, oral Mg^{2+} replacement (e.g. magnesium glycerophosphate 8 mmol tds) is adequate. However, this is often poorly tolerated owing to GI side effects.
- If $[Mg^{2+}]$ <0.6 mmol/l, the patient is symptomatic, or there is associated hypocalcaemia, then IV Mg^{2+} is required. Up to 10–20 mmol Mg^{2+} can be administered intravenously over 12–24 hours. Regular monitoring of Mg^{2+} levels is essential, especially in patients with renal failure.

Further reading

Lajer, H. and Daugaard, G. (1999). Cisplatin and hypomagnesaemia. *Cancer Treat. Rev.* **25**(1): 47–58.
Tong, G.M. and Rude, R.K. (2005). Magnesium deficiency in critical illness. *J. Intensive Care Med.* **20**(1): 3–17.

☼ Thyroid storm

Thyroid storm is a rapid deterioration of hyperthyroidism with:
- Hyperpyrexia
- Severe tachycardia
- Extreme restlessness

Although a rare complication, it can be life-threatening (mortality ~10%). In the treatment of hyperthyroidism with radioactive iodine-131, anti-thyroid drugs are discontinued prior to treatment. The subsequent radio-iodine can trigger a hyperthyroid flare and occasionally thyroid storm.

Precipitants include:
- Surgery
- Withdrawal of anti-thyroid drugs
- Radio-iodine treatment
- Iodine-containing contrast dye
- Sepsis
- Parturition
- DKA
- Trauma

Clinical features (see Table 4.4)
- Cardiovascular
  - Palpitations
  - Tachycardia/tachyarrhythmia
  - Cardiac failure
- Neurological
  - Anxiety/agitation
  - Psychosis
  - Seizures
  - Coma
- GI
  - Nausea and vomiting
  - Diarrhoea
  - Jaundice
- Other
  - Hyperpyrexia
  - Hyperventilation
  - Sweating
  - Dehydration
  - Rhabdomyolysis

Investigations
Bloods
- TFTs (TSH, fT_3, fT_4)
  - levels do not always correlate with severity
- U&Es
  - dehydration
  - hypokalaemia
- Ca^{2+} and Mg^{2+}
  - hypercalcaemia
  - hypomagnesaemia
- FBC
  - infection (often ↑ WCC but no infection)
- Glucose
  - hypoglycaemia
- LFTs
  - jaundice
- Blood cultures
  - infection

Urine
• MSU to rule out infection

ECG
• Tachycardia
• Arrhythmia, e.g. AF

CXR
• Pulmonary oedema
• Infection

Table 4.4 Assessment of severity of a thyrotoxic crisis

Temperature (°C)	Pulse (bpm)	Cardiac failure	CNS effects	GI symptoms	Score
Apyrexial	<90	Absent	Normal	Normal	0
>37.2	>90	Ankle oedema			5
>37.8	>110	Basal crepitations	Agitation	Diarrhoea, vomiting	10
>38.3	>120	Pulmonary oedema			15
>38.9	>130		Delirium	Unexplained jaundice	20
>39.4	>140				25
>40			Coma, seizure		30

• Add the scores for each column
• Add an extra 10 points for
  • AF
  • Definable precipitant
• Total score
  • >45   Thyroid storm
  • 25–44 Impending thyroid storm

Adapted from Ramrakhal and Moorel (eds) *Oxford Handbook of Acute Medicine*, 2nd edn. Oxford: OUP.

Management of thyroid storm

The patient may need to be transferred to ICU.

General measures

- CVP monitoring is often required, owing to cardiac decompensation and the need for substantial fluid replacement.
- Lower temperature with paracetamol and peripheral cooling (e.g. electric fan and tepid sponging. Do not use aspirin as it displaces T_4 from thyroid-binding globulin).
- Control AF rate with digoxin (requirements may be high as its metabolism is increased).
- Broad spectrum antibiotics (e.g. cefuroxime1.5 g IV tds) if infection is a possible precipitant.

Specific treatments

- Beta blockers to lower sympathetic tone
  - propanolol PO 10–40 mg 3–4 times daily as necessary or 1 mg IV over 1 minute, repeated every 2 minutes as required to a maximum dose of 10 mg. Beta blockers should help to control tachycardia, tremor, and rate-dependent cardiac failure.
- Anti-thyroid drugs
  - Propylthiouracil (PTU) 200–400 mg PO daily in adults and this dose is maintained until the patient becomes euthyroid; the dose may then be gradually reduced to a maintenance dose of 50–150 mg daily. This is more effective than carbimazole because of its ability to block peripheral conversion of T_4 to T_3. PTU also blocks *de novo* thyroid hormone synthesis within 2 hours but has no effect on release of preformed thyroid hormone.
- To block release of thyroxine from the thyroid gland
  - potassium iodide 60 mg PO qds.
  - alternatively give Lugol's iodine (5% iodine, 10% potassium iodide) 0.1–0.3 ml 3 times daily well diluted with milk and water.
  - these treatments should not be started until 2 hours after commencing PTU to prevent the iodine being used as a substrate for thyroid hormone synthesis.
- Hydrocortisone 300 mg IV stat, then 100 mg qds IV to reduce T_4 conversion to T_3.
- Monitor blood glucose carefully as hepatic glycogen stores are quickly depleted.
- If resistant to above treatments, may require plasmapheresis.

Further reading

Pimentel, L. and Hansen, K.N. (2005). Thyroid disease in the emergency department: a clinical and laboratory review. *J. Emerg. Med.* **28**(2): 201–209.

Rennie D. (1997). Thyroid storm. *JAMA.* **277**(15): 1238–1243.

⑦ **Refeeding syndrome**

Rapid correction of nutritional deficiencies can cause severe fluid and electrolyte shifts with micronutrient deficiencies and related metabolic disturbances. It can occur in any malnourished patient, including over-weight individuals who have had little food intake for protracted periods. Life-threatening problems can occur in patients

- with a BMI <16 kg/m^2.
- who have had very little or no food intake for >10 days.
- with weight loss >15% within the previous 6 months.

Cancer patients are often malnourished, e.g. loss of appetite, persistent vomiting, and are thus at risk of refeeding syndrome when nutritional support (enteral/parenteral) is commenced.

Other risk factors for developing refeeding syndrome:

- Chemotherapy
- Diarrhoea
- Alcoholism
- Major surgery

Pathophysiology

During starvation, insulin secretion decreases in response to low carbo-hydrate intake. Fat and protein are metabolized instead to produce energy. This leads to loss of intracellular electrolytes, particularly phos-phate. There can be whole body depletion of phosphate, K$^+$ and Mg^{2+} despite normal plasma levels.

As feeding commences, a sudden shift from fat to carbohydrate metabolism stimulates insulin secretion. This, in turn, leads to cellular uptake of phosphate, K$^+$ and Mg^{2+}, and a simultaneous shift of Na$^+$ and water out of cells. Thus, rapid or unbalanced nutritional support can precipitate dangerous changes in fluid and electrolyte balance along with micronutrient deficiencies. Hypophosphataemia is of particular importance because phosphate is needed for ATP generation.

Clinical features

- Hypophosphataemia
- Hypokalaemia
- Hypomagnesaemia
- Hypocalcaemia
- Hyperglycaemia
- Thrombocytopenia
- Leukocyte dysfunction
- Cardiac failure
- Pulmonary oedema
- Arrhythmias
- Muscle weakness
  - including diaphragm
- Rhabdomyolysis
- Paraesthesiae
- Tetany
- Seizures
- Coma

Management

- Identify at risk patients.
- Check K^+, Mg^{2+}, and phosphate prior to feeding.
- If all normal, feeding can be commenced at 20 kcal/kg for first 24 hours, then increase gradually during first week to full feeding rate.
- If electrolytes abnormal, then correct prior to feeding
  - $[K^+]$ <2.5 mmol/l
    — correct with IV K^+ e.g. 40 mmol K^+ in 1 litre 0.9% saline over 8 hours.
  - $[PO_4^{3-}]$ <0.3 mmol/l
    — correct with IV PO_4^{3-} e.g. 40 mmol PO_4^{3-} in 500 ml 5% dextrose over 6 hours.
  - $[Mg^{2+}]$ <0.5 mmol/l
    — correct with IV Mg^{2+} e.g. 20 mmol Mg^{2+} in 500 ml 5% dextrose over 6–12 hours.
  - Give IV thiamine (one pair pabrinex IVHP ampoules (250 mg thiamine)) at least 30 minutes before feeding starts.
  - Commence feeding at 20 kcal/kg for first 24 hours, then increase gradually during first week to full feeding rate.
  - During first 10 days of feeding, continue oral thiamine 100 mg bd, vitamin B and multivitamin supplementation, e.g. Forceval one capsule od.
  - Monitor fluid and electrolyte balance daily for 7 days and correct as necessary.

Further reading

Hearing, S.D. (2004). Refeeding syndrome. *BMJ*. **328**: 908–909.
Khardori, R. (2005). Refeeding syndrome and hypophosphataemia. *J. Intensive Care Med*. **20**(3): 174–175.

:+: **Pituitary apoplexy**

Life-threatening infarction of the pituitary gland due to either ischaemia or haemorrhage.

Causes

In patients with a pituitary adenoma (often undiagnosed)
- Spontaneous haemorrhage
- Pituitary radiotherapy
- Anticoagulant treatment
- Diabetes mellitus
- Following carotid angiography
- Head trauma

In patients with a normal pituitary gland
- Sheehan's syndrome
  - haemorrhagic infarction postpartum, usually owing to severe blood loss and hypotension

Clinical features

Symptoms and signs are either caused by rapid expansion of a pituitary lesion and compression of surrounding structures, or by leakage of blood and necrotic tissue into the subarachnoid space.
- Headache
  - 75% of cases
  - sudden onset
  - retro-orbital
- Nausea and vomiting
- Visual field defects (bitemporal hemianopia) or decreased visual acuity
- Ocular palsies, most commonly oculomotor nerve
- Meningeal irritation, fever, altered mental state
- Hemiplegia and seizures (rare)
- Symptoms of preceding pituitary tumour
- Acute hypopituitarism
  - Hypotension
  - Hypoglycaemia
  - Coma

Pituitary apoplexy is often difficult to differentiate from other intracranial haemorrhage, e.g. subarachnoid, bacterial meningitis or cavernous sinus thrombosis.

Investigations

Bloods
- U&Es
- Coagulation screen
- Endocrine tests for evidence of anterior pituitary dysfunction
  - Raised prolactin (majority of cases)
  - Check for other pituitary deficiencies (cortisol, TFTs, growth hormone, IGF-1, FSH, LH)

Imaging
- CT brain including pituitary
  - Will reveal tumour mass and intratumoural haemorrhage within 24–48 hours
- MRI brain
  - More useful in subacute stage (>4 days)

Management
- Stabilize airway, breathing, and circulation.
- If apoplexy suspected, start hydrocortisone IV 100 mg qds (as soon as anterior pituitary blood tests taken).
- Give IV fluids to restore the blood pressure if the patient is in shock.
- Give IV 10% dextrose if the patient is hypoglycaemic.
- Endocrine specialist team should be involved early.
- Monitor for diabetes insipidus
  - high urine output
  - high plasma Na^+ and osmolality
  - low urine osmolality.
- If significant visual deficit or deteriorating GCS, neurosurgical decompression of haemorrhage and/or tumour may be required.
- If no significant visual loss or other neurological defect, patient can be managed conservatively
  - glucocorticoid replacement
  - serial imaging.
- Once acute apoplexy resolves, the patient needs endocrine review to assess for pituitary hormone deficiencies and ensure adequate replacement.

Further reading
Ayuk, J., McGregor, E.J., Mitchell, R.D. and Gittoes, N.J. (2004). Acute management of pituitary apoplexy—surgery or conservative management? *Clin. Endocrinol. (Oxf)* **61**(6): 747–752.

Freeman, W.D., Maramattom, B., Czervionke, L. and Manno, E.M. (2005). Pituitary apoplexy. *Neurocritical Care,* **3**(2): 174–176.

Nielsen, E.H., Lindholm, J., Bjerre, P., Sandahl Christiansen, J., Hagen, C., Juul, S., Jorgensen, J., Kruse, A. and Laurberg, P. (2006). Frequent occurrence of pituitary apoplexy in patients with non-functioning pituitary adenoma. *Clin. Endocrinol. (Oxf)* **64**(3): 319–322.

Neurological emergencies

① Malignant extradural spinal cord compression

Spinal cord compression (SCC) occurs in 5–10% of all patients with a known diagnosis of malignancy but may be the first presentation of malignancy in up to 20%.

This common but devastating complication of metastatic cancer can result in paraplegia and sphincter dysfunction. Of patients who are ambulatory at diagnosis, 80–100% can preserve this level of function. Once lost, ambulation is regained in less than 25% of patients. The strongest predictor of post-treatment neurological function and survival is pre-treatment neurological function; therefore the most important intervention for improving the outcome from SCC is early detection of symptoms and the education of patients to report symptoms. One study has shown a median delay in diagnosis of 2 months from the onset of back pain and 10 days from developing symptoms of cord compression, during which one grade of bladder or neurological function was lost.

The spinal cord extends down to L1/2 in adults; below this is the cauda equina. Compression of the cord, cauda equina or nerve roots can all cause neurological symptoms and should be approached in a similar manner.

Causes
- Extrinsic compression of the thecal sac.
  - Metastases to the vertebral body with posterior expansion (see Figs 5.1–5.4).
  - Vertebral pathological fracture with posterior displacement of bony fragments.
  - Paraspinal mass gains access to the epidural space via the neural foramina (10%) (see Figs 5.5–5.7).
  - Epidural metastases (see Figs 5.8 and 5.9).
- Metastatic tumour from any site can produce SCC.
  - Breast   20%
  - Lung   20%
  - Prostate   20%
  - Unknown primary 10%
  - Myeloma   5%
  - Renal   5%
  - Colorectal   5%
  - Lymphoma   5%
  - Other   10%
- There are two phases of damage:
  - Reversible
    — obstruction of venous plexus and associated vasogenic oedema of the cord resulting in demyelination.
  - Irreversible
    — ischaemic damage and cord infarction.
- Site of compression
  - Thoracic   60%
  - Lumbar   30%
  - Cervical   10%
  - Multiple sites of compression in one-third of cases.

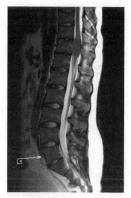

Fig. 5.1 Sagittal T2-weighted MRI scan showing disruption of the posterior cortex of the T11 vertebral body, with a soft tissue mass compressing the spinal cord at this level. Histology from a surgical resection and stabilization revealed a Ewing's sarcoma.

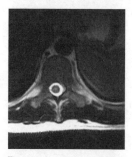

Fig. 5.2 Axial T2-weighted MRI at the T10 level, showing CSF surrounding the cord.

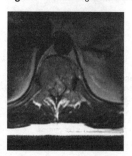

Fig. 5.3 Axial T2-weighted MRI at the level of cord compression at T11, showing the soft tissue mass compressing the cord. No CSF can be seen in the spinal canal.

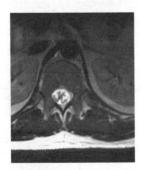

Fig. 5.4 Axial T2-weighted MRI at the T12 level, showing CSF surrounding the conus.

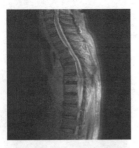

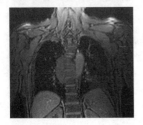

Fig. 5.5 Sagittal and coronal T2-weighted MRI shows a large paraspinal tumour mass extending from T6 to T9. This displaces the aorta and oesophagus, and invades the vertebral bodies extending into the spinal canal, where it compresses the cord at the T7 level.
• There is some high signal within the cord indicating oedema.
• Patient was known to have relapsed high grade non-Hodgkin's lymphoma.

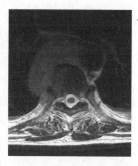

Fig. 5.6 Axial T2-weighted MRI shows a large paraspinal tumour, with no invasion into the spinal canal. CSF is evident surrounding the spinal cord.

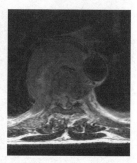

Fig. 5.7 Axial T2-weighted MRI shows a large spinal and paraspinal tumour, with direct tumour invasion into the spinal canal causing compression of the spinal cord. No CSF is present around the spinal cord.

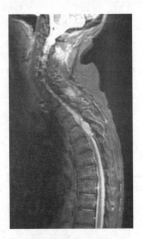

Fig. 5.8 Sagittal STIR MRI shows an extra-axial soft tissue metastasis, lying posteriorly at the level of T4 compressing the spinal cord, in a patient with previous melanoma.

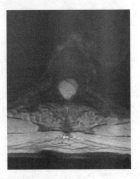

Fig. 5.9 Axial T2-weighted MRI shows an extra-axial soft tissue metastasis compressing and displacing the spinal cord anteriorly.

Clinical features

Symptoms

- Pain
  - Usually the first symptom
  - Present in 83–95% at diagnosis of SCC
  - Precedes neurological symptoms by median of 7 weeks
  - Type of pain
    - localized
      - midline
      - progressive
      - exacerbated by:
        - lying flat
        - Valsalva manoeuvre
        - eased by standing
      - constant
      - worse at night

        } opposite pattern of pain from degenerative disc disease
    - radicular
      - due to nerve root compression
      - cervical irritation radiates down upper limb
      - lumbar irritation radiates down lower limb
      - thoracic irritation often produces bilateral band-like tightness
- Neurological
  - Motor
    - present in 60–85% at diagnosis of SCC
    - usually precedes sensory changes
    - progression through:
      - weakness
      - ataxia/gait abnormality
      - paralysis
  - Sensory
    - ascending numbness and paraesthesia
    - cauda equina lesions produce dermatomal symptoms
  - Autonomic
    - late finding
    - present in about 50% at diagnosis of SCC
    - bladder dysfunction
      - urinary retention
      - incontinence
    - bowel dysfunction
      - incontinence
      - constipation
      - opioids may exacerbate constipation
    - impotence

Signs

- Percussion tenderness over spine
- Upper motor neurone (compression above conus medullaris)
  - flexors of lower extremities
  - extensors of upper extremities
  - hyperreflexia
  - extensor plantar response
- Lower motor neurone (cauda equina or nerve root compression)
  - flaccid weakness
  - hyporeflexia
  - loss of anal sphincter tone

- Sensory level
  - compression above conus medullaris
    - usually 1–5 levels below the lesion
    - sparing of sacral dermatomes to pin prick
  - compression of cauda equina
    - saddle anaesthesia
  - compression of nerve roots
    - radicular sensory loss

Differential diagnosis

- Musculoskeletal disease
  - intervertebral disc disease
  - spinal stenosis
- Spinal epidural abscess
  - *Staphylococcus aureus*
  - *Mycobacterium tuberculosis*
  - may only be distinguishable from malignant SCC on biopsy
- Vertebral metastases +/− nerve root compression
  - vertebral metastases may compress nerve roots resulting in neurological features. Treatment should be expedited to relieve symptoms, however, without the risks of paraparesis and bowel and bladder dysfunction inherent to SCC
  - radiotherapy and bisphosphonates may reduce the future development of SCC
- Radiation myelopathy
  - typically 9–15 months after radiotherapy to spine
- Intradural malignant pathology
  - intramedullary metastases
  - meningioma/neurofibroma
  - astrocytoma/ependymoma
- Epidural non-malignant pathology
  - cavernous haemangioma
  - sarcoidosis
  - spontaneous non-traumatic haematomas

Investigations

Bloods

- Ca^{2+}
  - hypercalcaemia
- Tumour markers
  - to aid diagnosis if unknown primary
- Coagulation screen
  - if biopsy is required
- FBC, U&Es, LFTs

Imaging

- MRI
  - gold standard
  - whole spine needs imaging to exclude multiple levels of compression
  - location of compression and extent of extraspinal disease
  - vital for radiotherapy planning
  - on axial T2-weighted images the absence of CSF surrounding the cord indicates SCC; if, however, there is CSF surrounding the cord this indicates, at worst, impending cord compression (see Figs 5.2–5.4, 5.6, 5.7, and 5.9–5.11)

- CT +/– myelogram
  - reconstructed spiral CT may be an alternative if the patient is unable to have an MRI

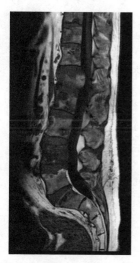

Fig. 5.10 Sagittal T1-weighted MRI showing multiple metastases in the lumbar spine. A large metastatic deposit in L1 vertebral body is protruding into the spinal canal, but is not cuasing cauda equina compression (see Fig. 5.11).

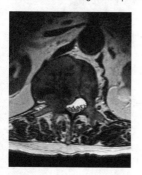

Fig. 5.11 Axial T2-weighted MRI showing a metastatic deposit in the right lateral aspect of the body of L1 and the right pedicle. This is causing some compression of the thecal sac, but no overt cauda equina compression at present. CSF is seen surrounding the nerve roots.

Management

- Aims of treatment
  - preserve/improve neurological function
  - pain control
  - avoidance of complications
- Analgesia
  - corticosteroids will usually improve pain within several hours
  - according to WHO pain ladder (see Pain 📖 p2)
- Corticosteroids
  - reduce vasogenic oedema
  - stabilize/improve neurological function
  - reduce pain
  - give dexamethasone 8 mg bd PO/IV
    — 0800 and 1400 to avoid nocturnal stimulation
    — cover with a PPI to reduce gastric irritation
  - high dose corticosteroid (96 mg/day)
    — may not improve functional outcome
    — increases the frequency of adverse events
      - GI bleeding   - hyperglycaemia
      - perforation
  - taper dose after definitive therapy (halve dose every 3 days)
  - patients without neurological impairment can be managed without corticosteroids although they should receive radiotherapy
- Bed rest
  - there is no requirement for strict bed rest
- Antithrombotic prophylaxis
  - high risk cohort of patients
  - TED stockings +/– LMWH
- Bowel care
  - patients are at high risk of constipation
    — autonomic dysfunction from neurological damage
    — opioid analgesia
    — immobility
  - use a regime combining oral laxatives and rectal suppositories (see Constipation 📖 p54)
- Rehabilitation
  - patients will need early referral to physiotherapist and occupational therapist
- Radiotherapy
  - the modality of choice in most patients with cord compression
  - aim to start as soon after diagnosis of SCC as possible, ideally within hours of diagnosis
  - planning
    — patient prone if possible
    — ideally use conventional or virtual simulation
    — clinical planning
      - locate painful area first
      - verify position using anatomical landmarks
      - simulate at first opportunity to verify field location

- treatment field
  - encompass one to two vertebral bodies above and below the site of compression
  - laterally cover the transverse processes (usually 8 cm wide)
  - field may need modification to encompass paraspinal soft tissue masses seen on diagnostic imaging
- dose range
  - 8 Gy in 1# to 40 Gy in 20#
  - no evidence for different outcomes with different regimes
  - most common regime in UK is 20 Gy in 5#
  - 8 Gy in 1# is usually reserved for pain control in patients with no real prospect of neurological recovery (total paraparesis for >24 hours)
- Surgery
  - surgery with postoperative radiotherapy is superior to radiotherapy alone for a subset of patients presenting with SCC
    - in one study, Patchell et al. (2005) reported that in patients undergoing surgery and radiotherapy:
      - more patients were ambulatory after treatment (p = 0.001)
      - more patients remained ambulatory for longer (p = 0.003)
      - more patients regained ambulatory status (p = 0.01)
      - pain control was improved (p < 0.05)
      - there was a trend towards longer survival (p = 0.08)
  - indications for surgery
    - good performance status
    - life expectancy >3 months
    - first presentation of malignancy
    - limited metastatic burden
    - bone fragment causing compression
    - spinal instability
    - recurrence in a previously irradiated site
    - neurological deterioration during radiotherapy
  - relative contraindications
    - radio/chemosensitive tumours
      - lymphoma   - germ cell tumours
      - myeloma
    - paraplegia >48 hours
  - it is important to select appropriate patients for surgery
    - surgery is associated with significant morbidity/mortality
      - 0–13% 30-day postoperative mortality
      - 0–54% postoperative complication rate
    - morbidity is increased in those patients proceeding to salvage surgery owing to neurological deterioration during radiotherapy
- Chemotherapy
  - rarely indicated apart from very chemosensitive tumours
    - lymphoma   - germ cell tumours
    - myeloma

Recurrent SCC

- 10% of patients will develop local recurrence of SCC
- 25–50% of patients surviving >1 year will experience local relapse

Management

- Surgery
  - treatment of choice   — may be inappropriate
- Re-irradiation
  - radiation myelopathy is an infrequent occurrence in studies, despite the cumulative dose exceeding accepted radiation tolerance of the spinal cord (45 Gy in 2 Gy per #)
  - this may be due to:
    - sublethal radiation damage repair
    - the short survival of patients with recurrent SCC (median 5 months) compared to the latency of radiation myelopathy
  - recurrence may be indicative of radioresistant tumour
- Supportive care and symptom relief

Prognosis

- Median survival is 3–6 months
- Prognostic indicators and median survival
  - Pre-treatment neurological state
    - ambulatory   8–10 months
    - non-ambulatory   2–4 months
  - Post-treatment neurological state
    - non-ambulatory   1 month
  - Primary tumour
    - good   6–9 months
      - myeloma   – breast
      - lymphoma   – prostate
    - poor   2–3 months
      - lung
  - Performance status
  - Disease burden
- Although the majority of patients will die within 3 months of their malignancy, there is a reasonable minority who will survive for a prolonged period of time (lymphoma 25% 3-year survival). Therefore it is vital to improve their functional outcome as much as possible to reduce the burden on their families, the social services, and health care systems

Reference

Patchell, R.A., Tibbs, P.A., Regine, W.F., Payne, R., Saris, S., Kryscio, R.J., Mohiuddin, M. and Young, B. (2005). Direct decompressive surgical resection in the treatment of spinal cord compression caused by metastatic cancer: a randomized trial. *Lancet* **366**: 643–648.

Further reading

Hardy, J.R. and Huddart, R. (2002). Spinal cord compression—what are the treatment standards? *Clin. Oncol.* **14**: 132–134.

Levack, P., Graham, J., Collie, D., Grant, R., Kidd, J., Kunkler, I., Gibson, A., Hurman, D., McMillan, N., Rampling, R., Slider, L., Statham, P. and Summers, D. (2002). Don't wait for a sensory level—listen to the symptoms: a prospective audit of the delays in diagnosis of malignant cord compression. *Clin. Oncol.* **14**: 472–480.

Loblaw, D.A. and Laperriere, N.J. (1998). Emergency treatment of malignant extradural spinal cord compression: an evidence based guideline. *J. Clin. Oncol.* **16**: 1613–1624.

Loblaw, D.A., Laperriere, N.J. and Mackillop, W.J. (2003). A population-based study of malignant spinal cord compression in Ontario. *Clin. Oncol.* **15**: 211–217.

Loblaw, D.A., Perry, J., Chambers, A. and Laperriere, N.J. (2005). Systematic review of the diagnosis and management of malignant extradural spinal cord compression: the cancer care Ontario practice guidelines initiative's neuro-oncology disease site group. *J. Clin. Oncol.* **23**(9): 2028–2037.

Schiff, D., Shaw, E.G. and Cascino, T.L. (1995). Outcome after spinal re-irradiation for malignant epidural spinal cord compression. *Ann. Neurol.* **37**(5): 583.

① **Raised intracranial pressure**

Raised intracranial pressure (↑ICP) in the cancer patient can be caused by the tumour or by the effects of treatment.

Causes
- Intra-axial tumours
  - brain metastasis (90%)
    — occur in 20–40% of adult cancer patients
    — common primary sites
      – lung   – melanoma
      – breast
    — may be intra-axial or leptomeningeal metastases
  - primary brain tumours (10%)
    — posterior fossa lesions are particularly likely to cause ↑ICP
- Leptomeningeal metastases
- Intracranial haemorrhage
  - haemorrhage into tumour (usually metastatic tumour)
    — melanoma   — germ cell tumours
    — renal cell cancer   — lung cancer
  - coagulopathy
    — especially haematological malignancies
  - thrombocytopenia
  - DIC
- Infection
  - abscess/meningitis
    — risk increased by treatment-related immunosuppression
- Cerebral infarction
  - accelerated atherosclerosis in irradiated vessels is a late effect of head and neck radiotherapy
- Venous sinus thrombosis

Clinical features
- Onset
  - sudden   acute event (e.g. haemorrhage)
  - insidious   tumours

Symptoms
- Headache
  - classically worse on waking and after activities which cause raised intrathoracic pressure
    — sneezing   — straining
    — coughing   — changing posture
  - can be associated with:
    — nausea and vomiting   — transient visual symptoms
  - commonly dull and continuous
- Nausea and vomiting   • Impaired consciousness
- Focal weakness   • Seizures
- Confusion

Signs
- Papilloedema
  - may only be seen in 50% of cases
- Focal neurology
  - diplopia/visual field defect
  - hemiplegia/hemiparesis
  - dysphasia
  - possible false localizing signs indicating brainstem shift
    — hemiparesis
    — VI nerve palsy
    — III nerve palsy
- Seizures
- Late signs suggestive of brain herniation
  - pupillary abnormalities
  - eye movement abnormalities
  - Cushing's reflex
    — bradycardia   — hypertension
  - respiratory abnormalities
    — slow deep breaths → Cheyne–Stokes → apnoea

Investigations

Bloods
- FBC
  - infection   • thrombocytopenia
  - leukopenia
- Coagulation screen
  - coagulopathy
- Blood culture

Imaging
- CT brain with contrast
  - acute haemorrhage   • oedema
  - mass effect   • hydrocephalus
- MRI brain
  - provides better anatomical detail and diagnostic information
    than CT

Management

Medical

Medical management is temporary until definitive management of the underlying cause can begin, where possible.

- Dexamethasone
  - reduces vasogenic oedema
    - especially seen in association with abscesses or neoplastic lesions
  - acts in hours, and effects last for several days
  - 16 mg/day in severe symptoms
    - 4–6 mg/day is usually sufficient in mild symptoms
    - can be increased up to 100 mg/day in rapidly progressive symptoms
  - orally well absorbed
    - consider SC/IV route if patient intolerant or develops refractory symptoms
  - consider co-administration of gastric protection (e.g. PPI)
- Mannitol
  - osmotic diuretic, produces osmotic gradient between the brain and blood, drawing water down the gradient
  - acts within a few minutes, and effects last for several hours
  - 1 g/kg 20% mannitol IV over 30 minutes
- Hyperventilation
  - most rapid method of reducing raised ICP
    - a decrease in pCO_2 causes cerebral vasoconstriction
      - aim for pCO_2 30–34 mmHg
  - effects only last for a few hours, owing to renal compensation
  - requires patient to be intubated
- Other
  - BP
    - in patients with intracerebral haemorrhage, treat blood pressure if mean BP >130 mmHg
    - use short-acting antihypertensive agents
      - labetolol   – esmolol
  - coagulation abnormalities
    - in patients with intracerebral haemorrhage correct platelets (if <50×10^9/l) and coagulation abnormalities
      - FFP (15 ml/kg)   – vitamin K (5–10 mg IV)
      - prothrombin complex concentrate (30–50 units/kg)

Surgical

- Decompression
  - debulking of mass lesions
  - evacuation of haematoma/abscess
  - ventriculoperitoneal shunt to relieve hydrocephalus

Intra-axial metastases

These account for the vast majority of all intracranial tumours. They are seen in 10–40% of all cancer patients (10% of children)

Their frequency is increasing due to:
- Better diagnostic tests (CT/MRI)
- Better control of extracranial disease with increasing use of systemic therapy (e.g. Herceptin)

Primary origin of metastases:
- Lung   50–60%
- Breast   10–20%
- Melanoma   5–10%
- Unknown primary   10%
- GI   4–6%
- GU   3–5%

Metastases result from haematogenous spread and therefore are most commonly seen at the junction of white and grey matter, and in watershed areas of arterial circulation.
- Cerebrum   80%
- Cerebellum   15%
- Brainstem   5%

Clinical features

The clinical features are caused by disruption of adjacent neural tissue
- Direct displacement
- Oedema
- Vascular disruption

The clinical features can be variable, but the occurrence of any neurological symptom in a patient with a known malignancy should raise the possibility of brain metastasis
- Headaches
  - seen in up to 50% of patients with brain metastases
  - more common if:
    — multiple lesions   — posterior fossa lesions
  - may localize to the side of the lesion or may be bilateral
- Neurological dysfunction
  - focal neurological dysfunction
    — presenting symptom in 20–40% of patients
    — may be slowly progressive or acute
    — type of dysfunction depends on the location of the lesion(s)
      - can be focal weakness or, commonly, a hemiparesis
    — 10% present with a stroke owing to:
      - embolization of tumour cells
      - arterial compression by the tumour
      - an intralesional bleed
        - melanoma   - renal cell carcinoma
        - germ cell tumour   - lung cancer
  - cognitive dysfunction
    — presenting symptoms in up to 35% of patients
    — commonly memory and personality changes
  - seizures
    — presenting symptom in 10–20% of patients

Investigations
Imaging
- Contrast-enhanced MRI is the gold standard imaging modality
  - it is more sensitive than un-enhanced MRI or CT scanning in detecting lesions and delineating metastases from other intracranial lesions
- Contrast-enhanced CT is an alternative in patients intolerant of an MRI (see Figs 5.12 and 5.13)
- Staging CT to define the extent of extracranial disease, to guide:
  - diagnosis (if *de novo* presentation)
  - treatment
  - prognosis

Stereotactic biopsy
- Consider in:
  - single lesions
  - *de novo* presentations with no systemic disease to biopsy

Management
Initial medical management
- Raised ICP
  - dexamethasone
    — slowly taper down dose after definitive treatment (e.g. radio-therapy) to lowest dose needed to control symptoms
    — Consider:
    – mannitol   – surgical referral
- Seizures
  - consider anticonvulsant medication in the presence of seizures
    — phenytoin (150 mg–300 mg od, titrated to phenytoin level)
    — carbamazepine (100–200 mg bd titrated up to control seizures)
  - prophylaxis is not recommended for patients with no history of seizures or in the postoperative phase in patients without a preoperative or perioperative history of seizures
  - status epilepticus
    — see Seizures 🕮 p78
- Analgesia
  - logically work through the WHO analgesic ladder (see Pain 🕮 p2)
  - steroids will also reduce headaches through decreasing peritumoural vasogenic oedema, thus reducing ICP

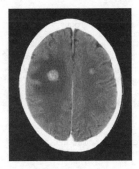

Fig. 5.12 CT scan shows cerebral metastases from a lung primary.
- An enhancing lesion in the right frontal lobe with significant oedema, and some mass effect but no midline shift.
- A further small enhancing lesion is seen in the left frontal lobe.

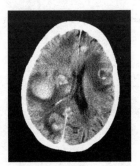

Fig. 5.13 Unenhanced CT brain shows multiple metastases in both hemispheres in a patient with melanoma.
- There is adjacent oedema and moderate midline shift to the left.

Further management

Stratification of patients into two broad prognostic groups is important to guide further patient management

- Poor prognosis patients
  - Any of the following:
    — PS ≥2
    — Multiple lesions
    — Uncontrolled systemic disease
    — Age >60 years
- Good prognosis patients
  - Isolated metastasis with all of the following:
    — PS ≤1
    — Age ≤60 years
    — Controlled systemic disease

Patients in the poor prognostic group can be stratified into treatment groups according to the following prognostic index. (see Table 5.1)

- Score one point for each factor
  - PS 0–1
  - Breast primary
  - Age <60 years
  - Dose of dexamethasone <8 mg

Patients in the good prognostic group should be considered for more invasive treatment

- Neurosurgery
  - Surgically accessible location
  - Postoperative whole brain radiotherapy (WBRT) 30–40 Gy in 10–20#
  - Median survival 9–12 months
- Radiosurgery
  - ≤4.5 cm diameter lesion and surgically inaccessible
  - Stereotactic multiple arc radiotherapy
  - Gamma knife (multisource cobalt unit)
  - Doses range from 15 to 25 Gy in a single fraction
  - No survival benefit from addition of WBRT, but reduced intracranial relapse
  - Side effects
    — dizziness
    — nausea
    — headaches
    — seizures in 1st week after treatment
      - especially in lesions located in motor cortex
  - Median survival 7.5–15 months
  - No randomized controlled trials have compared neurosurgery with radiosurgery
  - Most patients will die of systemic relapse rather than intracerebral recurrence
- Chemotherapy
  - can be considered in patients with chemosensitive disease.
    — lymphoma
    — germ cell tumour
    — SCLC
    — breast cancer
  - can control systemic disease and also have a limited impact on intracranial disease, therefore most meaningful in patients with small asymptomatic lesions and systemic disease, or patients relapsing after surgery/radiosurgery/WBRT.

Table 5.1 Management of poor prognosis patients with cerebral metastases

Score	Management	Median survival
0	Best supportive care	1–2 months
1–2	Whole brain radiotherapy 12 Gy in 2#	3 months
3–4	Whole brain radiotherapy 20–30 Gy in 5–10#	6 months

Further reading

Jyothirmayi, R., Saran, F.H., Jalali, R., Perks, J., Warrington, A.P., Traish, D., Ashley, S., Hines, F. and Brada, M. (2001). Stereotactic radiotherapy for solitary brain metastases. *Clin. Oncol.* **13**: 228–234.

Patchell, R.A., Tibbs, P.A., Walsh, J.W., Dempsey, R.J., Maruyama, Y., Kryscio, R.J., Markesbery, W.R., Macdonald, J.S. and Young, B. (1990). A randomised trial of surgery in the treatment of single metastases to the brain. *N. Engl. J. Med.* **322**(8): 494–500.

Patchell R.A., Tibbs P.A., Regine W.F., Dempsey, R.J., Mohiuddin, M., Kryscio, R.J., Markesbery, W.R., Foon, K.A. and Young, B. (1998). Postoperative radiotherapy in the treatment of single metastases to the brain: a randomised trial. *JAMA* **280**(17): 1485–1489.

Priestman, T.J., Dunn, J., Brada, M., Rampling, R. and Baker, P.G. (1996). Final results of the Royal College of Radiologists' trial comparing two different radiotherapy schedules in the treatment of cerebral metastases. *Clin. Oncol.* **8**: 308–315.

Vecht, C.J., Haaxma-Reiche, H., Noordijk, E.M., Padberg, G.W., Voormolen, J.H.C., Hoekstra, F.H., Tans, J.T.J., Lambooij, N., Metsaars, J.A.L., Wattendorff, A.R., Brand, R. and Hermans, J. (1993). Treatment of single brain metastases: radiotherapy alone or combined with neurosurgery? *Ann. Neurol.* **33**: 583–590.

Vecht, C.J., Hovestadt, A., Verbiest, H.B.C., Van Vliet, J.J. and Van Putten, W.L. (1994). Dose-effect relationship of dexamethasone on Karnofsky performance in metastatic brain tumours: a randomised study of 4, 8, and 16 mg per day. *Neurology* **44**(4): 675–680.

⑦ **Leptomeningeal metastases**

Leptomeningeal metastases (carcinomatous meningitis) are the spread of cancer cells into the CSF of the subarachnoid space. It is usually seen in patients with advanced systemic disease or who have had previous brain metastases treated. It is clinically apparent in 5% of all cancer patients; however, it is present in up to 20% of patients at autopsy.

Leptomeningeal metastases occur most commonly in:
- Breast cancer
  - especially lobular carcinoma
- Melanoma
- Lung cancer
- Acute lymphoblastic leukaemia
- Non-Hodgkin's lymphoma

Leptomeningeal metastases are often multifocal, and spread over the surface of the brain and spinal cord. However, some sites are particularly at risk owing to slow flow of CSF and in 'gravitational' sites.
- Base of skull
- Base of spine

Leptomeningeal metastases have a poor prognosis.
- The median survival:
  - untreated   1 month
  - treated   2–7 months

Clinical features

There are four key pathophysiological processes, producing signs and symptoms depending on the location and extent of disease.
- Direct invasion
  - brain parenchyma
    — focal dysfunction
    — diffuse dysfunction (encephalopathy)
  - cranial nerves
    — cranial nerve palsies
  - nerve roots
    — radicular pain
    — motor/sensory dysfunction
- Mass effect
  - producing obstruction of CSF flow
    — hydrocephalus and ↑ICP
- Disruption of blood–brain barrier
  - cerebral oedema
- Interruption of blood flow
  - infarction
    — focal dysfunction
    — seizures

Leptomeningeal disease is frequently multifocal, resulting in a wide array of neurological symptoms and signs.

- Spinal features
  - 75% of patients with leptomeningeal metastases
    — spinal/radicular pain   — asymmetrical reflexes
    — weakness (LMN)
- Cranial nerve features
  - 50% of patients with leptomeningeal metastases
    — diplopia   — hearing loss
    — facial numbness
        – 'numb chin syndrome'
- Cerebral/cerebellar features
  - 50% of patients with leptomeningeal metastases
    — headache   — seizures
    — cognitive changes   — nausea and vomiting
    — gait abnormalities

Investigations

Imaging

- Gadolinium-enhanced MRI of the entire neuroaxis is more sensitive than CT
  - leptomeningeal enhancement
  - multiple nodular deposits

CSF analysis

- Classic features
  - high opening pressure (>200 mmH$_2$O)
  - low glucose (CSF:serum ratio <0.6)
  - high protein (>40 mg/dl)
  - lymphocytosis
- CSF cytology
  - definitive test
  - high specificity with experienced cytologists
  - sensitivity optimized by:
    — repeated sampling if initially negative
        – 50% sensitivity after one sample
        – 90% sensitivity after three samples
    — analysis of ≥10 ml of CSF
    — prompt analysis
- CSF tumour markers
  - Ca 15.3   • α-FP
  - CEA   • β-HCG
  - low sensitivity
  - raised CSF tumour marker in comparison to serum values is highly suggestive of meningeal disease

- Differential diagnosis
  - infection
    - — bacterial
    - — viral
    - — fungal
  - inflammation
    - — rheumatoid arthritis
  - granulomatous infiltration
    - — TB
    - — sarcoidosis
  - subarachnoid haemorrhage

Management

Initial management

- Analgesia
  - according to the WHO analgesic ladder (see Pain 📖 p2)
  - consider early use of 'adjuvant' analgesics for neuropathic pain
  - steroids may have analgesic effects by reducing inflammation
- Reduce raised ICP
  - see Raised intracranial pressure 📖 p206
- Control seizures
  - see Raised intracranial pressure 📖 p206 and Seizures 📖 p78

Stratification of patients into two broad prognostic groups is important to guide further patient management
- Poor prognosis patients
  - PS 2–4
  - multiple fixed major neurological deficits
  - uncontrolled systemic disease with limited therapeutic options
  - bulky CNS disease
  - encephalopathy
- Good prognosis patients
  - PS 0–1
  - minimal fixed neurological deficits
  - systemic disease with reasonable therapeutic options

Management of poor prognosis patients

- Palliative radiotherapy (12 Gy in 2#) to sites causing symptoms

Management of good prognosis patients

- Radiotherapy
  - to sites of symptomatic or bulky disease
  - 20–30 Gy in 5–10#
  - craniospinal radiotherapy is not indicated as it does not eradicate the disease and is highly toxic
- Intrathecal chemotherapy
  - aims to deliver therapy to the craniospinal axis whilst minimizing systemic toxicity
  - most effective in non-bulky disease
  - efficacy limited by poor CSF flow
  - best delivered via a surgically placed subcutaneous reservoir and ventricular catheter (Ommaya reservoir) allowing administration directly into the lateral ventricle. Alternatively via lumbar puncture.

- drugs
  - methotrexate
    - 10–12.5 mg once or twice weekly
    - if responding at 4–6 weeks, change to a maintenance monthly regime for up to 6–9 months
    - if no response consider cytarabine 50 mg once a week
    - intrathecal methotrexate can cause significant systemic toxicity, particularly in the presence of:
      - reduced renal function
      - bone marrow impairment
      - 'third space' fluid collections
        - pleural effusions   • ascites
    - prophylactic folinic acid IV 15 mg qds for 24 hours can reduce systemic toxicity and does not enter the CSF
  - cytarabine and thiotepa are also used in haematological disease
  - monoclonal antibodies (trastuzumab and rituximab) have been used in small trials/case reports
- must be delivered
  - in a dedicated location
  - by an appropriately trained clinician
- side effects
  - aseptic meningitis
    - headache   – meningism
    - fever   – photophobia
    - nausea and vomiting
    - starts 1–2 days after treatment, peaks on the second or third day and usually resolves by day 5
    - treat with a 5-day course of oral dexamethasone
  - myelosuppression
  - infection
    - locally at injection site or in meninges
  - leukoencephalopathy
    - especially if patient has also had cranial radiotherapy
- Systemic chemotherapy
  - few drugs achieve adequate concentrations in the CSF when given intravenously
  - high dose methotrexate, thiotepa and cytarabine do achieve CSF penetration, but at the cost of significant toxicity
    - mucositis   — nephrotoxicity
    - myelosuppression   — neurotoxicity
    - hepatotoxicity
  - case reports suggest efficacy for temozolomide and capecitabine

Further reading

Platini, C., Long, J. and Walter, S. (2006). Meningeal carcinomatosis from breast cancer treated with intrathecal trastuzumab. *Lancet Oncol.* **7**(9): 778–780.

Schultz, H., Pels, H., Schmidt-Wolf, I., Zeelen, U. Germing, U. and Engert, A. (2004). Intraventricular treatment of relapsed central nervous system lymphoma with the anti-CD20 antibody rituximab. *Haematologica.* **89**: 753–754.

Updated national guidance on the safe administration of intrathecal chemotherapy HSC 2003/010. http://www.dh.gov.uk

Bone emergencies

⊕ **Bone pain and pathological fractures**

Bones can be affected by either primary or secondary malignancies.
- Primary bone tumours (1%)
  - These may arise from any cell type found in bones
    — Haematopoietic
      – lymphoma
      – myeloma/plasmacytoma
    — Osteoid
      – osteosarcoma
    — Cartilaginous
      – chondrosarcoma
    — Fibrous
      – fibrosarcoma
    — Others
      – Ewing's sarcoma
      – primitive neuroectodermal tumour
      – malignant giant cell tumour
- Secondary tumours (99%)
  - 90% are multiple
  - Mostly in the:
    — axial skeleton
      – vertebrae   – pelvis
      – ribs   – skull
    — femur
    — humerus
  - Rarely seen distal to elbow/knee
  - Common primary sites
    — breast   — lung
    — prostate   — renal
  - Median survival ranges from 3 to 6 months in NSCLC to 2 years in breast cancer
  - Osteoblastic
    — prostate   — carcinoid
    — medulloblastoma
  - Osteolytic
    — renal cell   — melanoma
    — thyroid
  - Mixed osteoblastic/osteolytic
    — breast   — GI cancers
    — most squamous cancers — lung cancer

Presenting features of bone emergencies
- Pain
- Pathological fracture
- Hypercalcaemia
  - see Hypercalcaemia 🕮 p164
- Bone marrow dysfunction
  - see Anaemia 🕮 p282, Thrombocytopenia 🕮 p288, Infections in the neutropenic patient 🕮 p326
- Nerve entrapment (spinal cord/nerve root compression)
  - see Malignant extradural spinal cord compression 🕮 p194

Investigations

Bloods
- FBC
  - bone marrow dysfunction
- U&E
  - renal impairment
    — hypercalcaemia   — myeloma
- ALP
  - ↑bone turnover
  - can use γ-GT to help distinguish from liver isoforms
- Ca^{2+}
  - hypercalcaemia
- PSA
  - prostate cancer
- ESR, serum electrophoresis, β_2 microglobulin
  - myeloma screen

Imaging
- Plain X-ray
  - fast and inexpensive, but insensitive
  - may need 30–50% of bone mineral to be lost before lesion is visible
  - good at showing structural integrity of bones
    — pathological or impending pathological fracture
- Bone scan
  - essential part of staging
  - most sensitive in osteoblastic lesions
  - will identify symptomatic and asymptomatic lesions earlier than plain films
  - may need correlation with other imaging modalities to exclude other processes (e.g. degenerative)
  - See Fig. 6.1
- MRI
  - more sensitive and specific than bone scanning
  - good at imaging axial skeleton and long bones
  - not helpful with rib lesions
  - gold standard for the diagnosis of spinal cord compression

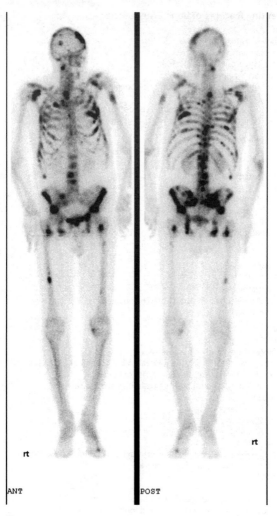

Fig. 6.1 Bone scan reveals multiple bone metastases in a patient with prostate cancer.

Biopsy
- May be useful if first presentation of malignancy
- Consider other imaging to search for:
  - primary site
  - alternative biopsy site to obtain a histological diagnosis

Pain

This is the most common initial symptom of bone involvement with either primary or secondary bone tumours.
- Biological factors
  - release of cytokines producing irritation of intraosseal nerves
- Mechanical factors
  - pressure effect with periostial stretching
  - loss of structural integrity, strength, and rigidity

Clinical features
- Focal dull ache
- Worse at night
- Eased with rest
  } opposite of degenerative pain
- Local tenderness to palpation/percussion
- Incident pain on movement, of greater severity than pain at rest

Gradually worsens over days to weeks.
   A sudden acute increase in pain, especially on activity, may herald an imminent pathological fracture.

Management
- Analgesia
  - Use WHO analgesic ladder (see Pain 📖 p2)
  - Opioids frequently required at an early stage
  - Regular opioids can be titrated to control the resting pain, but doses high enough to control the movement-related pain may cause side effects, e.g. sedation
  - To control movement-related pain
    — oral transmucosal fentanyl citrate 5–10 minutes before movement
- Radiotherapy
  - Produces effective pain control in 80–90% of patients, with complete resolution in 50–60%
  - Pain relief may take up to 2 weeks to occur. Over the first few days post-radiotherapy there may be an initial increase in pain
  - Focal
    — isolated/localized symptomatic lesions
    — a single fraction (8 Gy) is as effective as multiple fractions (20–30 Gy in 5–10#) for pain control and is more convenient for patients
    — See Fig. 6.2
  - Hemi-body
    — multiple symptomatic lesions
    — dose
      - 6 Gy to upper body and 8 Gy to lower body (treatments 4–6 weeks apart)

— patients need premedication with 5-HT₃ antagonists
- ondansetron 8 mg PO/IV or granisetron 1–2 mg PO/IV
- Systemic therapy
  - Bisphosphonates
    — reduce bone destruction
    — delay disease progression
    — can improve bone pain
    — pamidronate 90 mg IV 3–4 weekly
    — zoledronic acid 4 mg IV 3–4 weekly

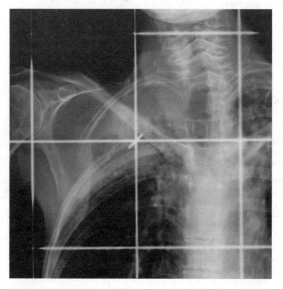

Fig. 6.2 Radiotherapy simulator field for palliative treatment (36 Gy/12#).

- This patient presented with severe chest wall pain and neuropathic pain radiating down the right arm
- CT scan and biopsy revealed a NSCLC Pancoast's tumour
- Simulator film reveals destruction of:
  - T3 vertebra
    — right half of the vertebral body
    — right lateral process
    — right pedicle
  - Destruction of right third rib
  - Partial destruction of right fourth rib.

- Hormonal therapy
  - in breast and prostate cancer is a useful adjunct to bisphosphonates with minimal morbidity
- Chemotherapy
  - should be considered in disease refractory to other systemic therapy
- Radioisotopes
  - Strontium-89
    - the only isotope licensed in the UK for treatment of multiple osteoblastic bone metastases from prostate or breast cancer that would not readily be encompassed within radiotherapy fields (samarium-153 is licensed in the USA)
    - β-emitter with range of 8 mm in soft tissue and 3 mm in bone
    - similar metabolism to calcium, so recent use of bisphosphonates (within 1 month) or calcium supplements (within 14 days) will reduce efficacy
    - preferentially taken up and retained at sites of increased bone turnover
    - contraindications
      - myelosuppression
        - Hb <10 g/dl
        - WCC <3.0 x10^9/l
        - platelets <125 x10^9/l
      - renal impairment (renal excretion of radioisotope)
        - urea >12 mmol/l
        - creatinine >150 μmol/l
      - urinary incontinence
        - risk of spillage of radioactive urine
      - impending cord compression
        - risk of causing neurological damage due to tumour 'flare'
      - life expectancy <3 months
    - dose 150 MBq IV
    - patients may experience 'flare' of pain within 48 hours of administration of radioisotope
    - response rate is 70–80% (complete response 10–20%)
    - follow up patient at 3–6 weeks
      - check FBC
      - assess response
    - avoid sequential chemotherapy for 12 weeks
    - dose can be repeated at 4–6-month intervals if tolerated

Pathological fractures

Pathological fractures occur:
- In 8–10% of patients with malignancy
- Most frequently in patients with osteolytic lesions
- Commonly in the femur (80% of pathological fractures)

- Most commonly in patients with:
  - breast cancer   50%
  - myeloma   12%
  - lung cancer   10%
  - prostate cancer   8%
  - renal cell carcinoma   5%
  - lymphoma   5%

Management
Goals of management
- Pain control
- Restoration/preservation of function
- Skeletal stability
- Tumour control

Factors determining fracture management
- Patient factors
  - co-morbidity
  - pre-morbid performance status
- Fracture location
  - Weight-bearing versus non-weight-bearing bones
- Fracture type
  - dislocated versus non-dislocated

Surgical intervention
- It is the most effective way to establish durable pain relief
- Should be considered in all fractures, except those in rib/scapula/pelvis
- Prognosis required for consideration of surgery
  - ≥1 month for weight-bearing bones
  - ≥3 months for non-weight-bearing bones
- Techniques
  - Reducing displaced fractures
  - Fixation
    — Internal or external
    — Most durable and effective method of achieving pain control
    — Internal fixation
      - most effective form of fixation
      - epiphyseal fractures, e.g. femoral head
        - fracture healing never occurs
        - replacement arthroplasty allowing immediate weight-bearing
      - diaphyseric fractures, e.g. subtrochanteric
        - intramedullary fixation with interlocking nails proximally and distally to control torsional forces
      - metaphyseal fractures, e.g. femoral shaft
        - fracture healing may occur
        - fixation is aimed at providing support and stability while the healing occurs
        - plate and screw fixation
    — External fixation
      - cast or brace immobilization
      - considered in:
        - pre-terminal patients with pain controlled by analgesics

- • extensive disease not suitable for internal fixation
- • patients medically unfit for surgery
- Amputation
  - — Has a limited but important role
  - — Considered in:
    - – intractable pain
    - – extremity lesions not amenable to stabilization/ reconstruction
    - – complications of tumour (fungation) or surgery (infection)
- Spinal fractures
  - May be difficult to distinguish from osteoporotic compression fractures
  - Patient must be assessed for evidence of spinal cord compression, with an urgent MRI whole spine if necessary
  - Pain
    - — tumour expansion/infiltration
      - – best managed by local tumour control
        - • radiotherapy
        - • chemotherapy
        - • hormone therapy
    - — mechanical pain +/– instability
      - – best managed by surgical intervention (if appropriate).
      - – consider cementoplasty
        - • cementoplasty is a generic term and includes vertebroplasty and sacroplasty
        - • injection of acrylic bone cement into malignant bone cavities
        - • useful for painful metastases and less commonly primary bone tumours
        - • it is only indicated for the axial skeleton (spine or pelvis) in patients who have failed conservative pain control
          - • analgesia
          - • radiotherapy
        - • major risk relates to cement injection
          - • epidural leak
          - • venous leak
          - • slightly higher risk in malignant cases owing to increased cortical destruction
  - For role of surgery in spinal cord compression see Malignant extradural spinal cord compression 📖 p194

Radiotherapy
- Radiotherapy is useful for pain control and promotion of bone healing in fracture sites not suitable for surgical intervention
- It is also recommended postoperatively (4–6 weeks)
  - to improve bone healing
  - to impede local tumour progression
    - — to improve pain control
    - — to reduce the risk of failure of the fixation device
- Fractionated courses (e.g. 20 Gy in 5#) are usually used postoperatively and in the presence of pathological fracture

Impending fractures

- Early identification and expedient management of impending fractures potentially reduces the pain and disability which would otherwise result from a fracture.
- Simple measures (e.g. avoiding weightbearing) may prevent fracture occurring whilst definitive management (surgery or radiotherapy) is planned.
- A scoring system has been developed based on site, size, and clinical and radiological features to assist in patient stratification (see Table 6.1).

Table 6.1 Mirels' criteria and scoring system for impending fracture

Variable	Points		
	1	2	3
Site	Upper extremity	Lower extremity	Peritrochanteric
Pain	Mild	Moderate	Severe
X-ray	Blastic	Mixed	Lytic
Size (% of shaft)	0–33	34–67	68–100

Score	Fracture rate (%)
0–6	0
7	5
8	33
9	57
10–12	100

A score ≤7 should be treated with radiotherapy.
A score ≥8 requires surgical intervention
(with postoperative radiotherapy).

Further reading

Bone Pain Trial Working Party. (1999). 8 Gy single fraction radiotherapy for the treatment of metastatic skeletal pain: randomised comparison with a multifraction schedule over 12 months of patient follow-up. *Radiother. Oncol.* **52**: 111–121.

Hillner, B.E., Ingle, J.N., Chlebowski, R.T., Gralow, J., Yee, G.C., Janjan, N.A., Cauley, J.A., Blumenstein, B.A., Albain, K.S., Lipton, A. and Brown, S. (2003). American Society of Clinical Oncology 2003 update on the role of bisphosphonates and bone health issues in women with breast cancer. *J. Clin. Oncol.* **21**: 4042–4057.

Mirels, H. (1989). Metastatic disease in long bones: a proposed scoring system for diagnosing impending pathologic fractures. *Clin. Orthop.* **249**: 256–264.

Percutaneous cementoplasty for palliative treatment of bony malignancies. Interventional procedure consultation document. (2006). National Institute for Health and Clinical Excellence. www.nice.org.uk

Robinson, R.G., Preston, D.F., Schiefelbein, M. and Baxter, K.G. (1995). Strontium-89 therapy of the palliation of pain due to osseous metastasis. *JAMA* **274**: 420–424.

Rosen, L.S., Gordon, D., Tchekmedyian, S., Yanagihara, R., Hirsh, V., Krzakowski, M., Pawlicki, M., De Souza, P., Ming Zheng, Urbanowitz, G., Reitsma, D. and Seaman, J.J. (2003). Zoledronic acid versus placebo in the treatment of skeletal metastases in patients with lung cancer and other solid tumors: a phase III, double-blind, randomized trial—the Zoledronic acid lung cancer and other solid tumors study group. *J. Clin. Oncol.* **21**: 3150–3157.

Gastrointestinal emergencies

☢ Gastrointestinal bleed

GI bleeding may be the presenting feature of malignancy (e.g. colorectal, oesophageal, gastric); however, it is more commonly related to the drugs used in the treatment of malignancy (e.g. NSAIDs, steroids) and other non-malignant causes.

GI bleeding can be a life-threatening event, with a 10–15% mortality in upper GI bleeds.

It is useful to subdivide GI bleeding into:

- Upper GI bleed (oesophagus → terminal ileum)
  - Haematemesis
    - fresh blood   — 'coffee ground' vomit
  - Melaena (>50 ml lost into UGI tract)
  - Rectal bleeding (massive UGI bleed)
- Lower GI bleed (caecum → anus)
  - Rectal bleed
    - fresh, on surface/toilet paper   — dark, mixed with stool

Causes

Upper GI

- Peptic ulcer disease
  - duodenal   • gastric
- Haemorrhagic gastropathy and erosions
- Varices
  - oesophageal   • gastric
- Oesophagitis
- Mallory–Weiss tear
- Malignancy
  - oesophageal   • gastric
- Other
  - hereditary haemorrhagic telangiectasia
  - Dieulafoy vascular malformation
  - portal hypertensive gastropathy
  - aorto-enteric fistula

Lower GI

- Colitis
  - infective
  - ischaemic
  - radiotherapy
  - IBD
    - Crohn's disease   — ulcerative colitis
- Diverticular disease
- Malignancy
  - colon   • rectum
- Benign colorectal polyps
- Haemorrhoids
- Anal fissure
- Angiodysplasia

Clinical features

- Pallor
- Tachycardia
- Postural hypotension
- ↓JVP
- Signs of chronic liver disease
- Abdominal mass
- Rectal examination
  - melaena
  - mass
  - fistula
  - fissure
  - thrombosed haemorrhoid

Investigations

Bloods

- FBC
  - acute bleed will not immediately lower Hb
  - thrombocytopenia
- U&Es
  - ↑urea:creatinine is suggestive of an UGI bleed
- LFTs
  - chronic liver disease increases the risk associated with UGI bleeds
- Coagulation screen
  - may be abnormal in chronic liver disease
  - if patient on warfarin, extent of bleeding will be exacerbated
- Crossmatch
  - 4 units
    — fresh melaena PR
    — postural hypotension
    — SBP <100 mmHg
  - 6 units
    — variceal bleed
  - Group & Save
    — all other patients

Re-bleed

20% of patients will have a re-bleed, usually within the first 48 hours.
Fresh haematemesis and/or melaena associated with one of:
- Shock (HR >100 bpm, SBP <100 mmHg)
- Fall in CVP greater than 5 mmHg
- Fall in Hb >2 g/dl over 24 hours
Re-bleeding should always be confirmed by endoscopy.
Re-bleeding is associated with a greatly increased acute mortality (40%).

Prognostic score

Rockall criteria for UGI bleed

Pre-endoscopy
- Age
  - <60 years   0
  - 60–79 yrs   1
  - ≥80 yrs   2

- Shock
  - None   0
  - HR >100 bpm and SBP >100 mmHg   1
  - SBP <100 mmHg   2
- Co-morbidity
  - None   0
  - Cardiac failure, IHD, or any major co-morbidity   2
  - Renal/liver failure or disseminated malignancy   3

Post-endoscopy
- Endoscopic diagnosis
  - MW tear or no lesion and no sign of recent haemorrhage   0
  - All other diagnoses   1
  - Malignancy of UGI tract   2
- Major stigmata of recent haemorrhage
  - None or haematin dark spot only   0
  - Blood in UGI tract, adherent clot, visible or spurting vessel   2

Predicted mortality

Pre-endoscopy score		Post-endoscopy score	
0	0.2%	0	0.0%
1	2.4%	1	0.0%
2	5.6%	2	0.2%
3	11.0%	3	2.9%
4	24.6%	4	5.3%
5	39.6%	5	10.8%
6	48.9%	6	17.3%
7	50.0%	7	27.0%
		≥8	41.1%

Management

☼ *UGI bleed*
- Resuscitate the patient
  - Lay the patient on their side to protect the airway
  - Give O_2
  - Large bore IV access ×2
  - Aggressive fluid resuscitation
    — If SBP <100 mmHg or HR >100 bpm
      – 500 ml–1 l colloid over 1 hour
      – further crystalloid as necessary to maintain circulating volume
      – If Hb<10 g/l also give 1 unit of blood per hour
      – If Hb low, SBP<80 mmHg despite colloid, and cardiovascular co-morbidity give O rhesus-negative blood whilst awaiting crossmatched blood
- Monitor the patient
  - Urinary catheter
    — aim for UO >0.5 ml/kg/hour
  - Consider central venous access for high risk patients
    – Rockall pre-endoscopy score ≥3
    – re-bleed
    – difficult access

— aim for CVP 5–10 cmH$_2$O
- Monitor for signs of fluid overload
  — ↑JVP   — Pulmonary oedema
- Monitor for signs of re-bleed
  — ↑HR   — ↓UO
  — ↓JVP or CVP   — ↓BP
  — further haematemesis or melaena
- Correct coagulopathy
  - FFP (12–15 ml/kg)
  - Vitamin K IV (5–10 mg)
    — low dose (0.5–1 mg) if anticoagulated for prosthetic heart valve
  - Platelets
    — if platelet count <50 × 10^9/l
- UGI endoscopy (OGD)
  - Patient to be kept NBM
  - Patient must be haemodynamically stable prior to endoscopy
    — if a patient cannot be stabilized consider emergency laparotomy
  - All patients should have an OGD within 24 hours
    — high risk patients within 4 hours
      – continued bleeding   – suspected varices
      – re-bleed
  - Diagnostic
    — site of bleeding   — nature of lesion (biopsy)
  - Estimate risk of re-bleeding
    — haematin   5%
    — adherent clot or ooze   30%
    — visible vessel   70%
    — bleeding vessel   90%
  - Therapeutic
    — inject epinephrine   — heater probe
    — band varices
- H$_2$-receptor antagonists and oral PPIs do not decrease the rate of re-bleeding nor do they reduce the mortality rate.
  - One study has suggested that omeprazole IV does reduce re-bleeding from actively bleeding ulcers after ulcer injected at OGD, and should therefore only be used after confirmation of the diagnosis by OGD.
  - Oral PPIs (+/– H. pylori eradication therapy) should be considered to treat the underlying cause of the bleed, but have no role in the acute management of an UGI bleed.
- Antifibrinolytic drugs and haemostatics
  - Tranexamic acid
    — 1–2 g PO tds   — pro-coagulant
    — weigh beneficial effect against increased risk of thrombosis
  - Etamsylate
    — 500 mg PO qds   — no effect on normal
    — may increase platelet   coagulation
      adhesiveness

- Management of a re-bleed
  - If the patient remains haemodynamically stable consider further endoscopy to confirm re-bleed and undertake endoscopic treatment; however, there must be a low threshold for proceeding immediately to surgical intervention, particularly in high risk patients.
- Surgical management
  - Discuss high risk patients with the surgical team at the earliest opportunity.
    — Pre-endoscopy Rockall score ≥4
    — Post-endoscopy Rockall score ≥5
    — Posterior duodenal ulcer
      - risk of erosion into gastroduodenal artery
  - Indications for surgery
    — Major UGI bleed
      - risk of exsanguination
      - persistent hypotension despite aggressive fluid resuscitation
      - >4 units of blood in 24 hours if >60 years old
      - >8 units of blood in 24 hours if <60 years old
    — Re-bleed in hospital
    — Lesion at OGD at high risk of rebleeding
  - Laparotomy
    — Over-sewing   — Resection

:Ọ: *Variceal haemorrhage*

Mortality is high (25–30%). The prognosis depends on the severity of the underlying liver disease (Child's grade) and not on the magnitude of the haemorrhage.
- Transfer to appropriate setting, e.g. HDU/ICU
- Resuscitate patient
- Monitor the patient
- Correct coagulopathy
- UGI endoscopy (OGD)
  - Diagnostic
    — 30% of patients with chronic liver disease have a non-variceal source of haemorrhage
  - Therapeutic
    — variceal banding
      - this should be repeated at 2-weekly intervals to obliterate the varices
    — injection sclerotherapy
    — endoscopic therapy is poor for gastric varices
- Medical therapy
  - Terlipressin
    — 2 mg IV, then 1–2 mg every 4–6 hours for up to 72 hours
    — causes splanchnic vasoconstriction
    — contraindications
      - IHD
    — side effects
      - abdominal colic

- Reduce the risk of encephalopathy
  - stop any drugs that may exacerbate encephalopathy
    - cerebral depressant drugs
  - empty the bowels
    - lactulose 15–30 ml tds and enemas
  - consider antibiotics to sterilize the gut of ammoniagenic bacteria
    - rifaximin   - metronidazole
- If the patient is currently drinking alcohol
  - reducing regimen of chlordiazepoxide to prevent delirium tremens (see Delirium 🕮 p304)
  - thiamine IV to prevent Wernicke's encephalopathy
  - dextrose IV to prevent hypoglycaemia
- Management of a re-bleed
  - 50% of patients will re-bleed within 10 days
  - If patient remains haemodynamically stable consider a further endoscopic therapeutic procedure
  - Sengstaken-Blakemore tube
    - controls bleeding by balloon tamponade
    - successful in 90% of patients
    - should only be inflated for a maximum of 12 hours
    - risks → 5% mortality
      - aspiration pneumonia   - mucosal ulceration
      - oesophageal rupture
  - Transjugular intrahepatic portocaval shunt (TIPS)
    - radiological insertion
    - short term measure, due to recurrent portal hypertension due to stent stenosis/thrombosis
  - Emergency surgery is seldom needed
    - oesophageal stapling
    - portosystemic shunt (high mortality)

① *Lower GI bleed*

Most lower GI bleeds stop spontaneously, allowing a more measured approach to the diagnosis and management of the causative lesion.
- Resuscitate the patient (as for UGI bleed)
- If the patient continues to bleed
  - UGI endoscopy (OGD)
    - exclude an UGI bleed
  - Proctoscopy
    - anorectal disease
      - haemorrhoids   - rectal cancer
  - Selective arteriogram
    - can selectively view the:
      - coeliac axis
      - superior mesenteric artery
      - inferior mesenteric artery
    - 'blush' apparent if bleeding >1–2 ml/minute
    - can be therapeutic by embolising feeding artery
  - Laparotomy +/– on-table colonoscopy or enteroscopy
    - causative lesion can be resected

- — if no causative lesion can be found, but the bleeding is severe and confirmed to be colonic in origin, subtotal colectomy may be considered
- Patient who has stopped bleeding
  - Colonoscopy
    - — colonoscopy is not advised in a patient who continues to bleed because
      - – the bowel contains blood and views are usually obscured
      - – risk of perforation is greater
- Once causative lesion is identified start definitive treatment
  - Infective colitis
    - — antibiotics
      - – metronidazole   – ciprofloxacin
  - Ischaemic colitis
    - — supportive care   — may require resection
  - Radiotherapy colitis
    - — steroids   — may require resection
  - IBD
    - — corticosteroids IV   — may require resection
    - — steroid enema
  - Diverticular disease
    - — supportive care   — may require resection
  - Colorectal cancer
    - — resection   — stenting
  - Benign colorectal polyps
    - — endoscopic snare polypectomy
    - — resection
  - Haemorrhoids
    - — banding   — resection
  - Anal fissure
    - — GTN ointment
  - Angiodysplasia
    - — endoscopic diathermy or laser photocoagulation
    - — may require resection
    - — embolization

Further reading

Palmer, K.R., on behalf of the British Society of Gastroenterology Endoscopy Committee. (2002). Non-variceal upper gastrointestinal haemorrhage: guidelines *Gut.* **51**(Suppl. IV): iv1–iv6.

Rockall, T.A., Logan, R.F.A., Devlin, H.B. and Northfield, T.C. (1996). Risk assessment following acute gastrointestinal haemorrhage. *Gut.* **38**: 316–321.

Savides, T.J. and Singh, V. (2006). How applicable is the Rockall score in patients undergoing endoscopic haemostasis? *Nat. Clin. Pract. Gastroenterol. Hepatol.* **3**: 378–379.

Vreeburg, E.M., Terwee, C.B., Suel, P. *et al.* (1999). Validation of the Rockall scoring system in upper gastrointestinal bleeding. *Gut* **44**: 331–335.

Clinical features

Symptoms

- Constipation
  - absolute (no faeces or flatus), if complete obstruction
  - there may be diarrhoea from faecal impaction in partial large bowel obstruction
- Nausea
  - which may build in waves and be relieved by vomiting
- Vomiting
  - which may be more frequent the higher the obstruction
- Colicky abdominal pain
  - may be present, especially in organic obstruction

Signs

- Dehydration
- Abdominal distension
- Palpable abdominal mass
  - tender bowel loops
  - tumour mass
- Bowel sounds
  - quiet or absent in a functional obstruction
  - hyperactive in an organic obstruction
- Succussion splash
  - may be present with a high obstruction
- Rectal examination may reveal faecal impaction
- Localized tenderness and peritonitis
  - bowel strangulation
  - GI perforation
- Surgical scars

Investigations

Bloods

- U&Es
  - electrolytes may be depleted
  - vomiting
  - fluid collects in intestinal lumen (third space)
  - abnormal electrolytes can cause a functional ileus
- Ca^{2+}
  - hypercalcaemia is a cause of constipation and ileus
- FBC, coagulation screen, crossmatch
  - preoperative bloods

Imaging

- Plain AXR
  - distended bowel loops
  - faecal impaction
  - fluid levels (erect AXR)
- CT scan with oral contrast or gastrografin follow-through
  - elucidate the level of obstruction
  - establish the extent of abdominal and pelvic disease
  - if the patient is able to swallow sufficient contrast
- Endoscopy (OGD, colonoscopy)
  - may allow visualization of the obstructing lesion

Management
Small bowel obstruction
- Resuscitate the patient
  - IV fluids (0.9% saline with K^+)
  - insert urinary catheter to monitor urine output
  - consider central venous line to monitor CVP
- Analgesia
  - diamorphine
    — 10 mg SC over 24 hours
      – increased dose will be needed in patients previously taking opioids
- Insert NG tube and allow free drainage
- Trial of conservative 'drip and suck' for 24–48 hours
  - more likely to be successful in patients with:
    — partial SBO
    — metastatic intra-abdominal malignancy
    — recurrent adhesive obstruction
    — obstructing radiation enteritis
    — during the early postoperative period

Medical management
- Oral absorption will be poor; give drugs by subcutaneous infusion
- There are two alternative approaches
  - Pro-kinetic regime
    — for functional or partial bowel obstruction
    — metoclopramide SC 30–100 mg/24 hours
      – dose can be titrated up over a few days
      – if nausea not adequately controlled add haloperidol SC 2.5–10 mg/24 hours
    — dexamethasone 8–12 mg SC od for 7 days
      – may reduce bowel oedema and improve transit
      – if effective, reduce dose by 2 mg per week
      – if ineffective stop after 7 days
      – it is most effective in tumours associated with local inflammation such as carcinoma of the ovary
    — docusate sodium 100–200 mg bd PO as a lubricating laxative if tolerated
    — IV/SC fluids
    — if this approach causes bowel colic, reduce the dose of metoclopramide or switch to an anti-kinetic regime
  - Anti-kinetic and anti-secretory regime
    — for:
      – organic or complete obstruction where surgery is not an appropriate option
      – failure of a pro-kinetic regime
    — hyoscine butylbromide SC 20–60 mg/24 hours
      – titrate the dose up over a few days (max. 120 mg/24 hours)
      – if vomiting volume and frequency is not significantly reduced add octreotide SC 300–600 µg/24 hours

    — cyclizine SC 100–150 mg/24 hours
      – if nausea not controlled change to levomepromazine SC
       5–25 mg/24 hours or as a SC stat dose at night
    — these measures may allow removal of the NG tube, which can
      become uncomfortable and cause rhinorrhoea
- If symptoms remain difficult to control then seek specialist palliative care advice

Surgery
- Must be considered
  - if there is no improvement
  - if symptoms or signs of strangulation develop
- The patient should be discussed at a multidisciplinary team meeting
- 50–75% of patients admitted for SBO require surgery
  - Laparotomy
    - division of adhesions   — small bowel resection
    - hernia repair   — palliative bypass
    - de-functioning stoma proximal to obstruction
  - Venting gastrostomy
- Not all SBO in cancer patients is due to cancer.
  - benign adhesions were responsible for the obstruction in 83% of patients with a history of adenocarcinoma of the colon without known recurrence, and 30% of patients with known recurrent malignancy.
- It is vital to select patients who are appropriate for surgery.
  - success of surgery in relieving obstruction in patients with cancer is 64–76% in most surgical series.
  - surgery for malignant obstruction has a high in-hospital mortality (28–45%).
  - non-operative therapy for malignant obstruction is also associated with high mortality (35–56%) and a high failure rate.
  - patients with no known recurrence or a long interval to the development of SBO should be aggressively treated with early surgery if non-operative treatment fails.
  - for patients with known abdominal recurrence in whom non-operative therapy fails, the results of surgical palliation are poor (median survival 3–6 months).
- While surgery must remain the primary treatment for malignant obstruction, there is a group of patients who are unfit for surgery and require alternative management to relieve distressing symptoms.
  - widespread intra-abdominal malignancy
  - multiple level obstruction
  - the patient's condition has deteriorated to the point where recovery from an abdominal operation is unrealistic
    - cachexia
    - severe hypoalbuminaemia
    - renal failure

Large bowel obstruction
- Resuscitate the patient
  - IV fluids (0.9% saline with K$^+$)
  - insert urinary catheter to monitor urine output
  - consider central venous line to monitor CVP
- Analgesia
  - diamorphine SC, e.g. 10 mg over 24 hours
    - increased dose will be needed in patients previously taking opioids
- If there is a competent ileocaecal valve then the plain X-ray will show only dilated large bowel and no dilated small bowel. This is closed loop obstruction and needs urgent surgical management to decompress the bowel
- If there is an incompetent ileocaecal valve then dilated small bowel loops will also show on the X-ray and the patient is likely to be vomiting. It is possible to decompress the bowel with a NG tube to buy a bit more time but the obstruction will not settle without further management
- Surgery
  - Colonic stenting
    - this will relieve the obstruction, allowing the dilated bowel to return to normal. An urgent elective resection of the obstructing lesion can then be performed with a primary anastomosis
  - Laparotomy with Hartmann's procedure
    - it is risky to anastomose obstructed dilated bowel, so an end colostomy is brought out proximal to the obstruction. If possible the lesion is resected and the distal end of the bowel closed off (Hartmann's procedure). At a later stage the colostomy can be reversed if appropriate

Further reading

Butler, J.A., Cameron, B.L., Morrow, M., Kahng, K. and Tom, J. (1991). Small bowel obstruction in patients with a prior history of cancer. *Am. J. Surg.* **162**: 624–628.

Tang, E., Davis, J. and Silberman, H. (1995). Bowel obstruction in cancer patients. *Arch. Surg.* **130**: 832–836.

⑦ **Malignant ascites**

Malignant ascites accounts for about 10% of cases of ascites. It is indicative of disseminated disease and is generally associated with a poor prognosis, with a median survival of 10–12 weeks. It is commonly caused by intra-abdominal tumours (especially ovary).

It is particularly important in women to achieve a tissue diagnosis (ascitic fluid cytology, USS-guided/transcutaneous/laparoscopic biopsy or debulking surgery), as optimally treated Stage III ovarian cancer presenting with ascites can result in a 30–40% 5-year survival.

Ascites is caused by changes in the rates of influx and efflux of fluid into and out of the peritoneal cavity. In malignant ascites these changes can be due to:
- Obstruction of the diaphragmatic lymphatics by tumour
- Obstruction of the main thoracic duct causes chylous ascites
- Increased permeability of microvessels
  - 'Vascular permeability factors', e.g. vascular endothelial growth factor, released by the tumour
- Raised hepatic venous pressure activates the renin–angiotensin–aldosterone pathway, resulting in salt and water retention
- Massive liver metastases

Malignant ascites is particularly resistant to spontaneous bacterial peritonitis owing to the high protein concentration of the ascitic fluid, which exhibits endogenous antimicrobial activity by acting as an opsonin. Peritonitis may develop secondary to paracentesis or intestinal perforation. Ascitic fluid and blood cultures should be sent to confirm the diagnosis and determine antibiotic sensitivities.

Common tumours causing malignant ascites
- Ovarian   30–54%
- Unknown primary   13–22%
- Pancreas
- Gastric
- Endometrial
- Hepatic
- Breast
- Lung
- Lymphoma

Clinical features
Symptoms
- Abdominal discomfort
- Anorexia and early satiety
- Indigestion
- Nausea and vomiting
- Dyspnoea
- Reduced mobility
- Altered body image
- Alteration in bowel motility and pseudo-obstructive symptoms

Signs

- Abdominal distension
- Shifting dullness and fluid thrill
- Bibasal dullness
  - raised splinted hemidiaphragms
- Look for underlying malignancy:
  - hepatomegaly
  - abdominal/pelvic mass
  - surgical scars, e.g. colectomy, TAH + BSO, mastectomy

- Everted umbilicus

- lymphadenopathy

Differential diagnosis for ascites
- See Table 7.1

Investigations

Bloods

- FBC and coagulation screen
- LFTs
- U&Es
- Amylase
- Glucose
- TFTs
- Tumour markers
  - αFP, CEA, Ca-125, Ca 19-9, Ca 15.3
    — these have low diagnostic specificity, but may assist in identifying the primary malignancy

- Liver screen
  - Hepatitis B and C serology
  - Autoantibodies
  - Iron, ferritin, and transferrin
  - Caeruloplasmin
  - α1-antitrypsin level

Urine

- Dipstick for protein
  - nephrotic syndrome

ECG

- CCF is highly unlikely in the presence of a normal ECG

Table 7.1 Differential diagnosis for ascites

Transudate (SAAG >11 g/l)	Exudate (SAAG <11 g/l)
Decompensated cirrhosis with portal hypertension	Disseminated malignancy
Congestive cardiac failure	Tuberculous peritonitis
Nephrotic syndrome	Acute pancreatitis
Constrictive pericarditis	Chronic pancreatitis
Myxoedema	Budd–Chiari syndrome

Imaging
- USS
  - Can detect 100 ml of ascitic fluid
  - May detect
    - pelvic mass
    - possible ovarian primary
    - multiple liver metastases (biopsy for tissue diagnosis)
    - intra–abdominal lymphadenopathy (biopsy for tissue diagnosis)
    - abnormal liver echogenicity
    - cirrhosis
  - Doppler USS can assess flow in the portal and hepatic veins
    - cirrhosis with portal hypertension, Budd–Chiari syndrome

Diagnostic paracentesis
- Send fluid for:
  - Cytology
    - 100% specific, 50–60% sensitive
    - up to 97% sensitive in cases of peritoneal carcinomatosis
  - Serum ascites albumin gradient (SAAG)
    - serum [albumin] – ascitic [albumin]
      - transudate   SAAG >11 g/l
      - exudate   SAAG <11 g/l
    - there is significant overlap so most causes of transudates can cause exudates and vice versa
  - Triglyceride
    - high in chylous ascites, chylomicrons in ascitic fluid
  - MC&S
    - to rule out bacterial peritonitis
  - Auramine or ZN stain and TB culture
    - tuberculous peritonitis
  - Amylase
    - pancreatitis

Further investigations
- CT scan of abdomen and pelvis
  - delineate abnormal tissue in abdomen and pelvis
  - consider biopsy for tissue diagnosis
- Laparoscopy
  - consider biopsy for tissue diagnosis
- Echo
  - CCF
  - constrictive pericarditis
- USS/CT-guided liver biopsy
  - cirrhosis

Management of malignant ascites
See Fig. 7.1.

Paracentesis
Paracentesis is the only treatment to provide immediate relief from symptomatic ascites (see Paracentesis ☐ p250).

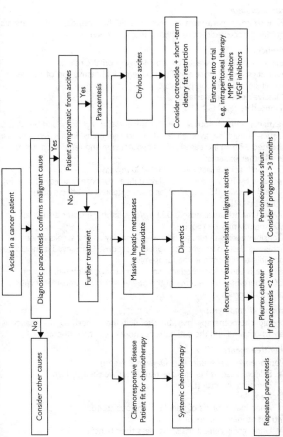

Fig. 7.1 Management of malignant ascites.

Pleurex catheter

This long term peritoneal catheter should be considered for patients requiring paracentesis more often than every 2 weeks.

Diuretics

Diuretics may take 4 weeks to provide symptomatic relief.

Diuretics are of most benefit in patients with activation of the renin–angiotensin–aldosterone pathway:

- Massive hepatic metastases
- Transudate (SAAG >11 g/l)

In patients with chylous ascites, positive ascitic cytology and exudates, diuretics should be avoided as they are generally ineffective and are associated with an increased risk of hypotension and renal impairment.

In all other patients:

- Start with spironolactone PO 100–200 mg/day
- Increase by 100 mg every 5–7 days until a response is achieved (aim for a weight loss of 0.5–1 kg/day) or unacceptable side effects occur (monitor U&Es)
- Typical maintenance dose is 300 mg/day, although doses as high as 600 mg/day may be required
- Consider adding in furosemide 40–80 mg/day after 2 weeks if not achieving desired weight loss. Once a response is achieved it should be possible to discontinue the furosemide
- If there is above-knee oedema secondary to hypoalbuminaemia or CCF there may be oedema of the bowel which can impair absorption of oral diuretics

Systemic chemotherapy

Systemic chemotherapy may be useful if the underlying malignancy is likely to respond and the patient is fit enough for chemotherapy.

Other treatments

- Peritoneovenous shunts (e.g. Denver, LeVeen)
  - Seldom used as benefits are usually outweighed by high complication rate (DIC)
- Octreotide
  - Anecdotal reports of benefit in chylous ascites
- Intraperitoneal treatment
  - Undergoing clinical trials to assess their benefit
  - Chemotherapy
  - Immunotherapy (e.g. TNFα, IFNα, IFNβ)
  - Matrix metalloproteinase inhibitors
  - VEGF inhibitors

Further reading

Adam, R.A. and Adam, Y.G. (2004). Malignant ascites: past, present and future. *J. Am. Coll. Surg.* **198**(6): 999–1011.

Aslam, N. and Marino, C.R. (2001). Malignant ascites: new concepts in pathophysiology, diagnosis and management. *Arch. Intern. Med.* **161**(22): 2733–2737.

Parsons, S.L. (1996). Malignant ascites. *Br. J. Surg.* **83**(1): 6–14.

Smith, E.M. and Jayson, G.C. (2003). The current and future management of malignant ascites. *Clin. Oncol.* **15**(2): 59–72.

⑦ **Paracentesis**

Preparation

- The only indication for paracentesis is the presence of symptoms requiring palliation
- In patients with advanced cancer cachexia, particularly if there is liver failure, paracentesis may precipitate a rapid deterioration in their condition. This risk must be carefully weighed against possible symptomatic benefit. Abdominal discomfort from ascites in this context may be managed with adequate analgesia
- Check FBC, coagulation screen and U&Es, especially in patients with:
  - Liver disease/abnormal LFTs
  - Anticoagulated
  - Possibility of neutropenia/bone marrow failure
- Blood results
  - Consider delaying procedure if patient neutropenic
  - Consider IV hydration if patient dehydrated or has renal impairment
  - Consider vitamin K if INR >1.5
  - Consider platelet transfusion if platelet count <50 ×10^9/l
- Explain procedure and possible complications (major complication rate <1%)
  - Complications
    — Transient fatigue and abdominal discomfort
    — Bleeding
    — Hypotension
    — Infection
    — Visceral injury
    — Leak post-procedure
    — Protein depletion (recurrent paracentesis)
    — Cutaneous seeding
- Seek consent for procedure
- If there is substantial ascites clinically it is usually safe to proceed with drainage without diagnostic imaging. Consider USS evaluation prior to procedure when:
  - Diagnostic uncertainty
  - Suspected loculated ascites
  - High risk procedure
    — e.g. distended bowel
  - Previous complicated or difficult paracentesis
- IV hydration is unnecessary unless clinically indicated
  - Clinically dehydrated
  - Renal impairment
  - Symptomatic hypotension
- No evidence for the use of IV albumin in malignant disease, use 0.9% saline

Procedure

- Position patient supine, and ensure patient is comfortable.
- Strict aseptic technique should be maintained at all times.
- Select site for drainage clinically
  - LIF>RIF
  - Avoid
    - Scars
    - Tumour masses
    - Distended bowel
    - Bladder
    - Liver
    - Inferior epigastric arteries (5 cm lateral to anterior midline)
- Clean site, infiltrate with 5–10 ml of warmed bupivacaine/lignocaine.
- Aspirate with syringe used for infiltrating local anaesthetic, until ascites is obtained. If blood is obtained, remove the needle and apply pressure to the puncture site for 2 minutes and try at a different site.
- Wait for 2–5 minutes for local anaesthetic to work.
- Insert 8-F pigtail catheter, aspirate fluid for laboratory tests if necessary.
- Connect to overnight urinary catheter bag.
- Secure catheter in place with a dressing; it is not necessary to suture.
- Monitor observations every 2 hours; changes in BP are more important than absolute values.
- Allow free drainage as long as patient remains well and observations stable.
- Tailor drainage to clinical situation.
- Clamping drains to control the drainage rate is unnecessary.
- In patients with advanced cachexia or liver failure, removing large volumes of fluid can lead to a rapid deterioration. In these patients controlled drainage, e.g. drain 2 litres over 1 hour, up to a further 3 litres over 3–4 hours, and larger volumes over 12–24 hours, may be appropriate.
- Drainage will often tail off after a few hours and symptomatic benefit is most marked after the first few litres have been removed.
- If there are large abdominal or pelvic tumour masses, extensive paracentesis may remove 'cushioning fluid' and lead to an increase in abdominal pain. In this context consider removing just enough ascites to relieve distension and repeating this at more frequent intervals.
- Ascites can accumulate at several hundred ml/day, so a drain left in indefinitely is likely to continue draining until it becomes blocked.
- Remove the drain within 6 hours.
- Withdraw pigtail catheter and apply a dressing pad.
- If there is significant leakage following removal of the drain, apply a stoma bag over the drain site.
- If there is persistent leakage for >72 hours consider a single suture to the drain site.

⊕ Gastrointestinal perforation

In the cancer patient this most commonly occurs at the site of the tumour; however, perforation can also occur in the caecum proximal to an obstructing colonic tumour. Tumour necrosis during chemotherapy or radiotherapy can also cause perforation.

Causes
- Malignant infiltration of GI wall
- Non-malignant causes
  - Peptic ulceration (NSAIDS, steroids)
  - Surgical dehiscence
  - Colonoscopy
  - Upper GI endoscopic dilatation +/− biopsy
  - Radiation enteritis
  - Diverticular disease
  - Infective colitis
  - IBD toxic megacolon
  - Typhlitis

Clinical features
Symptoms
- Sudden onset
  - Abdominal pain (worse on movement)
  - Nausea
  - Vomiting
  - Fever

Signs
- Peritonism
  - Abdominal tenderness
  - Abdominal guarding
  - Abdominal rebound
  - Abdominal rigidity
- Absent bowel sounds
- Tachycardia
- Tachypnoea
- Hypotension
- Febrile

The symptoms and signs may be reduced or absent if the patient is on corticosteroid treatment.

Investigations
Bloods
- FBC
  - Neutropenia/thrombocytopenia post-chemotherapy
- Amylase
  - Acute pancreatitis
- U&Es, coagulation screen, crossmatch
  - Preoperative work-up

ECG
- Preoperative work-up

Imaging
- Erect CXR
  - Free gas under diaphragm diagnostic of perforation
  - Absent in 50% of perforations
- Lateral decubitus AXR
  - Free gas

- CT abdomen and pelvis
  - Free gas, site of perforation
- Water-soluble contrast study
  - Suspected UGI perforation
  - Indicates whether perforation has sealed
  - Useful if considering conservative management

Management

Despite surgery 40% of cancer patients with GI perforation will die in the perioperative period, mostly due to bacterial peritonitis. Selecting patients for surgery is, therefore, particularly important. Patients with potentially curable cancer should have aggressive management of their acute condition and be admitted to an intensive care unit if necessary. In patients with incurable disease discuss the risks and benefits of surgery in light of their predicted life expectancy, quality of life, performance status, and suitability for surgery.

- Resuscitate the patient
  - Oxygen
  - IV fluids
    - to maintain urine output >0.5 ml/kg/h
- Insert urinary catheter to monitor urinary output
- Analgesia
  - IV/SC morphine or diamorphine
- IV antibiotics to cover bowel flora
  - Cefuroxime 1.5 g tds + metronidazole 500 mg tds
- Consider an NG tube if vomiting is a significant problem
- If surgery is appropriate refer urgently to a GI surgeon for consideration of a laparotomy and definitive management of the perforation
- If surgery is not appropriate (patient's wishes, risks of surgery too great), conservative measures should be continued, with sedation as appropriate. A self-sealed perforation may resolve spontaneously with conservative management (NBM, NG tube, IV fluids, IV antibiotics, analgesia). However, the majority of conservatively managed perforations will be the terminal event in the patient's life.

Typhlitis

This is a necrotizing enterocolitis of the caecum, which is fatal in 30% of cases. It is associated with chemotherapy-induced neutropenia, particularly in children and those being treated for acute leukaemia.

It classically presents with:
- RIF pain
- Diarrhoea (may be bloody)
- Fever

Imaging with AXR, USS or CT may demonstrate dilatation of the caecum with thickening of the caecal wall.

Management involves aggressive management with IV fluids and antibiotics to try to prevent bowel necrosis, perforation, and septicaemia; however, surgery may be needed if these conservative measures fail.

! **Acute pancreatitis**

Pancreatitis is an inflammatory condition of the pancreas.

The inflammation can range from a mild self-limiting oedematous inter-stitial pancreatitis to a fulminant necrotizing haemorrhagic process involving the pancreas and surrounding tissues with multiple organ failure.

Pancreatitis is a common cause of an acute abdomen and accounts for approximately 1% of general surgical admissions.

Overall mortality has remained at 10% despite advances in medical treatment, with mortality up to 30% in severe cases.

Oncology patients can be at particular risk of pancreatitis due to their disease (e.g. pancreatic duct obstruction by pancreatic tumours) and its treatment (e.g. ERCP, chemotherapy).

Causes

- Gallstones
- Alcohol
- Iatrogenic
    - ERCP+/− stenting +/−
      sphincterotomy
    - Post-abdominal surgery
- Drugs
    - Thiazides
    - Sulphonamides
    - Valproate
    - ACE inhibitors
    - Metronidazole
    - Octreotide
    - Oestrogens
    - Steroids

- Trauma
- Infections
- Systemic vasculitis
    - SLE
    - PAN

    - Azathioprine
    - Interferon
    - Cytarabine
    - Methotrexate
    - Bleomycin
    - Cisplatin
    - Cyclophosphamide
    - Ifosfamide
    - Fluorouracil
    - Mitomycin C
    - Vinca alkaloids

- Hypertriglyceridaemia
- Hypercalcaemia

- Hypothermia
- Idiopathic

Clinical features

Symptoms
- Severe pain
- Epigastric
- Radiates to the back

- Relieved by sitting forward
- Vomiting

Signs
- Mild pyrexia
- Epigastric tenderness
- Absent bowel sounds
- Distended abdomen
- Ecchymoses (if haemorrhagic pancreatitis)
    - Flank – Grey Turner's sign
    - Periumbilical – Cullen's sign

- Tachycardia
- Hypotension
- Jaundice

Differential diagnosis
- Perforated duodenal ulcer
- Mesenteric infarction
- Myocardial infarction
- Leaking abdominal aortic aneurysm
- Acute cholecystitis
- Ascending cholangitis

Investigations
The investigations are used to:
- Confirm pancreatitis
- Exclude other causes of epigastric pain
- Measure prognostic factors for pancreatitis

Bloods
- Amylase
  - sensitive, not specific unless >4× upper limit of normal, no prognostic information
- Plasma lipase
  - more sensitive and specific
- FBC
- U&Es
- Glucose
- Ca^{2+}
- LFTs
- LDH
- CRP
- ABG

} Patient's general condition
  Prognostic information

Imaging
- CXR
  - exclude GI perforation
  - pulmonary infiltrates
- Abdominal USS
  - may confirm pancreatitis and detect biliary cause
- Contrast-enhanced CT
  - pancreatic necrosis
  - grading of severity (most accurate 6–10 days after onset)
- MRCP
  - degree of pancreatic damage and detect biliary cause (stones, tumours)

Prognostic indicators
It is critical to manage pancreatitis according to the severity of the disease. Many patients may on initial inspection appear well; however, many pancreatitic patients deteriorate over the next 24 hours. Prognostic indicators have been developed to enable patients to be managed appropriately (e.g. transfer to HDU/ICU).

Modified Glasgow prognostic criteria
- Age   >55 years
- Albumin   <32 g/l
- Arterial pO_2 (room air)   <8 kPa (60 mmHg)
- Ca^{2+} <2.0 mmol/l
- Glucose   >10 mmol/l
- LDH   >600 IU/l
- Urea   >16 mmol/l
- WCC   >15 × 10^9/l

These criteria are assessed over the 48 hours following presentation. The presence of ≥3 of these criteria indicates severe acute pancreatitis.

0–2 <5% mortality
3–4 20% mortality
5–6 40% mortality
7–8 100% mortality

If the CRP >150 mg/l in the first 48 hours this also constitutes severe acute pancreatitis.

Management

The principles of management are:
- Supportive care
- Identifying and treating the cause
- Careful observation for the development of complications

Supportive care

- Admit to an appropriate bed
  - HDU/ ICU for severe cases
  - Patients must be repeatedly assessed in the first 48 hours to monitor the progress of the disease, as the severity of the attack may only become apparent after admission
- Aggressive fluid resuscitation
  - A CVP line may be necessary
    — aim for CVP 5–10 cmH$_2$O
  - Insert a urinary catheter to monitor urinary output
    — aim UO >0.5 ml/kg/h
- Oxygen as required to maintain oxygen saturations
- NBM +/– nasogastric suction
  - If the attack is severe consider early enteral nutrition via a nasojejunal tube to provide adequate nutrition whilst avoiding pancreatic stimulation
- Analgesia
  - Strong opioid analgesia is indicated; pethidine is the drug of choice as it causes less sphincter of Oddi spasm
  - PCA is preferable to repeated IM injections
- Antibiotics
  - Should not be given routinely in mild cases
  - A broad spectrum antibiotic such as cefuroxime should be given in cases where there is confirmed or a high suspicion of infection and before invasive procedures, e.g. ERCP
  - 50% of patients with pancreatic necrosis develop infection in the pancreas. These patients should receive antibiotics, e.g. tazocin and metronidazole
- Metabolic complications
  - Monitor blood glucose regularly and treat with an insulin sliding scale if high
  - Correct abnormalities in serum Ca^{2+} level

Identifying and treating the cause
- ERCP
  - In patients with pancreatitis and a dilated biliary system secondary to gallstones, ERCP with sphincterotomy and removal of the stone, ideally in first 72 hours, has been shown to decrease complications and mortality in patients with severe gallstone pancreatitis

Complications of acute pancreatitis
Systemic complications
- Respiratory
  - ARDS
  - Pleural effusion
- Cardiac failure
  - Myocardial depression
  - Capillary leakage
- Renal failure
  - Hypovolaemia
  - Splanchnic vasoconstriction
- DIC
- Metabolic complications
  - Hypocalcaemia
  - Hyperglycaemia
  - Hypomagnesaemia
  - Metabolic acidosis
- Sepsis

Local complications
- Pancreatic necrosis
- Pancreatic infection
  - Occurs in 50% of patients with necrosis
  - Infection typically caused by Gram-negative and anaerobic bacteria
  - May rapidly lead to overwhelming sepsis
- Pancreatic pseudocysts
  - Collection of pancreatic fluid surrounded by granulation tissue
  - Occur in ~20% of cases, more common in alcoholic pancreatitis
  - They present as:
    — persisting abdominal pain
    — an epigastric mass
    — a persistently raised amylase
  - They are confirmed with an USS or CT scan
  - Those <6 cm in diameter tend to resolve within 6 weeks
  - Those >6 cm are unlikely to resolve and they can:
    — become infected and form an abscess
    — cause rupture of splenic vessels
    — obstruct the duodenum and bile duct
  - Pseudocysts can be drained
    — percutaneously under USS or CT guidance
    — endoscopically by forming a cyst-gastrostomy
    — open cyst-gastrostomy
- Pancreatic abscess
  - These can form in pseudocysts or in areas of pancreatic necrosis that has become infected
  - These can also be drained radiologically or by open surgery
- Colonic infarction
- Fistula formation

Surgical management
The indications for surgery are:
- Necrotic infected pancreas
- Complications of pancreatitis
  - Pseudocyst
  - Abscess

The types of procedures performed are:
- Laparotomy with debridement of necrotic pancreas
- Laparotomy and peritoneal lavage
- Laparostomy—abdomen left open with sterile packs in the ICU

Further reading
UK Working Party on Acute Pancreatitis (2005). UK guidelines for the management of acute pancreatitis. *Gut.* **54** (Suppl. III); iii1–iii9.

ⓘ **Ascending cholangitis**

Ascending cholangitis is a surgical emergency. Cholangitis is an ascending infection in the biliary system secondary to biliary obstruction. Biliary obstruction is not sufficient on its own; the biliary tree must already contain bacteria prior to the onset of the obstruction.

Instrumentation of the biliary system (e.g. ERCP) risks introducing infection and therefore should always be covered by appropriate antibiotics (e.g. ciprofloxacin).

Causes
- Gallstones impacted in the common bile duct
- Malignancy
  - Pancreatic carcinoma
  - Secondary deposits in lymph nodes at porta hepatis
  - Cholangiocarcinoma
- Postoperative stricture
- Parasitic infections, e.g. onchocerciasis
- Congenital biliary anomalies

Clinical features
Symptoms
- Characterized by Charcot's triad (in 70% of patients)
  - Pain
  - Rigors
  - Jaundice

Signs
- Fever (95%)
- RUQ tenderness (90%)
- Jaundice (80%)
- Peritonism (15%)

Differential diagnosis
- Acute cholecystitis
- Acute acalculus cholecystitis
- Biliary colic
- Acute pancreatitis

Investigations
Bloods
- FBC
  - ↑ WCC
- U&Es
  - dehydration
  - prerenal uraemia
- LFTs
  - ↑bilirubin
  - ↑↑ALP
  - ↑↑γ-GT
  - ↑AST and ALT

- Amylase
  - rule out concomitant pancreatitis
- CRP
- Blood cultures
  - often multiple organisms, e.g. *E. coli*, *Klebsiella*, *Enterococci*, *Bacteroides*, *Proteus*, *Pseudomonas*

Imaging
- AXR
  - Aerobilia
    — gas-forming organism   — enterobiliary fistula
    — recent instrumentation
- USS
  - dilated ducts   • gallstones
- ERCP
  - biliary pathology, e.g. at ampulla   • stones in CBD
- MRCP
- PTC

Management
- Fluid resuscitation
- IV antibiotics, e.g. cefuroxime +/– metronidazole +/– gentamicin
- NBM
- Analgesia
- If there is no clinical improvement within 12 hours, emergency decompression of the common bile duct is required, with removal of the obstruction where possible
  - ERCP +/– sphincterotomy +/– stenting
  - Percutaneous drainage
  - Surgical decompression
- For ascending cholangitis secondary to gallstones, once the patient is stabilized and the biliary system decompressed (e.g. ERCP) they will need definitive management, usually by laparoscopic cholecystectomy +/– bile duct exploration

! **Hepatic bleeding**

Hepatic bleeding is an uncommon problem in oncology patients. However, primary benign or malignant liver tumours may cause spontaneous bleeding, while this is less frequent with metastatic lesions. Bleeding can also occur following trauma.

Hepatic bleeding can be classified as:
- Intrahepatic—bleeding within the liver or liver lesion without resulting haemodynamic instability.
- Abdominal bleeding—localized intraparenchymal haematomas can rupture through the liver capsule and cause either a localized collection or free intraperitoneal haemorrhage

Clinical suspicion is important in diagnosing a localized haematomata prior to rupture.

Clinical features
- RUQ pain
- Nausea and vomiting
- Drop in Hb
- Peritonism
- Circulatory collapse
  - Hypotension
  - Tachycardia
  - Peripheral shutdown

Investigations

Bloods
- FBC
  - drop in Hb and haematocrit
- Coagulation screen
- Crossmatch

Imaging
- USS
  - may show free fluid/blood
  - may show liver lesions
- CT scan
  - will show liver morphology in more detail
- Hepatic angiography
  - identify source of bleeding
  - embolize specific vessel

Management

The principles of management are:
- Resuscitate the patient and maintain circulating volume
- Treatment to stop the bleeding

Resuscitation
- Oxygen
- Two large bore IV cannulae
- Aggressive IV fluid resuscitation (crystalloid or colloid)
- Correct coagulation deficiencies, e.g. vitamin K
- Give blood or plasma products (e.g. FFP)
- Institute appropriate monitoring (urinary catheter, CVP measurement)
- Transfer to an appropriate area of care (HDU/ICU)

Treatment to stop the bleeding

Following adequate resuscitation, conservative management may be used unless the patient is haemodynamically unstable.

The patient should be regularly reviewed by the surgical team, with repeat scanning to ensure resolution.

For patients who require intervention, hepatic angiography and embolization may be considered. Complications include: hepatic abscess, sepsis, and gallbladder ischaemia.

If the patient remains haemodynamically unstable with ongoing blood loss and the haematoma continues to expand on serial imaging, a laparotomy is indicated following optimization of the patient. The surgeon may use diathermy, topical haemostatic agents, suturing, packing, vascular ligation or resection to control the bleeding. Postoperative complications include: rebleeding, DIC, cardiopulmonary complications, and sepsis.

⑦ **Budd–Chiari syndrome**

Budd–Chiari syndrome is the combination of clinical symptoms and signs caused by obstruction to the venous outflow of the liver.

Obstruction may be at the level of the hepatic venules, large hepatic veins, IVC or right atrium. Classically it is caused by obstruction by acute thrombus at the junction of the IVC and the hepatic veins.

Obstruction to the venous outflow of the liver results in intrahepatic congestion with resulting hepatocellular ischaemia and necrosis. This process leads to portal hypertension and liver insufficiency/failure.

Causes

- Tumours
  - hepatoma
  - renal cell carcinoma
  - Wilm's tumour
  - adrenal carcinoma
  - sarcoma
  - atrial myxoma
- Haematological disorders
  - primary polycythaemia
  - leukaemia
  - paroxysmal nocturnal haemoglobinuria
  - essential thrombocythaemia
- Coagulation disorders
  - antiphospholipid syndrome
  - antithrombin deficiency
  - protein C or S deficiency
- Pregnancy or the post-partum period
- Drugs
  - oral contraceptive pill
- Inflammatory disorders
  - SLE
  - Behçet's disease
  - sarcoidosis
  - inflammatory bowel disease
- Infections
  - hepatic abscess
  - hydatid cyst
- Trauma to the liver
  - hepatobiliary surgery

Clinical features

The classic triad is:
- Ascites
- Abdominal pain
- Hepatomegaly

Other features include:
- Jaundice
- Collateral formation over the flanks and back
  - if obstruction is at the level of the IVC
- Lower limb oedema
- Renal failure
- Portal hypertension
  - splenomegaly
  - oesophageal varices

Patients may present with:
- Chronic Budd–Chiari
  - less common in cancer patients
  - cirrhosis with venous collaterals
- Subacute Budd–Chiari
- Acute Budd–Chiari
- Fulminant hepatic failure
  - rapidly deteriorating liver function and encephalopathy

A high index of suspicion is required to make the diagnosis.

Investigations
Bloods
- FBC
  - primary haematological cause
- LFTs
  - ↑↑ AST, ALT
  - ALP, bilirubin can be ↑
- Thrombophilia screen
  - not in the acute phase
  - once anticoagulation has been stopped
- Antiphospholipid antibody
- Antinuclear antibody
- SAAG
  - usually <11 g/l (exudate)

Imaging
- Doppler ultrasonography
  - investigation of choice
  - 85% sensitivity
  - shows abnormal flow in hepatic vein
- Contrast-enhanced CT or MRI
  - shows hepatic vein occlusion or IVC obstruction and diffuse abnormal liver parenchyma on contrast enhancement
- Echo
  - constrictive pericarditis
  - right-sided heart failure

Liver biopsy
- Centrilobular necrosis with venous congestion and possibly fibrosis

Management
- Medical management
  - Liaise with a hepatologist
  - Na$^+$ restriction to reduce formation of ascites
  - Spironolactone and furosemide to reduce ascites
  - Consider paracentesis with albumin infusion when ascites is tense or refractory to medical therapy
  - If encephalopathic:
    — search for, and treat, any underlying sepsis
    — stop any drugs that may have precipitated the encephalopathy
    – cerebral depressant drugs

- — give laxatives to empty the bowel of nitrogenous substances
  - – lactulose 30 ml tds   – enemas
- — consider antibiotics to sterilize the gut of ammoniagenic bacteria
  - – rifaximin   – metronidazole
- — monitor electrolytes carefully, adjust IV fluids and diuretics as necessary
  - Anticoagulation with LMWH followed by warfarin
    - — INR 2–3 if evidence of thrombosis involved in the obstruction
- Invasive management
  - Thrombolysis
    - — urokinase or recombinant tissue plasminogen activator may be infused directly into the hepatic vein for 24 hours via a transjugular or transfemoral approach
    - — the success rate is generally low and there is a substantial risk of bleeding
  - Transjugular intrahepatic portosystemic shunt (TIPS)
    - — this may relieve hepatic congestion in selected patients and allows the development of collaterals
    - — if liver transplantation is being considered, liaise with a transplant surgeon as the presence of TIPS may interfere with surgery
  - Surgical portosystemic shunt
    - — outcome is generally good if the patient is fit for surgery
    - — it is recommended for patients with an underlying cause that carries a good long term prognosis
      - – essential thrombocythaemia
  - Liver transplantation
    - — is an option for those with fulminant hepatic failure
      - – and deterioration after shunting procedures
      - – when the underlying condition is associated with a good prognosis
    - — long term survival is seen in up to 95% of such cases
  - Lifetime anticoagulation
    - — is usually required after definitive treatment because of the high risk of recurrent thrombosis

Further reading

Narayanan Menon, K.V., Shah, V. and Kamath, P.S. (2004). The Budd–Chiari syndrome. *N. Engl. J. Med.* **350**(6): 578–585.

Urological emergencies

:✪: **Acute renal failure**

Acute renal failure (ARF) may cause sudden, life-threatening biochemical disturbances and is therefore a medical emergency.

Acute uraemia can conveniently be classified as:

- Prerenal
  - impaired perfusion of the kidneys
- Postrenal
  - obstructive uropathy
- Renal
  - renal parenchymal damage

More than one category may be present in an individual patient. Whether acute uraemia progresses to ARF, with the need for dialysis/haemofiltration, depends on the initial management of the patient. With a ~50% mortality for ARF, correct management of acute uraemia is of vital importance.

An acute deterioration in renal function (e.g. secondary to nephrotoxic drugs, dehydration) often occurs on the background of a chronic process of renal impairment (e.g. chronic retention due to prostatic hypertrophy).

Cancer patients are at increased risk of renal impairment owing to both their underlying disease (e.g. pelvic tumours) and also through their treatment (e.g. nephrotoxic drugs, e.g. cisplatin).

Causes

Prerenal

- Hypovolaemia
  - Vomiting
  - Diarrhoea
  - Dehydration
  - Haemorrhage
  - Diuretics
- Hypotension
  - Septic shock
  - Cardiogenic shock
- Renal hypoperfusion
  - Drugs
    - NSAIDs
    - angiotensin II receptor antagonists
    - COX-II inhibitors
    - ACE inhibitors
  - Renovascular disease
  - Hepatorenal syndrome

Postrenal

- Intraluminal
  - Urinary tract calculi
    - ureteric
    - bladder
- Intramural
  - Urothelial tumours (most commonly TCC)
    - renal pelvis
    - ureteric
    - bladder
  - Ureteric or urethral stricture
    - infection
    - post-surgical
  - Neuropathic bladder

- Extramural
  - Retroperitoneal fibrosis
    - idiopathic
    - post-surgical
    - post-radiotherapy
    - post-chemotherapy
  - Benign prostatic hypertrophy
  - Tumours in the pelvis
    - prostate
    - cervical
    - ovarian
    - vulval
    - colon
  - Metastatic tumours in retroperitoneal and pelvic lymph nodes

Renal
- Acute tubular necrosis (ATN)
  - Ischaemia due to prerenal uraemia
  - Septicaemia
  - Myoglobinaemia/haemoglobinaemia
  - Drugs
    - cisplatin
    - ifosfamide
    - radiological IV contrast
    - high dose methotrexate
    - streptozocin
    - gentamicin
    - NSAIDs
- Glomerulonephritis
  - Wegener's granulomatosis
  - Goodpasture's syndrome
  - SLE
  - PAN
  - Malignancy-associated, e.g. membranous glomerulonephritis
    - colon cancer
    - lung cancer
- Thrombotic microangiopathy
  - Accelerated hypertension
  - HUS/TTP
- Interstitial nephritis
  - Drugs
    - NSAIDs
    - allopurinol
    - phenytoin
    - antibiotics
      - cephalosporins
      - penicillins
- Tubular deposition nephropathy
  - Tumour lysis syndrome
  - Bence Jones protein in myeloma
  - Urate nephropathy

Clinical features
- Biochemical and fluid balance abnormalities
  - malaise
  - confusion
  - nausea and vomiting
  - anorexia
  - seizures
  - peripheral oedema
  - pulmonary oedema
  - high JVP
  - Kussmaul's breathing
  - oliguria/anuria
- Prerenal uraemia
  - postural hypotension
  - tachycardia
  - dry mucous membranes
  - low JVP
  - ↓ skin turgor

- Postrenal uraemia
  - loin pain
  - fever (if secondary infection)
  - lower urinary tract symptoms
    - — hesitancy
    - — weak stream
    - — terminal dribble
    - — nocturia
  - haematuria
  - palpable hydronephrotic kidney
  - rectal and vaginal examination for pelvic malignancies
- Renal uraemia
  - arthralgia
  - rash
  - sinusitis
  - neurological signs

Investigations
Bloods
- U&Es
  - uraemia
  - hyperkalaemia
- Ca^{2+}, Mg^{2+} and phosphate
- Urate
- Bicarbonate
- FBC and blood film
  - haemorrhage/anaemia
  - ↓ and dysfunctional platelets
  - sepsis
  - HUS/TTP
- Serum Ig and electrophoresis
- LFTs
- Coagulation screen
- Blood cultures
- ABGs
  - metabolic acidosis
- Vasculitic screen
  - ANCA
  - ANA
  - anti-GBM antibodies

Urine
- Microscopy
  - haematuria
  - proteinuria
  - crystalluria
  - pyuria
  - urinary casts
  - eosinophils
- MC&S
  - infection
- Bence Jones protein
- Myoglobin/haemoglobin

ECG
- Hyperkalaemia
  - loss of P wave
  - broad QRS complexes (sinusoidal)
  - peaked T waves

Imaging
- USS renal tract
  - obstruction
    - — dilated upper renal tract with hydronephrosis
  - chronic component
    - — small kidneys with increased echogenicity

- CXR
  - fluid overload/pulmonary oedema
  - pulmonary infiltrates
- IVU/CTU
  - identifies the site of obstruction, but requires contrast medium, therefore avoid in patient with compromised renal function

Biopsy
- For renal causes of ARF (liaise with nephrologist)

Management
Hyperkalaemia
- If there are ECG changes give calcium gluconate
  - 10 ml of 10% calcium gluconate IV over 2 minutes
  - repeat until ECG normalizes
  - protects the heart from pro-arrhythmic effect of high $[K^+]$
  - no effect on $[K^+]$
- To lower extracellular $[K^+]$
  - Actrapid insulin 10 units plus 50 ml of 50% dextrose
    — infusion over 30 minutes
    — monitor blood glucose and K^+ regularly
    — repeat as necessary
  - Correct acidosis if insulin + dextrose failing to lower $[K^+]$
    — 400 ml 1.26% $NaHCO_3^-$ IV
    — can be repeated
  - Deplete body K^+ (takes 24 hours to work)
    — calcium resonium
      - 15 g PO 3–4 times daily (with laxative)
      - 30 g PR retained for 9 hours and then irrigation to remove resin from colon
- Consider dialysis if $[K^+]$ >7 mmol/l and refractory to other measures

Indications for dialysis/haemofiltration
- Symptomatic uraemia (usually >45 mmol/l)
  - Tremor
  - confusion
  - coma
  - seizures
  - pericarditis
- $[K^+]$ >7 mmol/l and refractory to other measures
- Metabolic acidosis (arterial pH <7.1, HCO_3^- <12 mmol/l)
- Fluid overload (e.g. refractory pulmonary oedema) unresponsive to diuretics

Prerenal uraemia
For the majority of cancer patients prerenal uraemia is due to hypovol-aemia and hypotension, and prompt fluid replacement is vital to prevent the development of ischaemic renal injury (ATN) and ARF.
- Clinical assessment of fluid balance
- Careful fluid balance charts
- Stop all nephrotoxic drugs
  - renal perfusion pressure autoregulation is impaired by NSAIDs and ACE inhibitors, therefore increasing the tendency to develop prerenal uraemia.

- Catheterize patient to monitor urine output
- Insert central venous line and measure CVP
- Aggressive fluid resuscitation
  - give 500 ml 0.9% saline or colloid over 30 minutes
  - monitor the response of urine output and venous pressure
  - continue fluids (colloid or crystalloid) until CVP is 5–10 cm
  - monitor patient for development of pulmonary oedema
  - if oliguria/anuria persists despite an adequate CVP (>10 cm), and uraemia is worsening, discuss with renal team for further advice and consideration of initiation of dialysis/haemofiltration for ARF
- In the presence of cardiogenic or septic shock, the patient should be managed in an HDU/ICU, for consideration of inotropic support

Postrenal uraemia

Prompt relief of the obstruction is the key to preservation of renal function. Obstructive uropathy coexisting with infection (pyonephrosis) is a urological emergency, as this leads to accelerated destruction of renal tissue.

- In the presence of infection treat with broad spectrum IV antibiotics, e.g. cefuroxime IV 1.5 g tds (750 mg bd in the presence of renal impairment), until blood and urine culture sensitivities are known.
- Insertion of a urinary/suprapubic catheter may be all that is required in the case of lower urinary tract obstruction
- In the presence of hydronephrosis despite catheterization, upper tract drainage is required
  - insertion of a retrograde ureteric stent
    — frequently impossible in cancer patients owing to the presence of anatomical deformities, bleeding, or ureteric compression
  - insertion of a percutaneous nephrostomy tube
    — required in the majority of cases of 'malignant' obstructive uropathy causing hydronephrosis
- Patients with significant biochemical abnormalities owing to obstructive uropathy may require dialysis/haemofiltration prior to consideration of upper tract drainage
- Post-obstructive diuresis usually follows relief of obstruction, and the patient's urine output and electrolytes must be monitored and replaced
  - oral fluid and supplements
  - IV fluids and electrolytes (if UO >200 ml/hour)
- Temporary relief of the obstruction provides time for further investigation of the cause and definitive management
- Inserting a percutaneous nephrostomy in patients with advanced malignancy may not always be in the patient's best interest
  - in patients with malignant obstructive uropathy where further treatment options are available, Lau *et al.* (1995) report a median survival of 20–27 weeks, and a 10–20% 5-year survival
  - in patients with malignant obstructive uropathy with no further antineoplastic treatment option, Lau *et al.* (1995) report the median survival to be 6.5 weeks, with no patient surviving beyond 1 year
  - we must be honest with our patients where no further treatment is available, and ascertain their wishes as to their further management

Reference

Lau, M.W., Temperley, D.E., Mehta, S., Johnson, R.J., Barnard, R.J. and Clarke, N.W. (1995). Urinary tract obstruction and nephrostomy drainage in pelvic malignant disease. *Br. J. Urol.* **76**: 565–569.

Further reading

Walsh, P.C., Retik, A.B., Vaughn, E.D. and Wein, A.J. (eds) (2002). *Campbell's Urology,* Chapter 12: 414–432. Saunders.

Weiss, R.M., George, N.J.R. and O'Reilly, P.H. (eds) (2001). *Comprehensive Urology.* Chapter 23: 333–346. London: Mosby.

Priapism

Priapism is a relatively uncommon disorder and refers to a persistent penile erection, not accompanied by sexual desire or stimulation, lasting greater than 6 hours.

Ischaemic priapism is a urological emergency, as erectile dysfunction is a common sequel of its inappropriate management.

Subtypes
- Low flow priapism (ischaemic, veno-occlusive)
  This is characterized by fully rigid corpora cavernosa, as a result of 'sludging' of blood, the glans penis and corpus spongiosum are soft and uninvolved. This results in pain arising from tissue ischaemia and smooth muscle hypoxia which, if untreated, result in muscle necrosis and cavernosal fibrosis.
- High flow priapism (non-ischaemic, arterial)
  Typically the penis is neither fully rigid nor painful. This does not generally require emergency treatment.

Causes
Primary
- Idiopathic (60% of cases)

Secondary
- Haematological
  - Leukaemia
  - Lymphoma
  - Myeloma
  - Sickle cell disease
  - Thalassaemia
- Neoplastic
  - Metastatic renal cell cancer
  - Prostate cancer
  - Bladder cancer
  - Melanoma
- Neurogenic
  - Autonomic neuropathy
  - Cauda equina compression
  - Spinal cord lesion
  - Spinal cord injury
- Trauma
  - Genital trauma
  - Perineal trauma
- Iatrogenic
  - Intracavernosal prostaglandin E1 (for erectile dysfunction; risk <1%)

Drugs
- Neuroleptics
  - Chlorpromazine
  - Trifluoperazine
  - Thioridazine
  - Haloperidol
- Antidepressants
  - Fluoxetine
  - Sertraline
- Anticoagulants
  - Heparin
- Recreational drugs
  - Cocaine/marijuana
  - Alcohol

Investigations

Bloods

- FBC
  - to rule out leukaemia
- Haemoglobin S
- Blood gas measurement from a cavernosal sample
  - to differentiate low flow priapism and high flow priapism
  - low flow
    - pO_2 <4 kPa (30 mmHg)
    - pCO_2 >8 kPa (60 mmHg)
    - pH <7.25
  - high flow
    - values for arterial blood
    - pO_2 10–13.3 kPa (75–100 mmHg)
    - pCO_2 4.8–6.1 kPa (36–46 mmHg)
    - pH 7.35–7.45

Urine

- MSU
  - to rule out UTI

Colour doppler USS

- Used to assess the presence or absence of arterial flow if doubt exists after cavernosal blood gas measurement

Management

Low flow priapism

- Most patients will regain potency if the priapism is aborted within 12–24 hours; beyond 36 hours the prognosis for future erections is poor.
- Haematological malignancies may cause altered viscosity, and malignant infiltration (e.g. prostatic carcinoma) may obstruct venous drainage, leading to stasis and thrombosis in the tissues.
- Correct any underlying causal factor if possible (e.g. sickle cell disease).
- Analgesia and anxiolytic.
- Initial treatment involves aspiration of 50 ml blood from the corpora via a 21-G butterfly needle; repeat once if necessary.
- Inject α-adrenergic agonist via intracavernous irrigation.
  - Continuous BP and HR monitoring.
  - Caution in patients with IHD, HT, CVD, patients on MAOIs.
  - Phenylephrine 100–200 µg in 0.5–1 ml. Repeat every 5–10 minutes as necessary. Maximum dose 1 mg.
  - Epinephrine 10–20 µg in 1 ml (1:200 000). Repeat as necessary. Maximum dose 100 µg.
  - Metaraminol 100 µg in 5 ml. Repeat every 15 minutes as necessary.
- Shunt surgery
  - To create a fistula between the corpora and a venous structure.
  - Cavernosal–glandular fistula (Winter procedure)
    - Trucut needle is pushed through the glans into the underlying corporal tissue.
    - Limited success and causes ugly deformity of the glans.

- • Cavernosal–spongiosal shunt.
- • Cavernosal–saphenous shunt (Grayhack procedure).
- Insertion of a penile prosthesis early after failure of shunt surgery prior to the development of penile fibrosis and shortening.

High flow priapism
- Ice packs/ice cold enema.
- Angiography and selective embolization of the responsible vessels.
- Surgical ligation may be required.

Further reading

Keoghane, S.R., Sullivan, M.E. and Miller, M.A.W. (2002). The aetiology, pathogenesis and management of priapism. *BJU Int.* **90:** 149–154.

Walsh, P.C., Retik, A.B., Vaughn, E.D. and Wein, A.J. (eds) (2002) *Campbell's Urology*, Chapter 45; 1661–1663. Saunders.

Haematological emergencies

⚠ **Disseminated intravascular coagulation**

Disseminated intravascular coagulation (DIC) is a clinical syndrome characterized by widespread intravascular activation of the coagulation cascade, with fibrin deposition and consumption of clotting factors and platelets.

Causes

DIC is a syndrome and therefore always has an underlying cause. In a cancer patient, the most common causes include:

- Sepsis (60% of cases)
- Malignancy
  - Solid tumours
    — especially mucin-secreting adenocarcinoma
  - Haematological malignancies
    — especially acute promyelocytic leukaemia
- Transfusion reaction
- Severe hepatic failure
- Pancreatitis
- Other causes
  - obstetric emergencies
  - severe trauma/burns
  - haemangioma
  - recreational drug use

Pathophysiology

Coagulation system activation is caused by an accelerated generation of fibrin and simultaneous impairment of fibrinolysis. Generation of fibrin is because of abnormally high levels of tissue factor expression resulting in factor VII activation. Impaired fibrinolysis is caused by a sustained increase in plasma levels of plasminogen activator inhibitor-1 (PAI-1). A reduction in plasma levels of the natural anticoagulants antithrombin and protein C also potentiate coagulation activation. Excessive fibrin formation results in thrombosis of small and medium sized vessels, resulting in tissue ischaemia and organ dysfunction. Clotting factor and platelet consumption leads to increased risk of bleeding.

Malignancy causes DIC by a number of different mechanisms:

- Expression of tissue factor
- Expression of a 'cancer procoagulant'
  - which has factor X-activating properties
- Hyperfibrinolysis
  - particularly seen with acute promyelocytic leukaemia and some forms of prostate cancer
- Sepsis resulting from immunodeficiency as a direct result of the malignancy or due to its treatment

Presentation

DIC may present with:
- Thrombosis
  - large vessel deep vein thrombosis, with or without embolic phenomena
  - small vessel thrombosis with tissue ischaemia and dysfunction, e.g. renal impairment, adult respiratory distress syndrome (ARDS)
- Bleeding
  - extensive bruising
  - mucosal bleeds
    - especially venepuncture/cannulation sites
  - intracranial bleeds
- Subclinical
  - 50–70% of patients with disseminated cancer will show laboratory markers of abnormal activation of the coagulation cascade with no overt evidence of DIC

Investigations

Diagnosis of DIC

No single test is sufficiently sensitive and specific to diagnose DIC (see Table 9.1). It is important to take into account the clinical condition of the patient, any underlying disorders present and all available laboratory tests. The following results are frequently observed (see Table 9.1)
- Prolonged APTT and PT
- Prolonged thrombin time (TT)
- Reduced plasma fibrinogen level
- Raised D-dimers
- Falling platelet count (owing to peripheral consumption)

Table 9.1 Laboratory findings in DIC

Laboratory test	Expected result in DIC	Problems with test
APTT	Prolonged	May also be prolonged in liver disease, vitamin K deficiency, heparin therapy
PT	Prolonged	May also be prolonged in liver disease, vitamin K deficiency, warfarin therapy
TT	Prolonged	Very sensitive to contamination with heparin
Fibrinogen	Reduced	Acute phase protein so may be artificially elevated, often elevated in cancer therefore a normal level does not rule out DIC
D-dimers	Raised	Very non-specific; raised postoperatively and in the presence of active thrombus or infection
Platelet count	Reduced	May also be low due to drug reaction, myelosuppressive therapies or sepsis

Serial laboratory tests are more useful than isolated measurements. In particular, a falling platelet count is a sensitive (but not specific) sign of DIC.

A blood film may be helpful in diagnosing DIC as it may show one or a combination of the following:
- Thrombocytopenia
- Occasional red cell fragments
- Toxic neutrophils
- Leukoerythroblastic change

Diagnosis of underlying cause

It is vital to try to identify an underlying cause in any patient with DIC. It should not be assumed that, in a cancer patient, DIC is due to the underlying malignancy. A vigorous search for other causes (particularly sepsis) should be undertaken.

Bloods
- Serial blood cultures
- CRP
  - systemic inflammatory change
- Amylase
  - pancreatitis
- LFTs
  - biliary sepsis
- If the patient has recently received a blood transfusion
  - repeat antibody screen
  - direct antiglobulin test
  - serum bilirubin
  - serum LDH
  - blood film
- U&Es
  - renal impairment
- ABG if signs of respiratory compromise
  - ARDS

Urine
- MC&S

Imaging
- CXR
  - source of sepsis
- CT
  - occult sepsis
    — prostatitis
    — biliary sepsis
    — paracolic abscess

Management
- The treatment priority in DIC is vigorous treatment of the underlying disorder. However, in malignancy-associated DIC this can be difficult
- Supportive measures to correct shock, acidosis and hypoxia
  - aggressive fluid resuscitation
  - O_2 therapy

- DIC-directed treatment is not indicated unless the patient is symptomatic or requires an interventional procedure
  - If the patient is bleeding
    - Fresh frozen plasma (FFP)
      - to correct a prolonged APTT and PT (dose of 12–15 ml/kg)
      - potential complications
        - fluid overload
        - viral transmission (in UK)
        - transfusion-related acute lung injury (TRALI)
    - Platelet transfusions
      - to bring the platelet count to >50×10^9/l
      - potential complications
        - allergic reactions to the suspending plasma
        - development of HLA antibodies with subsequent refractoriness to subsequent transfusions
        - TRALI
    - Cryoprecipitate if the fibrinogen level is <1.0 g/l after FFP and bleeding persists
      - potential complication
        - viral transmission
- Anticoagulation
  - theoretically this may be helpful by interrupting the activated coagulation system. However, no controlled trial has ever demonstrated a clinically meaningful benefit in patients with DIC
  - therapeutic doses of unfractionated heparin (infusion, aim for APTT ratio 1.5–2.0) are still sometimes used in the following situations:
    - clinically overt thromboembolism
    - purpura fulminans
    - acral ischaemia
- Activated protein C (aPC)
  - levels of the naturally occurring anticoagulant and anti-inflammatory protein aPC are low in DIC
  - a phase III trial of recombinant aPC in patients with sepsis was terminated prematurely owing to the demonstration of a mortality benefit. The benefit was particularly apparent in those patients with DIC. Any patient with sepsis-associated DIC should be considered for aPC according to local policy

Further reading

Bernard, G.R., Vincent, J.-L., Laterre, P.-F., LaRosa, S.P., Dhainaut, J.-F., Lopez-Rodriguez, A., Steingrub, J.S., Garber, G.E., Helterbrand, J.D., Ely, E.W. and Fisher, C.J. (2001). Efficacy and safety of recombinant human activated protein C for severe sepsis. *New Engl. J. Med.* **344**: 699–709.

British Committee for Standards in Haematology (2004). Guidelines for the use of fresh frozen plasma, cryoprecipitate and cryosupernatant. *Br. J. Haematol.* **126**: 11–28.

Levi, M. (2004). Current understanding of disseminated intravascular coagulation. *Br. J. Haematol.* **124**(5): 567–576.

⑦ **Anaemia**

Anaemia is a reduced oxygen-carrying capacity of the blood.
Male   Hb <13.5 g/dl   Female   Hb <11.5 g/dl

Causes

There are many causes of anaemia in the cancer patient and it is convenient to classify them according to the mean cell volume (MCV).

- Microcytic (MCV <80 fl)
  - Iron deficiency
    - usually due to chronic blood loss
  - Underlying thalassaemia trait
- Normocytic (MCV 80–100 fl)
  - Anaemia of chronic disease (can be microcytic)
  - Chemotherapy- or radiotherapy-induced marrow suppression
  - Marrow infiltration
    - haematological malignancy
    - secondary malignancy
  - Acute blood loss
  - Mixed vitamin deficiency
- Macrocytic (MCV >100 fl)
  - Haemolysis
    - lymphoproliferative condition
    - drugs, e.g. fludarabine
    - mismatched blood transfusion
  - Vitamin B_{12} and/or folate deficiency
  - Myelodysplasia
    - primary
    - secondary to chemotherapy or radiotherapy
  - Myeloma

Clinical features

- Shortness of breath on exertion
- Fatigue
- Headaches
- Palpitations
- Exacerbation of angina
- Heart failure (in severe cases)

Investigations

Bloods

- FBC
  - WCC and platelets will also be low in marrow suppression or infiltration
  - Platelets often elevated in:
    - acute blood loss
    - haemolysis
    - iron deficiency
  - WCC may be high or low in sepsis
- Blood film
  - Leukoerythroblastic change and tear drop poikilocytes suggest marrow infiltration

- Iron deficiency and vitamin B_{12}/folate deficiency produce specific changes
- Spherocytes with polychromasia is suggestive of an immune haemolysis
- Usually unremarkable in anaemia of chronic disease
- Haematinics
  - Sample not to be taken soon after a blood transfusion is administered
  - Iron deficiency
    — low serum iron   — low serum ferritin
    — high transferrin
  - Folate deficiency
    — low serum and red cell folate
    — serum folate reflects recent intake
    — red cell folate reflects tissue stores
- Haemolysis screen
  - blood film   • haptoglobin level (absent)
  - ↑ serum LDH   • ↑ unconjugated bilirubin
  - direct antiglobulin test (positive if immune cause)
- Inflammatory markers (CRP, ESR) to screen for chronic inflammatory or infectious disorder. If raised, full septic screen indicated
- Anti-gastric parietal cell (GPC) and anti-intrinsic factor (IF) antibodies if vitamin B_{12} deficiency proven (pernicious anaemia)
  - GPC antibodies are sensitive but not specific
  - IF antibodies are specific but not sensitive
- Bone marrow aspirate
  - Diagnostic for many primary haematological disorders
    — leukaemia   — myelodysplasia
    — myeloma
- Bone marrow trephine
  - diagnostic for marrow infiltration by secondary malignancy or lymphoma

Endoscopy

- Upper and lower GI endoscopy +/− biopsy to ascertain cause of iron deficiency, e.g. GI malignancy

Management

- Correct any reversible factors
  - Iron deficiency
    — ferrous sulphate PO 200 mg tds or iron sucrose IV
  - Folate deficiency
    — folic acid PO 5 mg od
  - Vitamin B_{12} deficiency
    — hydroxocobalamin IM 1 mg every 3 months
- Blood transfusion
  - Usually required if Hb <8 g/dl or if symptomatic.
  - Aim for Hb >10 g/dl
    — for radical radiotherapy to cervix and head and neck cancers aim for Hb >12 g/dl

- Indications for irradiated blood products in adults
  — any patient with a current or previous diagnosis of Hodgkin's disease
  — any patient who has ever received a purine analogue (e.g. fludarabine, cladribine)
  — all transfusions from first or second degree relatives
  — all granulocyte transfusions
  — all HLA-matched platelet transfusions
  — all recipients of allogeneic stem cell transplantation from the time conditioning chemotherapy commences until graft-versus-host disease prophylaxis is finished and the lymphocyte count is $>1.0 \times 10^9/l$
  — any patient who is planning to donate stem cells
    – before and during the time of harvest
  — any patient who is planning to store autologous stem cells
    – from 7 days before the stem cell harvest up to the time of the harvest
  — any patient who is undergoing autologous stem cell transplantation
    – from the time conditioning chemotherapy starts to 3 months after the transplant (6 months if total body irradiation used)
- Indications for CMV-negative blood products vary between hospital trusts.
  — some trusts do not advocate CMV-negative products for any of their patients as they argue that leukocyte depletion of all products makes transmission of CMV very unlikely
  — other trusts use CMV-negative products for any patient who is seronegative for CMV (or in whom a result is pending) and is being considered for an allogeneic stem cell transplant at some future point in their treatment
- Side effects of blood transfusion
  — formation of alloantibodies
  — haemolytic transfusion reactions
  — transmission of viral infection
  — unknown risk of transmission of variant Creutzfeldt–Jakob disease
  — volume overload is a risk in patients with poor cardiac function
- Erythropoiesis-stimulating agents (epoetin alfa, epoetin beta or darbepoetin)
  - Effective in raising the Hb in approximately 50% of cancer patients undergoing treatment
  - Should be considered in patients with chemotherapy-associated anaemia with a Hb <10 g/dl
  - Side effects
    — mild flu-like illness during the first few days of treatment
    — hypertension
    — thrombosis (rare)
    — development of pure red cell aplasia due to anti-erythropoietin antibody formation (very rare)

- Cytotoxic chemotherapy
  - If patient has evidence of bone marrow suppression due to infiltration by secondary malignancy, e.g. breast cancer, consideration must be given to treatment with cytotoxic chemotherapy, e.g. epirubicin 20 mg/m^2 weekly. Care must be taken because of the poor marrow reserve and the myelosuppressive nature of cytotoxic chemotherapy

Further reading

Littlewood, T. and Collins, G. (2005). Epoetin alfa: basic biology and clinical utility in cancer patients. *Expert Rev. of Anticancer Ther.* **5**: 947–956.

Rizzo, J.D., Lichtin, A.E., Woolf, S.H., Seidenfeld, J., Bennett, C.L., Cella, D., Djulbegovic, B., Goode, M.J., Jakubowski, A.A., Lee, S.J., Miller, C.B., Rarick, M.U., Regan, D.H., Browman, G.P. and Gordon, M.S. (2002). Use of epoetin in patients with cancer: evidence-based clinical practice guidelines of the American Society of Clinical Oncology and the American Society of Hematology. *J Clin Oncol* **20**: 4083–4107.

British Committee for Standards in Haematology, Blood Transfusion task force. (1996). Guidelines on gamma-irradiation of blood components for the prevention of transfusion-associated graft-versus-host disease. *Transfusion Medicine* **6**: 261–271.

⑦ Polycythaemia

A haematocrit of >0.48 for women and >0.52 for men which persists for >2 months can be considered abnormal.

Causes
Absolute polycythaemia
- Erythropoietin-dependent
  - Malignant or benign tumours
    — renal cell carcinoma
    — hepatoma
    — parathyroid adenoma or carcinoma
    — adrenal adenoma or carcinoma
    — cerebellar haemangioblastoma
  - Chronic hypoxia due to lung disease or heart disease
  - Benign renal lesion
    — hydronephrosis
    — cystic disease
  - Congenital high affinity haemoglobins
- Erythropoietin-independent
  - Primary polycythaemia
  - Excess testosterone
    — exogenous
    — endogenous
  - Congenital erythropoietin receptor truncations

Relative polycythaemia
- Dehydration
  - Vomiting
  - Diarrhoea
  - Diuretics
- Apparent erythrocytosis
  - Stress
  - Diabetes
  - Obesity
  - Alcohol

Clinical features

Polycythaemia may present as an emergency with:
- Stroke
- Myocardial infarction
- Pulmonary embolism
- Hepatic or portal vein thrombosis

General features
- Fatigue
- Headaches
- Confusion
- Plethoric complexion

Primary polycythaemia is associated with pruritus in the absence of rash and there may be a palpable spleen.

Investigations
Bloods
- ABG
  - pO_2 persistently <92% may cause polycythaemia
- U&Es, LFTs, serum Ca^{2+}
- Serum erythropoietin
  - Is polycythaemia erythropoietin-dependent or independent?

- Red cell mass
  - Is polycythaemia absolute or relative?
- Further specialist tests can be used to seek high affinity haemoglobin – liaise with a haematologist. A new test can look for a mutation in the *Jak2* gene which is associated with primary polycythaemia

Imaging
- CXR
  - Cardiac disease
  - Pulmonary disease
- Abdominal USS
  - Renal disease
  - Liver disease
  - Splenomegaly

Treatment
- If the patient presents with active thrombosis
  - Urgent venesection of 500 ml blood
  - Consider replacement with 500 ml 0.9% saline if patient unlikely to tolerate reduced intravascular volume, e.g. in the presence of aortic stenosis or ischaemic heart disease
  - Repeat daily until PCV <0.45
  - Venesection should be more cautious in patients with a hypoxia-driven erythrocytosis – liaise with a haematologist in this situation
- In secondary polycythaemia, the underlying cause should be sought and treated if possible. A chronic venesection programme may need to be undertaken
- In primary polycythaemia, aspirin 75 mg od should be prescribed in the absence of contraindications, as evidence suggests this lowers the rate of thrombosis in these patients

Further reading
British Committee for Standards in Haematology. (2005). Guidelines for the diagnosis, investigation and management of polycythaemia/erythrocytosis. *Br. J. Haematol.* **130**: 174–195.

ⓘ **Thrombocytopenia**

A platelet count less than the lower limit of normal (typically <150x10^9/l). Thrombocytopenia is a common occurrence in cancer patients and is caused both by the underlying disease and as a result of cancer treatment.

Causes

There are many causes of thrombocytopenia, and the cause is often multifactorial.

- Reduced production of platelets
  - Myelosuppressive drugs
    - carboplatin
    - topotecan
    - cyclophosphamide
    - ifosfamide
    - mitomycin C
    - lomustine
    - carmustine
    - gemcitabine
    - methotrexate
    - etoposide
  - Radiotherapy
    - particularly pelvic radiotherapy
  - Infiltration by malignancy
    - haematological
    - secondary solid tumours
  - Alcohol
  - Primary marrow failure syndromes
    - myelodysplasia
  - Sepsis
  - Viral infections
    - HIV
    - EBV
    - rubella
    - mumps
- Increased peripheral consumption
  - Sepsis (with or without DIC)
  - Drugs
    - heparin (HIT)
    - vancomycin
  - Idiopathic thrombocytopenic purpura (ITP)
    - can be associated with:
      - Hodgkin's disease
      - NHL
      - CLL
      - lung cancer
      - breast cancer
      - gastrointestinal cancer
  - Thrombotic thrombocytopenic purpura (TTP)
  - Haemolytic uraemic syndrome (HUS)
  - Post-transfusion purpura (PTP)
- Altered distribution
  - Massive blood transfusion
  - Splenomegaly with sequestration

Investigations

In a cancer patient undergoing chemotherapy or radiotherapy (especially pelvic radiotherapy), a degree of temporary thrombocytopenia is to be expected and further investigations are often not required. Knowledge of the patient's current chemotherapy (drug, dose, and timing), as well as any previous chemotherapy and/or radiotherapy history, is therefore vital. However, if the thrombocytopenia is unexplained (severity, timing, duration), further tests are frequently helpful.

Bloods
- FBC
  - Coexisting leukopenia and anaemia suggest marrow failure or splenic sequestration
  - Raised MCV may indicate myelodysplasia or occasionally marrow infiltration
- Blood film
  - Tear drop poikilocytes (dacrocytes) are suggestive of marrow infiltration or fibrosis
  - A leucoerythroblastic film is suggestive of marrow infiltration, fibrosis or sepsis
  - Features of a primary haematological malignancy may be seen, e.g. blasts in acute leukaemia
  - Frequent red cell fragments suggest microangiopathic disease, e.g. TTP, HUS
- Coagulation
  - Prolonged APTT, PT, TT, and low fibrinogen suggests DIC (see Disseminated intravascular coagulation ☐ p278)
  - Coagulation tests are normal in ITP and TTP

Bone marrow aspirate
- Increased numbers of megakaryocytes suggest peripheral consumption or altered distribution
- May show primary marrow disorder or marrow infiltration

Further tests
These will depend on the clinical context and frequently require involvement of a haematologist.
- HIV antibody
- Heparin/platelet factor 4 antibody test if heparin-induced thrombocytopenia (HIT) is suspected
- Specific tests for the detection of beta-lactam or glycopeptide-induced antibodies
- Anti-HPA 1A antibody test if post-transfusion purpura is suspected
- LDH if a microangiopathic process such as TTP is suspected

Clinical features
- Bleeding, bruising and/or purpura
  - Spontaneous bleeding or purpura is uncommon until the platelet count is $<10\times10^9$/l
  - Examine for retinal haemorrhages
- Thrombosis
  - Certain conditions present characteristically with thrombocytopenia and thrombosis
    — TTP
    — HIT
    — some cases of DIC

Management

- Treat the underlying cause where possible
  - refer to haematologist for primary haematological causes
  - consider cytotoxic chemotherapy when due to marrow infiltration by secondary malignancy. Care must be taken owing to the poor marrow reserve and the myelosuppressive nature of chemotherapy
- Stop any anti-platelet medication, including aspirin. Stop NSAIDs
- Avoid intramuscular injections
- If minor mucosal bleeding, consider tranexamic acid mouthwash (10 ml of a 5% solution qds) or tablets (15–25 mg/kg tds PO but reduce in renal failure)
- If the patient is bleeding consider reversing any anticoagulation
- Platelet transfusions (1 bag of platelets = full adult dose) should only be used if:
  - the patient is actively bleeding in the presence of a low platelet count (<100x10^9/l)
  - the platelet count is <10x10^9/l (↑ risk intracerebral haemorrhage)
  - the platelet count is <20x10^9/l and the patient has a coexisting coagulopathy or evidence of active infection, e.g. fever
  - the platelet count is <50x10^9/l and the patient is due to undergo an invasive procedure (e.g. central line insertion, biopsy, lumbar puncture, epidural insertion)
  - check the platelet count the day after the platelet transfusion. If the rise in platelet count is <5x10^9/l without good cause, contact the haematologist for further advice
- If the thrombocytopenia is because of an immune cause such as ITP and the count needs to be increased owing to:
  - active bleeding
  - level <10x10^9/l
  - impending invasive procedure
  - consider giving IV immunoglobulin (0.25–1.0 g/kg infusion) and/or corticosteroids (60 mg PO od) (liaise with a haematologist). In this situation platelet transfusions are generally not effective and are only given in the presence of major haemorrhage

Note: platelet transfusions are contraindicated in TTP and HIT.
- Side effects of platelet transfusions
  - allergic transfusion reactions
  - alloimmunization

Further reading

British Committee for Standards in Haematology (2003). Guidelines for the use of platelet transfusions. *Br. J. Haematol.* **122**: 10–23.

Schiffer, C.A., Anderson, K.C., Bennett, C.L., Bernstein, S., Elting, L.S., Goldsmith, M., Goldstein, M., Hume, H., McCullough, J.J., McIntyre, R.E., Powell, B.L., Rainey, J.M., Rowley, S.D., Rebulla, P., Troner, M.B. and Wagnon, A.H. (2001). Platelet transfusion for patients with cancer: clinical practice guidelines of the American Society of Clinical Oncology. *J. Clin. Oncol.* **19**(5): 1519–1538.

⑦ **Thrombocytosis**

A platelet count higher than the upper limit of normal (typically $>400\times10^9/l$).

Causes
- Reactive causes (80–90%)
  - Underlying malignancy
  - Sepsis (especially abscesses)
  - Inflammatory conditions
  - Bleeding
  - Iron deficiency
  - Haemolysis
  - Previous splenectomy
- Primary causes
  - Essential thrombocythaemia
  - Other myeloproliferative conditions
  - Unusual cases of myelodysplastic syndrome (such as the 5q⁻ syndrome)

Investigations
These should be primarily to investigate an underlying cause. An underlying malignancy should not be automatically assigned as the reason for thrombocytosis without exclusion of other causes. If a primary cause is suspected, liaise with a haematologist.

Bloods
- FBC
  - ↑ Hb
    — polycythaemia rubra vera
  - ↓ Hb
    — bleeding   — iron deficiency
  - ↑ WCC
    — chronic myeloid leukaemia   — sepsis
- CRP, ESR
  - sepsis   • inflammatory conditions
- Blood cultures
- Blood film
  - in reactive cases the platelets are usually small and uniform
  - in primary cases the platelets are frequently morphologically abnormal

Urine
- MC&S

Imaging
- CXR
- CT scan (chest, abdomen, pelvis)
  - for occult infection
    — paracolic abscess   — prostatitis
- Echo
  - endocarditis

Management

In cases of reactive thrombocytosis, treat the underlying cause. No specific treatment is required for the high platelet count as the risk of thrombosis is not thought to be increased. In particular, there is no evidence that antiplatelet agents are beneficial.

For primary causes of thrombocytosis, liaise with a haematologist for definitive treatment (e.g. hydroxycarbamide).

Further reading

Schaeffer, A.I. (2004). Current concepts: thrombocytosis. *N. Engl. J. Med.* **350**: 1211–1219.

⊕ **Hyperviscosity syndrome**

The clinical manifestations caused by increased viscosity of either the plasma or cellular component of blood.

Causes

These can be divided into causes of a high plasma viscosity or causes of a high red or white cell count.

- High plasma viscosity
  - Waldenström's macroglobulinaemia: most common cause
  - Myeloma (usually IgA subtype): much less common cause of hyperviscosity
  - Connective tissue disorders: a rare cause due to immune complexes
- High red cell count (polycythaemia)
  - See Polycythaemia 📖 p286
- High white cell count
  - Acute leukaemia (myeloid or lymphoid)
  - Chronic myeloid leukaemia

Note: chronic lymphocytic leukaemia almost never causes the hyperviscosity syndrome even when the WCC is extremely high (>300×10^9/l).

Clinical features

- Due to raised immunoglobulins (paraprotein)
  - Mucosal bleeding
    — gum bleeding   — GI blood loss
    — epistaxis
  - Visual loss
    — retinal haemorrhages   — central retinal vein thrombosis
  - Neurological involvement
    — headaches   — ataxia
    — confusion   — seizures
  - Renal impairment
- Due to raised red cell count
  - Lethargy
  - Itch
  - Hypertension
  - Plethora
  - Arterial thrombosis
    — myocardial infarction   — stroke
    — hepatic or portal vein thrombosis
- Due to raised white cell count
  - Pulmonary leukostasis
    — dyspnoea   — pulmonary haemorrhage
    — cough
  - Cerebral leukostasis
    — confusion   — decreased conscious level
    — cranial nerve palsies   — intracranial haemorrhage

Investigations
Bloods
- FBC
  - polycythaemia
  - leukocytosis
- Blood film
  - rouleaux if high immunoglobulin level
- ESR
  - ↑ in the presence of raised immunoglobulins
- Protein : albumin ratio
  - ↑ in the presence of raised immunoglobulins
- Plasma viscosity
  - >4 mPa/s to cause symptoms (1.5–1.7 mPa/s)
- Cryoglobulins
  - if an immunoglobulin has features of a cryoglobulin
    (i.e. if it precipitates in the cold), normal laboratory measurements
    of immunoglobulin will be falsely low. Cryoglobulins should be
    assayed at 37°C and the cryocrit determined

Treatment
- Due to raised immunoglobulins
  - Arrange for urgent plasmapheresis, usually 1–1.5 × blood volume
    exchange. Repeat daily until symptoms have resolved.
  - Aim to start chemotherapy soon.
  - In the absence of a plasma exchange machine, venesect 500 ml
    blood with replacement by 0.9% saline unless Hb <7 g/dl when
    packed red cells should be used.
- Due to raised red cell count
  - Urgent venesection of 500 ml blood.
  - Consider replacement with 500 ml 0.9% saline if patient unlikely to
    tolerate reduced intravascular volume, e.g. in the presence of aortic
    stenosis or ischaemic heart disease.
  - Repeat daily until PCV <0.45.
- Due to raised white cell count
  - Urgent leukopheresis, replacing volume with 0.9% saline unless Hb
    <7 g/dl when packed red cells should be used.
  - In the absence of a suitable machine, venesect 500 ml blood from a
    peripheral vein, replacing fluid as above.
  - Commence tumour lysis preventative measures (see Tumour lysis
    syndrome 📖 p166).
  - Commence chemotherapy as soon as it is safe to do so.
  - Leukopheresis should be continued until symptoms have resolved
    or WCC <50 × 10^9/l.
- Blood transfusions may be dangerous in the context of the
  hyperviscosity syndrome as they can lead to an acute deterioration.
  Only initiate a transfusion if anaemia symptoms are severe and steps
  have been taken to control the viscosity
- In the presence of a cryoglobulin or cold agglutinin, blood and fluids
  should be warmed before infusion into the patient

ⓘ Stem cell transplant

High dose therapy followed by stem cell transplantation is now common practice for certain disorders such as myeloma, relapsed lymphoma and high risk acute leukaemias. The source of stem cells may either be from the patient themselves (autologous transplantation) or from another individual (allogeneic transplantation).

The transplant-related complications may be caused by the conditioning chemotherapy and/or radiotherapy, the stem cell infusion or post-transplant complications.

Conditioning-related complications

These depend on the type of conditioning treatment administered (see Table 9.2).

Table 9.2 Side effects associated with commonly used stem cell transplant conditioning protocols or specific agents

Regimen	Potential acute toxicities
High dose melphalan (200 mg/m^2)	Severe mucositis and diarrhoea
	Anaphylactoid reactions: hypotension, tachycardia, urticaria, bronchospasm
	Pneumonitis
	Renal impairment
B – bleomycin	Fevers and chills
E – etoposide	Pneumonitis
A – ara-C (cytarabine)	Anaphylactoid reactions
M – melphalan	Mucositis and diarrhoea
High dose cyclophosphamide	Haemorrhagic cystitis
	Nausea, vomiting, diarrhoea
	Pneumonitis
	Haemorrhagic myocarditis
Total body irradiation	Nausea, vomiting, diarrhoea
	Severe mucositis
	Pneumonitis
	Dermatitis
Monoclonal antibodies, e.g. CAMPATH (alemtuzumab) or rituximab	Infusion reactions: fevers, chills, rigors, bronchospasm
Anti-thymocyte globulin (ATG) or anti-lymphocyte globulin (ALG) – used in some transplant protocols	Fevers and chills (very common)
	Thrombocytopenia (early)
	Anaphylactoid reactions
	Serum sickness (fever, urticaria, arthralgia, haematuria with renal impairment)

Stem cell infusion-related complications

Stem cells may come in the form of bone marrow or, more commonly, from cells harvested from the peripheral circulation after stimulation with G-CSF +/– chemotherapy and selected on the basis of expression of the marker CD34. Stem cells are frequently stored in DMSO which is infused into the patient along with the stem cells at time of transplant. Potential stem cell infusion-related complications are listed in Table 9.3.

Post-transplant complications
Acute graft-versus-host disease (GvHD)

Acute GvHD results from the allogeneic recognition and attack on host tissues by donor T cells. Acute GvHD occurs <100 days post-SCT.

Risk factors include:
- CMV reactivation
- Increasing age of patient and donor
- Sex mismatch
- Poor HLA match

Table 9.3 Stem cell infusion-related complications

Complication	Clinical features	Management
Infusion reaction	Itch	If mild:
	Urticaria	Oxygen
	Bronchospasm: breathlessness and wheeze	Intravenous fluids
		Hydrocortisone 100 mg IV
	Hypotension and tachycardia	Chlorphenamine 10 mg IV
		If severe:
		As for anaphylaxis (see Hypersensitivity reaction 🕮 p342.)
Fluid overload	Breathlessness	Slow or stop infusion
	Raised JVP	Furosemide 40–80 mg IV
	Crackles in chest	If severe: consider diamorphine 2.5 mg IV and a GTN infusion
Transfusion reaction (if blood group mismatch)	Rare as major group mismatches are red cell-depleted:	Stop infusion
		Intravenous fluids
	Fever	Monitor renal function and fluid balance
	Loin pain	Check PT, APTT, fibrinogen and platelet count for DIC
	Breathlessness	
	Bleeding	
	Jaundice	
	Renal failure	
DMSO toxicity	Headache, lethargy	Slow infusion
	Rarely renal or liver impairment	If multiple bags to infuse, split infusion over more than 1 day
		Otherwise, supportive care

Clinical features
- Skin
  - erythema progressing to generalized erythroderma and bullae
- Liver
  - jaundice progressing to liver failure
- GI
  - diarrhoea progressing to abdominal pain and ileus

Each feature of acute GvHD is staged (see Table 9.4) and the stage of involvement contributes to the overall clinical grade (see Table 9.5).

Investigations
- LFTs
  - bilirubin and ALP usually increase more than the transaminases
- U&Es
  - severe disease may lead to dehydration and renal failure or the hepatorenal syndrome with derangement of electrolytes
- Glucose, albumin, PT, and APTT
  - become deranged in severe liver disease
  - albumin may fall owing to loss from the GI tract
- Full septic screen, including stool, for *Clostridium difficile* toxin
  - many features of GvHD may be similar to those produced by infection
- An attempt at obtaining a tissue diagnosis should be made, but initiation of treatment should not be delayed if the grade of GvHD ≥2
  - Skin biopsy
  - Rectal biopsy
    — risk of bleeding, particularly if thrombocytopenic and abnormal coagulation
  - Upper GI endoscopy
    — in the setting of persistent nausea
  - Liver biopsy
    — normally transjugular owing to bleeding risk
    — seek advice of a hepatologist

Management
Mild forms of GvHD may not need any specific treatment and confers a reduced risk of relapse of malignancy because of concomitant graft-versus-malignancy effect.
- Grade 1 skin involvement usually only requires topical steroids
- Treatment of grades 2–4 involves:
  - Supportive care
    — Careful fluid balance monitoring and clinical estimation of fluid status of patient.
    — Regular electrolyte monitoring with correction of derangements.
    — Diarrhoea may be initially treated with loperamide up to 2 mg every 2 hours with initiation of octreotide if refractory (100–150 µg SC every 8 hours initially, increasing to 500–1500 µg if required). Octreotide should be stopped within 24 h of cessation of diarrhoea to prevent ileus formation and should be continued for a maximum of 7 days.

- Infection prophylaxis with co-trimoxazole and aciclovir should continue in all patients with GvHD unless contraindicated owing to enhanced immunosuppression associated with this complication. Where there is a history of previous fungal infection, consider prophylaxis with amphotericin or voriconazole and monitor CMV PCR for evidence of reactivation.
- Broad spectrum antibiotics should be administered for suspected infection, with early addition of antifungal therapies if fever persists.
- Definitive treatment
  - Continue GvHD prophylaxis.
  - Commence methylprednisolone IV 1 mg/kg bd.
  - Assess response at day 5.
  - For responders, reduce methylprednisolone to 0.5 mg/kg bd for a further 5 days and then taper over the next 20 days (can be converted to PO prednisolone if patient eating and drinking).
  - If no response, increase to 5 mg/kg bd and re-assess after 3–5 days. If responding at this point, reduce to 2.5 mg/kg bd for a further 5 days and then taper down over 20 days.
  - If still not responding the disease is considered steroid-resistant and secondary treatments should be considered, e.g. antilymphocyte globulin, pentostatin, daclizumab (anti-IL2 receptor antibody), infliximab (anti-TNF antibody), alemtuzumab (anti-CD52 antibody).
  - If acute GvHD flares up during steroid withdrawal, reinstate previous dose and re-assess in 5 days.

Table 9.4 Staging of acute GvHD

Stage	Skin	Liver	GI
1	Rash <25% body	Bilirubin 34–51 µmol/l	Diarrhoea 0.5–1 l/day or persistent nausea
2	Rash 25–50% body	Bilirubin 52–102 µmol/l	Diarrhoea 1–1.5 l/day
3	Generalized erythroderma	Bilirubin 10–256 µmol/l	Diarrhoea >1.5 l/day
4	Desquamation and/or bulla formation	Bilirubin >256 µmol/l	Severe abdominal pain +/– ileus

Table 9.5 Grading of acute GvHD

Grade	Skin	Liver	GI
0	Stage 0	Stage 0	Stage 0
1	Stage 1 to 2	Stage 0	Stage 0
2	Stage 1 to 3	Stage 1	Stage 1
3	Stage 2 to 3	Stage 2 to 3	Stage 2 to 3
4	Stage 2 to 4	Stage 2 to 4	Stage 2 to 4

CMV reactivation and disease

Past infection with CMV is common in the general population and results in a latent infection. In immunocompromised individuals, the virus can re-activate and after a period cause CMV disease such as pneumonitis, colitis, oesophagitis, hepatitis, and retinitis. The mortality from overt CMV disease in post-allogeneic transplant patients is high and it used to be a major killer of such patients. However, since the introduction of sensitive surveillance monitoring and pre-emptive therapy to detect and treat CMV reactivation before the onset of disease, the death rate from CMV disease is now very low.

CMV surveillance
- Every allogeneic stem cell transplant patient and donor should be tested for the presence of CMV IgG indicating previous infection.
- If the patient and/or the donor are seropositive, PCR monitoring of the patient's peripheral blood should be performed once or twice weekly until at least 120 days post-transplant (longer if on steroids, in the presence of active GvHD or previous CMV reactivation).
- Two consecutive weekly positive PCR results indicate reactivation and pre-emptive antiviral treatment should be commenced.
- A CMV-negative recipient with a CMV-negative donor transplant does not need surveillance but CMV PCR should be performed in the event of the occurrence of GvHD or a non-specific illness. Autologous stem cell transplant patients do not require monitoring.

Prevention of CMV

All CMV-seronegative recipients should receive CMV-negative blood products. The risk of transmission of CMV from leukodepleted products is, however, very low and, in an emergency, CMV-unscreened products can be administered. In addition, a seropositive recipient or a seronegative recipient receiving a seropositive donor transplant should receive aciclovir prophylaxis. A typical regimen is:
- Aciclovir 500 mg/m^2 IV tds from the day of the transplant until discharge, then 400 mg PO twice daily until day 100.

Treatment of CMV reactivation
- Ganciclovir 5 mg/kg IV bd until two consecutive CMV PCR results are negative. Frequent side effects include myelosuppression, renal dysfunction, abnormal liver function tests and GI upset. Dose should be adjusted in renal impairment.
- Foscarnet is used in ganciclovir-intolerant or -resistant patients. It is dosed according to creatinine clearance and side effects include genital irritation owing to excretion of toxic metabolites (adequate hydration reduces this side effect), renal impairment, hypocalcaemia, and hypomagnesaemia. Electrolytes must be regularly monitored and the drug should only be administered through a central line.

Investigation of CMV disease

CMV disease is best diagnosed by biopsy of affected tissue. Broncho alveolar lavage may also be useful diagnostically in patients with a pneumonitis of unknown aetiology.

Treatment of CMV disease

- As for CMV reactivation, ganciclovir followed by foscarnet if poorly responsive.
- Intravenous immunoglobulin treatment is also often used although the evidence base supporting this intervention is thin.

Veno-occlusive disease of the liver (VOD)

Hepatic veno-occlusive disease results from the obstruction of small intrahepatic venules with resulting damage to surrounding centrilobular hepatocytes and sinusoids. It usually occurs as a complication of chemo-irradiation, particularly following allogeneic stem cell transplantation. Risk factors include:

- Elevated pre-transplant transaminases
- Intensive cytoreductive conditioning regimens
- Persistent fever post-conditioning therapy
- Mismatched or unrelated donor transplants
- Previous treatment with regimens containing the monoclonal antibody Mylotarg

Clinical features

VOD can be diagnosed when there is onset within 21 days after stem cell transplant of:

- Bilirubin >34 µmol/l plus two of the following:
  - Hepatomegaly
  - Ascites
  - Weight gain >5% from baseline

Additional investigations

- Liver biopsy (usually transjugular)
- Liver USS

The following tests should also be performed:

- Regular tests of hepatic synthetic function
  - blood glucose
  - PT and APTT
- Regular assessment of renal function

Treatment

- Supportive care
  - Ascites present
    — salt restriction and consider fluid restriction
    — avoid saline infusion
    — cautious use of loop diuretics to achieve negative Na$^+$ balance

- Encephalopathy present
  - avoid sedatives and opioid analgesia
  - correct known precipitants
    - hypokalaemia   – infection
    - constipation
- Avoid nephrotoxic drugs and ensure cyclosporin levels are within the therapeutic range
- Definitive treatment
  - Defibrotide
    - initial dose 10 mg/kg/day in four divided doses infused over 2 h
    - dose is then slowly escalated to 60 mg/kg/day for a minimum treatment duration of 14 days
  - Other options include:
    - recombinant tissue plasminogen activator with heparin
    - prostaglandin E1
    - glutamine with vitamin E

Psychiatric emergencies

① **Delirium**

Acute confusional state
- Rapid onset
- Impairment of consciousness
- Global cognitive impairment
- Fluctuating course (often worse at night)

Delirium is common in patients with cancer (up to 25% of hospitalized patients and 85% of terminal patients). It is probably the most common psychiatric emergency in oncology.

It occurs:
- As a result of the cancer
- As a result of treatment
- At the end of life

Nearly all cancer patients will experience at least one episode of delirium during their illness.

Delirium must always be treated promptly as:
- It implies environmental and physiological pressure upon the brain such that it is unable to support normal conscious functioning
- It may signal impending multi-organ failure (or death) and it is associated with high mortality
- It impairs the patient's ability to participate in, and benefit from, treatment
- It is associated with significant distress and suffering for the patient (and others)
- Delirium-related behaviours can rapidly escalate into a more urgent situation with risk of harm to the patient or the assault of others

Presentation

Delirium usually presents acutely, and the physiological or environmental trigger is often clearly linked to the onset of symptoms. Although classic delirium is easier to diagnose, it is important to realize that subtle disturbances in the following symptoms can herald a developing delirium.

Cardinal symptoms
- Impaired cognition
  - Disorientation: time, place, and person
  - 30-point MMSE
  - Impaired clock or star drawing
- Impaired attention: poor concentration or distractibility
- Altered level of consciousness, from hyper-alert to difficult to rouse. The majority of delirium is hypoactive/lethargic delirium and is more frequently missed. Hyperactive/agitated delirium is more likely to attract attention
- Altered sleep/wake cycle
- Delusions, hallucinations (perceptions in the absence of stimuli), and illusions (misinterpretations of external stimuli) that are typically frightening

Investigations

Use a 'delirium screen' to identify reversible medical factors that may be precipitating or perpetuating the delirium.

Bloods

- FBC, coagulation screen
  - infection
  - bleeding
  - DIC
- U&Es
  - renal failure
  - electrolyte imbalance
- TFTs
  - hypothyroidism
  - thyrotoxicosis
- ABGs
  - hypoxia
  - hypercapnia
- LFTs
  - hepatic encephalopathy
- Blood cultures
  - infection
- Glucose
  - hypoglycaemia
- Ca^{2+}
  - hypercalcaemia
- Cardiac enzymes
  - cardiac ischaemia
- Toxicology
  - drug toxicity

Urine

- MSU
  - UTI

ECG

- Cardiac ischaemia

Imaging

- CXR
  - chest infection
  - heart failure
- AXR
  - constipation
  - bowel obstruction
- CT head/MRI brain
  - subdural haematoma
  - metastasis
  - acute stroke
- Skeletal X-ray
  - occult fracture

Management

Immediate management

Contain any risks associated with agitated behaviour.

- Ensure help is available appropriate to the situation, e.g. nursing staff, hospital security.
- Protect your own and others' safety first. Other patients may need to be moved if the patient will not move to a safe, quiet area.
- Attempt to defuse the situation verbally. People that are familiar or trusted by the patient may be more successful, e.g. a family member.

- If medication is necessary to end the need for physical restraint or reduce the risk of harm from agitated behaviour, try to persuade the patient to take medication. If this is refused consider covertly or forcibly giving medicine. The most effective medication is haloperidol 2–10 mg PO or IM (elderly 0.5–2 mg) repeated every 15–30 minutes as necessary.
- If acute alcohol withdrawal is suspected treat with a reducing regimen of chlordiazepoxide (adjusted for symptoms) PO and thiamine.
  - Chlordiazepoxide
    - Day 1–2   20 mg qds   10 mg prn   max. 200 mg/day
    - Day 3   20 mg tds
    - Day 4   20 mg bd
    - Day 5   10 mg bd
  - Thiamine
    - 1 pair Pabrinex IVHP ampoules (250 mg thiamine) IV od for 3 days
- Rule out potentially treatable medical emergencies such as a myocardial infarction, hypoxia, metabolic crises or haemorrhage by reviewing the recent history, examining the patient and carrying out appropriate investigations.

Subsequent management

- Identify the precipitating factors, remove them or ameliorate their effects. Almost any acute medical or surgical condition can trigger an episode of delirium, as well as many medications (especially opioids, steroids, and benzodiazepines).
- Medications should be rationalized to prevent high dose polypharmacy. Swapping opioids can be a useful strategy for opioid-related delirium.
- Identify any potential protecting factors and initiate or enhance them, such as providing treatment in a familiar, quiet, unambiguous environment with key staff and family rather than many different people. Calm, frequent reassurance, and reorientation is critical.
- Consider regular medication until the delirium is fully resolved (e.g. haloperidol 0.5–10 mg bd, lower doses in the elderly). Haloperidol is relatively contraindicated in Parkinsonism or other extrapyramidal syndromes (EPS). In children or adolescents it can cause an acute dystonia or oculogyric crisis. However, since anticholinergic drugs can worsen delirium, benzatropine (1–2 mg) or procyclidine (2.5–5 mg) should only be given if such complications occur. Risperidone or quetiapine may be used as alternatives to haloperidol, with a lesser risk of EPS.
- In hypoactive delirium, there may be no need for medication because these medicines do not treat the underlying delirium, rather they reduce distressing symptoms.
- Distressing terminal delirium may be treated with haloperidol, midazolam and levomepromazine delivered subcutaneously in divided doses or via an infusion pump (see The distressed dying patient ⏢ p30).
- Provide education and support for the patient and their carers.

Special considerations

- Be alert for patients with hypoactive delirium. Although they may not need medication to reduce agitation they still need investigation for an underlying cause and appropriate treatment.
- Delirium can persist for days or weeks after the trigger is removed.
- Missing or minimizing delirium in the presence of pre-morbid dementia.
- Misdiagnosing dementia when there is no such syndrome.
- Misdiagnosing challenging behaviour from other causes such as that related to intellectual impairment, autism or other psychiatric illness; behaviour related to extremes of coping; or because cultural barriers exacerbate clinical misinterpretation.

Further reading

Breitbart, W. and Cohen, K.R. (1998) Delirium. In: Holland, J.C. (ed.) *Psycho-oncology*, Chapter 48: 564–575. New York: Oxford University Press.

Breitbart, W. and Cohen, K.R. (2000) Delirium in the terminally ill. In: Chochinov, H.M. and Breitbart, W. (eds). *Handbook of Psychiatry in Palliative Medicine*, Chapter 6: 75–90. New York: Oxford University Press.

Wasan, A.D., Artamonov, M. and Nedeljkovic, S.S. (2004). Delirium, depression, and anxiety in the treatment of cancer pain. *Techniques in Regional Anesthesia & Pain Management* **9**(3): 139–144.

⑦ Anxiety

Anxiety is part of the human condition, a combination of frightening or worrying thoughts, the bodily sensations that go with them, and perhaps a 'feeling' element that is more than the sum of these parts. The heart of anxiety is a response to a perceived threat. When anxiety disturbs patients' abilities to conduct their lives in the way that they might normally wish or that others deem normal, it is pathological. Different manifestations of anxiety can give rise to panic, treatment refusal or other emergencies in oncology.

Presentation

Panic

Panic has a relatively acute onset, with severe somatic manifestations of anxiety exacerbated by hyperventilation:

- Dyspnoea
- Chest tightness
- Awareness of tachycardia
- Paraesthesiae of the digits or peri-orally
- Nausea or awareness of gastrointestinal hyperactivity
- Visual changes
- Pre-syncope or light-headedness
- Tremor
- Urgency (or incontinence) of bowel or bladder

The patient may not be aware of the trigger; for example, a bodily sensation (e.g. a palpitation) or a thought (e.g. imagining one's death) rather than an external stimulus such as entering an MRI scanner. The subjective experience is feeling out of control with an intense need to escape the situation that is associated with the panic. There is often a non-specific sense of impending doom or a specific conviction that one is dying, for example, from a heart attack. Panic arises in oncology because of the intensity of thoughts about death or harm that the cancers can give rise to, unpleasant physical symptoms of the cancers or treatments, and because the other emotional and psychiatric difficulties that can arise in cancer increase the propensity for anxiety. Direct cancer-related panic is very rare (NB. phaeochromocytoma).

Specific phobias (e.g. needle phobia)

Phobias typically give rise to panic if the trigger stimulus is present. They give rise to significant avoidance of the trigger(s) and often troublesome generalized worry in other settings. For oncology patients, fear of necessary procedures (e.g. bone marrow aspirates, blood tests) gives rise to a particular set of management problems. This is especially common in children, possibly because they are cognitively less able to respond to imagined or real harm with rationalization.

Social phobia and agoraphobia

Syndromes of phobic avoidance of social contact can arise in various anxiety disorders, especially fears centred upon aspects of social contact itself (such as concerns about being scrutinized by others) and agoraphobia (fearful avoidance of any situation in which it is conceivable that one might panic). When severe, these can prevent cancer patients attending for treatment and follow up appointments.

Generalized anxiety

Chronic severe worry, either relatively unfocused or specific to physical illness and symptoms (somatoform), has a marked disabling effect. This occurs frequently with depression (both as a cause and as an effect of depression) and impairs patients' decision-making capacity and motivation for difficult treatments. Generalized anxiety will seldom lead to a true emergency without other symptoms such as suicidal ideation. A particular situation of which to be aware is the pulmonary embolus presenting as sudden-onset generalized anxiety with incomplete features of panic.

Immediate management

Panic

- Attempt to calm the person with reassurance in a quiet and private environment. A familiar person will be more effective (e.g. a key nurse or a family member).
- Encourage the person to breathe more slowly (count out breaths with them) and relax their shoulders.
- Do not give oxygen.
- Breathing into a paper bag. This also helps the patient to focus on something other than the reinforcing physical symptoms of panic and their panicky thoughts.
- Tell the patient what is happening. A diagnosis of panic can be very reassuring to a patient who is convinced they are dying from a myocardial infarction.
- If the panic does not respond to the above measures after a few minutes, give a short-acting potent benzodiazepine, e.g. lorazepam 2 mg PO or IM. Repeat as necessary after 30 minutes; adjust the dose for the young, old or those in renal failure. Longer acting agents such as clonazepam may be considered if the anti-panic effect is desired for many hours.
- For very severe panic associated with more significant behavioural problems such as violence or dissociative symptoms (e.g. hallucinations or altered levels of consciousness), the threshold for using medicine at reasonable doses is lower, and combination with an antipsychotic may be considered (see Delirium 🕮 p304).

Treatment refusal

The keys to managing anxious refusal for treatments that are felt to be necessary are to avoid recrimination, defer the intervention, and deal with the underlying problem as soon as possible. In this way, the patient does not feel coerced or ignored, increasing their sense of control and thus the possibility that they can accept treatment in the future. Early treatment may also forestall a cycle of escalating anxiety. Incompetence to reject treatment on the basis of anxiety alone would be a very unusual situation indeed and should not be invoked as a rationale for treating forcibly without serious consideration and senior input, usually including a psychiatrist (see The Mental Capacity Act 2005 📖 p406).

Subsequent management

- The key to subsequent management is to take a careful history to attempt to understand fully why the patient is experiencing the particular symptom of concern at the current time. With anxiety the hidden triggers of thoughts and bodily sensations are peculiar to the individual and only once these have been elucidated can appropriate management be undertaken.
- Unrelieved pain is a significant trigger for anxiety in the context of cancer, highlighting the need for optimum pain control in cancer patients.
- Anxiety secondary to the dyspnoea of respiratory failure in patients with terminal cancer can respond well to opioid drugs.
- Rule out other psychiatric disorders that could be lowering the threshold for anxiety and treat as appropriate:
  - Depression
  - Substance withdrawal (nicotine, alcohol, benzodiazepines, antidepressants)
  - Cognitive impairment
- Psychotherapy, particularly cognitive behaviour therapy, is frequently effective for the anxiety disorders mentioned above.
- Relaxation training or progressive muscle relaxation is a specific intervention that can be coupled with breathing training, music, meditation, and imagery techniques to enhance patients' mastery over their anxiety symptoms.
- Longer term treatment with a benzodiazepine (with longer acting compounds, e.g. clonazepam or diazepam) and/or an antidepressant (e.g. SSRI, TCA) may be warranted. A specialist opinion may be useful if these treatments are being considered in the absence of depression.
- Reconsider the oncology-related treatment being offered in case there are realistic alternative treatments (e.g. chemotherapeutic agents with more tolerable side effect profiles for the patient) or delivery methods (e.g. surgery under GA rather than regional or local anaesthesia).

Special considerations

- Needle phobia
  - The gold standard treatment for a specific phobia is systematic desensitization (e.g. to needles, blood) in a supportive therapeutic space and at a pace that does not exceed the patient's capacity to tolerate the anxiety generated.
  - Management must also focus on the particular symptom of hypotensive syncope that is a hallmark of this condition.
  - Psychologists are adept at tailoring such treatments to the situation and individual involved, and should be approached at an early stage for assistance.

- Post-traumatic stress disorder can follow experiences that a patient has found to be particularly traumatic. Symptoms of sleep disturbance, flashbacks, numbing, and lowered mood should signal the need for closer enquiry and referral on as required.
- Acute, disabling but transient anxiety may be termed an 'acute anxious adjustment reaction' and is usually best thought of as an extreme of normal coping. However, it must be watched because it may become pathological and therefore associated with the risks covered above.
- Anticipatory anxiety, as well as anticipatory nausea and vomiting, are common in the context of chemotherapy. This responds well to lorazepam 1–2 mg PO taken before the patient attends for treatment and also responds to psychotherapy. This anticipatory anxiety can also generalize beyond the specific setting of chemotherapy to any visit to hospital, with the resultant impact on the wellbeing and care for the patient.

Further reading

Acierno, R.E., Herson, M. and Van Hasselt, V.B. (1993). Interventions for panic disorder: a critical review of the literature. *Clin. Psychol. Rev.* **13**: 561–578.

Payne D.K. and Massie, M.J. (2000). Anxiety in palliative care. In: Chochinov, H.M. and Breitbart, W. (eds) *Handbook of Psychiatry in Palliative Medicine*, Chapter 5: 63–74. New York: Oxford University Press.

Noyes, R., Holt, C. and Massie, M.J. (1998). Anxiety disorders. In: Holland, J.C. (ed.) *Psycho-oncology*. Chapter 47: 548–563. New York: Oxford University Press.

⑦ **Depression**

Depression is a syndrome of low mood that occurs most of the day for most days for at least 2 weeks, and is severe enough to significantly impair a person's ability to function normally and impairs their quality of life.

Depression is relatively common for patients with cancer and particularly common following certain oncology treatments, e.g. formation of a colostomy, disfigurement following head and neck surgery, infertility following chemotherapy.

In oncology depression is important as it:
- Disturbs the patient's ability to participate in, and adhere to, treatment, e.g. treatment refusal, lowering motivation for treatment or reducing physical or emotional tolerance for difficult treatments.
- Is associated with poorer cancer outcomes, e.g. worse pain tolerance, increased handicap for particular disabilities.
- Carries its own morbidity/mortality, e.g. poor nutritional state, suicide.
- Causes significant suffering and distress for patients and their families.

Sudden onset depressed mood in the context of a crisis can be associated with significant risk or suffering, and is termed an 'acute depressive adjustment reaction'.

Clinical features
Cardinal symptoms
- Subjective lowered mood with predominant feelings of sadness, irritability, anxiety, guilt, jealousy and/or hopelessness, and an inability to experience pleasure.
- Pervasive negative thoughts about oneself, others or the world at large, and the future (Beck's 'cognitive triad of depression').
- Suicidal ideation, from fleeting thoughts to full intent with planning.
- Lowered motivation and impaired self-care.
- In melancholic depression, slowed thinking, slowed and attenuated behaviour (including speech and all movements), poor sleep with early morning wakening, tiredness and low energy, diurnal variation (mornings typically worst), and poor appetite with weight loss.
- In psychotic depression, auditory or other hallucinations may occur, typically accompanied by mood-congruent delusions, including persecutory, nihilistic, guilty or hypochondriacal delusions.
- In agitated depression, restlessness with marked anxiety and other negative emotional states predominates.
- In atypical depression, excessive sleeping and increased eating may be present.

Diagnosis
A core challenge in oncology is to detect depression in the first place. Depression's biological symptoms, e.g. poor sleep, tiredness, poor appetite with weight loss, may be duplicated or masked by the symptoms of the cancer and by its treatments, particularly for inpatients or people with terminal stage disease. Depression's emotional and cognitive symptoms

may also be present as part of normal coping or adjustment to various challenges during an individual's treatment journey.

A good screening question to ask patients is 'Are you depressed most of the time?'. This should be followed by a full history and mental status examination, placing relatively more weight upon the cognitive and affective symptoms rather than the biological symptoms (unless their time course fits a depression better than the underlying cancer or its treatment). Also ask colleagues involved in the patient's care whether they think that the patient is depressed. There will always be difficult cases that require specialist review.

Besides a suggestive symptoms list, the time course, symptom pervasiveness and impact upon functioning and quality of life are key features that not only help to delineate a clinical major depressive episode from other causes of lowered mood but also help to guide management.

Investigations
Bloods
- FBC
  - occult subacute infection
  - anaemia
- TFTs
  - hypothyroidism
  - thyrotoxicosis
- Ca^{2+}
  - hypercalcaemia

Imaging
- CT head/MRI brain
  - white matter disease
  - metastasis

Risk factors
Cancer factors
- More severe disability
- Certain cancers, especially pancreatic
- Cerebral tumours or tumour-related infarction/anoxia, especially in frontal regions
- Diagnosis phase, relapse of cancer, terminal phase
- Cachexia

Patient factors
- Previous depression
- Family history of depression
- History of generalized coping difficulties
- Particular dread of cancer or disability in general
- Other psychiatric illness, e.g. substance misuse, personality disorder

Treatment factors
- Treatment resistance in respect of current or previous depression
- Certain oncology drugs, especially steroids, interferon, tamoxifen
- Infertility
- Disfigurement, especially to the head and neck
- Treatment-resistant pain

Immediate management

Some manifestations of depression do require immediate management. Psychotic depression can lead to other emergencies and is dealt with elsewhere (see Psychosis 🕮 p318).

Suicidal ideation

- Assess suicide risk
  - Severity and frequency of suicidal thoughts
  - Presence of definite suicide plans
  - History of psychiatric disorder or previous suicide attempts
  - Substance misuse
  - Lack of social support
- Identify factors that heighten and lower suicide risk for this person
- Build up the best therapeutic alliance possible to deal with this risk
- Collaboratively decide upon the best setting to manage the risk, e.g. at home, compulsory admission to a psychiatric ward; and the level of monitoring necessary, e.g. community psychiatric nurse input, 24-hour one-to-one nursing.
- Agree upon supports that can be put in place to assist the person and mobilize protective factors and coping resources
- Remove potential means of suicide; consider the toxic potential of all prescribed medication
- Decide upon treatment for underlying low mood
- Instill hope
- Treat underlying severe agitation, anxiety (see Anxiety 🕮 p308) or psychosis (see Psychosis 🕮 p318) that may be impacting upon risk, as well as any medical factors that may be raising risk, such as pain or delirium (see Delirium 🕮 p304)
- ECT may be indicated for depression associated with morbid suicidal ideation and high, unremitting risk of death that is difficult to contain

Treatment refusal

- Not all treatment refusals are an emergency or reflect an incompetent decision, even in the context of depressed mood.
- The key is to establish the patient's level of competency to refuse treatment. Listening, discussing, and reflecting enables you to understand respectfully what the patient is thinking and why. Specialist help may be required to assist in capacity assessments in which psychiatric illness seems to be present and interfering with thinking.
- Legally a competent patient must be able to:
  - Understand information about their condition and treatment
  - Remember this information
  - Deliberate about the therapeutic choices posed by the information
  - Believe that the information applies to them
- See The Mental Capacity Act 2005 🕮 p406.

Severe malnutrition
- Severe depression, especially melancholia, can lead to dehydration and serious weight loss as a result of failure to eat and drink. This may result from loss of appetite, loss of motivation, hopelessness, psychosis or a combination of factors. In the setting of cancer, a patient's medical risk factors for cachexia and their vulnerability to the negative effects of poor nutrition may be greatly heightened.
- Refeeding may require a range of measures, from encouragement and monitoring to nasogastric feeding. Metabolic indices, infection risk, bowel activity, renal function, and weight all require close monitoring.
- Treat any underlying agitation, anxiety (see Anxiety 📖 p308), psychosis (see Psychosis 📖 p318) or any medical factors that may be raising risk, e.g. pain.
- ECT may be indicated for depression associated with morbid cachexia.

Subsequent management
- Offer antidepressant therapy.
- If the patient has previously been treated for depression, use the agent that was effective.
- Otherwise, first line treatment should be with a:
  - Tricyclic antidepressant (TCA), e.g. amitriptyline
  - Selective serotonin re-uptake inhibitor (SSRI), e.g. fluoxetine
  - Serotonin norepinephrine re-uptake inhibitor (SNRI), e.g. venlafaxine
- Side effect profiles and pharmacokinetics should be matched to the patient and their current treatments.
- The highest tolerable dose within the standard therapeutic range should be achieved.
- A treatment trial should be at least 3 weeks. If there is no response and symptoms are severe, consider switching to an antidepressant from a different class. In less severe cases, waiting for a 6-week trial or increasing the dose could be considered.
- Consider psychotherapy of some kind, depending upon local availability, cost, severity of depression, and characteristics of the person and their depressive symptoms. Specialist help may be useful to recommend a therapy or therapist.
- Assist patients to mobilize their own coping resources and supports.
- Attend to the need for positive experiences for the patient in overall treatment, not just primary cancer-related treatment goals. This may lead to different weighting or time courses for oncology treatment options.
- Review risk of suicide and other depression-related harms regularly.

Special considerations

- The desire to die does not imply pathological suicidal ideation. Views about euthanasia and the right to die are diverse in society, probably more so among doctors. 'Rational suicide' may be a legitimate ending for some people's lives, although the law is fairly clear about the doctor's role in respect of this. In the UK, 'physician-assisted suicide' is illegal. What clinicians must do is listen.

- Death wishes are more common in periods of uncontrolled symptoms, from pain or vomiting to depressive symptoms themselves, and can change following good treatment, even in the end stages of terminal care.

- Self-limiting depressive adjustment reactions are relatively common compared with clinical depression, and are distinguished on the basis of a clear link to a stressor, short time course (less than 2 weeks) and often less pervasive symptoms. They may still be associated with significant risk from suicide when severe. They often occur relatively suddenly in the context of a crisis such as cancer diagnosis or treatment setbacks.

- 'Minor depression' and 'Dysthymia' are states that are also relatively common. These syndromes are less severe, less pervasive and present with a smaller number of symptoms. Duration is still lengthy and the impact upon a person's cancer treatment may still be significant. However, they are less likely to be associated with an emergency.

- Depression is often recurrent irrespective of the context, including with cancers of long duration and cancers in remission.

- End-stage terminal illness is frequently associated with significant depressive symptomatology. An antidepressant may not be indicated because of the lagtime of weeks before clinical efficacy. Psychostimulants have been successfully used for symptomatic relief of low energy and motivation, psychomotor retardation, and low mood. Trial methylphenidate 5 mg bd, increasing up to 20–30 mg per day as tolerated (monitor for arrhythmia, anorexia, delirium, and psychosis in particular). Benzodiazepines (e.g. midazolam, lorazepam) have a role for agitation, anxiety and sleeplessness, and antipsychotics (e.g. haloperidol) for psychosis, delirium, and agitation (as well as nausea and intractable hiccupping) (see The distressed dying patient 📖 p30).

Further reading

Block, S.D. (2000). Assessing and managing depression in the terminally ill patient *Ann. Intern. Med.* **132**: 209–218.

Chochinov, H.M. (2001). Depression in cancer patients. *Lancet Oncol* **2**: 499–505.

Lloyd-Williams, M., Spiller, J. and Ward, J. (2003). Which depression screening tools should be used in palliative care? *Palliat. Med.* **17**: 40–43.

ⓘ **Psychosis**

Psychosis is a syndrome of disorganized thinking and behaviour, delusions, hallucinations, and so-called 'negative symptoms' such as reduced speech or motivation.

Acute psychotic illness or psychotic symptoms are not common in oncology patients. When they do occur, the 'positive symptoms' cause alarm and raise the risk of adverse outcomes for the patient or others. There may be a heightened risk of suicide, violence, disruption to the medical care of the patient or others, and treatment refusal. Psychosis is often very frightening or distressing to the patient, their family and to other patients.

Presentation

Psychosis arises in four main ways in the context of cancer and its treatment.

- As a symptom of the cancer itself, e.g. cerebral tumours.
- As a side effect of treatment, e.g. following high dose steroid use.
- As part of another psychiatric syndrome, e.g. delirium (see Delirium 📖 p304), depression (see Depression 📖 p312).
- In the context of a pre-existing psychotic illness that is exacerbated by aspects of the cancer or its treatment, including psychosocial aspects.

Investigations

In acute psychosis of unexplained cause the main use of investigations is to identify reversible medical factors that may be precipitating or perpetuating a delirium (see Delirium 📖 p304).

Management

Immediate management

- Identify any acute risks and contain them with as much collaboration with the patient as possible, abiding by the protocols of the health provider. Treatment under Mental Health Act legislation may be necessary when compulsory treatment is required but should be invoked with the guidance of the duty psychiatry service (see Delirium 📖 p304).
- Reassurance and reorientation should routinely and explicitly become part of the management plan, offered by trusted staff or others known to the patient.
- An overstimulating environment is usually best avoided, either in hospital or at home – less activity, less change, less in the way of unfamiliar people. This does not mean ceasing to involve the patient in decisions about their treatment, but may change the manner in which treatment is offered.
- Antipsychotic medicine is indicated for troubling or dangerous symptoms. If acute control of behaviour is required, use a combination of an antipsychotic with a short-acting benzodiazepine, e.g. haloperidol 10 mg and lorazepam 2 mg (higher doses may be required than those used in delirium), parenterally if necessary (with appropriate consent or proper legal basis).

- Attempt to rule out delirium and psychosis due to depression or mania, as the presence of these conditions might alter management.
- Seek psychiatric help at an early stage if psychosis is giving rise to an emergency situation.

Subsequent management

- Seek psychiatric help to clarify the diagnosis and fine-tune medium and longer term treatment with psychiatric medicine and other treatment approaches.
- Never lose sight of the fact that psychosis is usually extremely distressing for the patient at a time when their resources are needed for coping with their cancer and its treatment.
- The aims of subsequent treatment are to relieve suffering, manage risks, achieve remission from the psychosis, and monitor for relapse or the presence of factors associated with relapse so as to enable early treatment.
- Psychotic depression is a particular indication for ECT, especially in the elderly, as it is particularly effective and rapidly acting for this condition.

Special considerations

- Not all psychosis constitutes an emergency, especially transient relatively mild psychotic symptoms related to phases in treatment, such as over-valued grandiose ideas at peaks of steroid use. However, psychosis does indicate significant brain malfunction and should be regarded as a sentinel symptom for close observation in case severity, suffering or risks escalate.
- In the terminal phase, delirium and attendant psychosis are very common and may be treated with haloperidol, midazolam and levomepromazine delivered subcutaneously in divided doses or via an infusion pump (see The distressed dying patient 📖 p30).

Dermatological emergencies

⑦ **Paraneoplastic pemphigus**

The pemphigus family of skin disorders is a collection of autoimmune blistering conditions affecting the skin and/or mucous membranes. Paraneoplastic pemphigus occurs in patients with a known or occult neoplasm. It is a very rare phenomenon associated with autoantibodies to various antigens contained in desmosomes and hemi-desmosomes. The antibodies attack the desmosomes of keratinocytes via a type II hypersensitivity reaction, causing them to separate. The gaps between the cells then fill with fluid, causing the skin to blister or peel off, leaving raw areas. Treatment of an underlying malignancy does not appear to affect the outcome, but treatment of benign conditions (e.g. thymoma) can lead to resolution.

Conditions associated with paraneoplastic pemphigus
- Non-Hodgkin's lymphoma
- Giant cell lymphoma
- Chronic lymphocytic leukaemia
- Waldenström's macroglobulinaemia
- Poorly differentiated sarcoma
- Follicular dendritic cell sarcoma
- Bronchogenic squamous cell carcinoma
- Castleman's disease
- Thymoma

Clinical features
- Painful, denuded areas of mouth, lips, throat, and skin
- Other mucosal surfaces may also be affected
  - nose
  - genitals
  - respiratory membranes
  - intestinal membranes
- Skin lesions can be very variable in appearance
  - diffuse erythema
  - scaly plaques
  - papules
  - fluid-filled blisters
  - erosions
  - ulcerative lesions
- Skin involvement can be widespread and variable
  - palms and soles may be affected
- Large areas of denudation with a positive Nikolsky's sign may occur
- Some patients complain of pruritus
- Eye involvement may also occur
  - conjunctivitis

Differential diagnosis
- Pemphigus vulgaris
- Erythema multiforme
- Bullous pemphigoid
- Cicatricial pemphigoid
- Lichen planus
- Drug eruptions
- Stevens-Johnson syndrome and toxic epidermal necrolysis
- Epidermolysis bullosa/bullosa acquisita

Investigations
- Skin biopsy
  - from fresh blister and perilesional skin
  - this may show
    - acantholysis — keratinocyte necrosis/dyskeratosis
    - interface dermatitis
  - direct immunofluorescence reveals antibodies and complement (C3) within the intercellular spaces and at the basement membrane
- Circulating immunoglobulins specific for stratified squamous or transitional epithelium can also be detected by indirect immunofluorescence and immunoprecipitation analysis
- If the patient is not known to have an underlying neoplasm, then diagnosis of paraneoplastic pemphigus may prompt the search for such a condition

Management
General measures
- Skin care
  - daily examination for new lesions
  - aspiration of intact blisters
  - non-adherent dressings
  - nursing on a suitable bed
- Prevention and treatment of supra-added infection
  - antibacterial washes and emollients
- Prophylactic LMWH for immobile patients
- Monitor fluid and electrolyte balance carefully

Systemic treatments
Seek specialist dermatological advice.
- High dose prednisolone 80–100 mg PO od
- Cyclophosphamide
- Alemtuzumab or Rituximab
- Intravenous immunoglobulins
- Plasmapheresis

Complications
- Involve appropriate specialists at the earliest opportunity
  - ophthalmologist
  - otolaryngologist
  - respiratory physician
  - gastroenterologist

Prognosis
Between 75 and 80% of patients die as a consequence of the paraneoplastic pemphigus or their underlying cancer. Involvement of the respiratory or gastrointestinal mucosa and secondary sepsis significantly increases the chance of death from the condition itself.

Further reading

Anhalt, G.J., Kim, S.C., Stanley, J.R., Korman, N.J., Jabs, D.A., Kory, M., Izumi, H., Ratrie, H., Mutasim, D., Ariss-Abdo, L. *et al.* (1990). Paraneoplastic pemphigus. An autoimmune mucocutaneous disease associated with neoplasia. *N. Engl. J. Med.* **323**: 1729–1735.

Joly, P., Richard, C., Gilbert, D., Courville, P., Chosidow, O. Roujeau J.C., Beylot-Barry, M., D'Incan, M., Martel, P., Lauret, P. and Tron F. (2000). Sensitivity and specificity of clinical, histologic, and immunologic features in the diagnosis of paraneoplastic pemphigus. *J. Am. Acad. Dermatol.* **43**: 619–626.

Chemotherapy-related emergencies

:O: Infections in the neutropenic patient

Neutropenia and infection are major dose-limiting side effects of chemotherapy. The risk of initial infection and subsequent complications is directly related to the severity and duration of neutropenia (see Table 12.1), which is dependent on the intensity of the chemotherapy regimen.

All patients should be advised to consider themselves at risk from neutropenia from day 1 of their first cycle of chemotherapy until 4–6 weeks after their last cycle of chemotherapy. All patients must be advised of the risk of neutropenic fever and be encouraged to report any fevers or symptoms of infection via a 24-hour telephone contact number.

A number of host- and disease-related factors may also influence the risks from neutropenia in the patient receiving chemotherapy. High risk features include:
- expected prolonged (>10 days) neutropenia
- profound (<0.1×10^9/l) neutropenia
- age >65 years
- uncontrolled primary disease
- pneumonia
- hypotension
- multi-organ dysfunction
- invasive fungal infection
- being hospitalized at the time of the development of fever

Febrile neutropenia

ANC <0.5 ×10^9/l or <1.0 ×10^9/l and expected to fall.
AND

Temperature ≥38.0°C on two separate occasions >1 hour apart or one reading ≥38.5°C (temperature >37.5°C in any bone marrow transplant patient).

Neutropenic sepsis is a medical emergency requiring prompt treatment (IV antibiotics within 30 minutes of presentation) and can progress within hours to shock and death.

Clinical features

Have a low threshold for suspecting febrile neutropenia in anyone who has had chemotherapy within the last 4–6 weeks.

Symptoms
- General deterioration and non-specific symptoms (e.g. confusion in the elderly)
- Rigors
- Cough
- Sore throat
- Diarrhoea
- Central venous access device
  - soreness
- Dysuria
- Skin lesions
- Perianal pain

  - discharge

Table 12.1 Risk of infection is related to absolute neutrophil count (ANC)

Neutrophil count (x10^9/l)	Risk of life-threatening infection
1.0	10%
0.5	19%
0.1	28%

Signs
- Pyrexia
  - may be absent or mild
- Hypotension (SBP <100 mmHg)
- Tachycardia (HR >100 bpm)
- Tachypnoea (RR >30 bpm)
- Hypoxia
- Peripherally shut down
- Focus of infection
  - central venous access device
  - intravenous cannula
  - throat
  - chest
  - abdomen
  - perianal area
  - skin lesions

Investigations
Bloods
- FBC
  - to confirm neutropenia, thrombocytopenia, anaemia
  - should be repeated daily until ANC >1.0 x10^9/l
- U&Es and LFTs
- CRP
- Coagulation screen
- Blood cultures
  - central (from each lumen)
  - peripheral
- Avoid ABG if patient may be thrombocytopenic

ECG
- If cardiac co-morbidity

Urine, stool, sputum
- Urine MC&S if dysuria
- Sputum MC&S if productive cough
- Stool MC&S and *Clostridium difficile* toxin if diarrhoea

Imaging
- CXR
  - urgent if respiratory signs or hypoxia

Management

Many patients developing neutropenic sepsis will be receiving potentially curative high dose chemotherapy and therefore should be aggressively managed, with ICU admission if required.

- O₂ as required
- Intravenous access
- Aggressive fluid resuscitation to maintain circulatory volume
  - Aim for UO >0.5 ml/kg/hour do not catheterize unless absolutely required for monitoring of fluid balance;
- Treatment with antibiotics should be commenced within 30 minutes of presentation, without waiting for confirmation of neutropenia, if the patient is:
  - Hypotensive (SBP <100 mmHg)
  - Tachycardic (HR >100 bpm)
  - Febrile ≥38.0°C (within 4 weeks of a course of cytotoxic chemotherapy)
  - Clinically unwell even in the absence of fever
- Monitor observations hourly until clinically stable, then 4-hourly
  - Temperature
  - Blood pressure
  - Pulse
  - Respiratory rate
  - O₂ saturation
  - Urine output

Antibiotics

Chemotherapy and radiotherapy damage the membranes of the oropharynx, GI tract and lung, and thereby allow predominantly Gram-negative organisms to enter the systemic circulation more readily.

Every hospital trust should have a 'Neutropenic Sepsis Policy', and local protocol should be followed.

- First line antibiotics
  - Meropenem IV 1000 mg every 8 hours (2 g tds if CNS infection suspected) + gentamicin IV 7 mg/kg od
    — the dose of gentamicin may need to be reduced or omitted in patients with significant renal impairment
  - Alternatives to meropenem + gentamicin
    — Tazocin IV 4.5 g qds + gentamicin IV 7 mg/kg od
    — Ceftazidime IV 1 g tds
      – 2 g tds if CNS infection suspected
      – dose must be reduced if renal impairment is present
      – may be indicated in patients at risk of renal impairment owing to current treatment with cisplatin or ifosfamide chemotherapy, as high dose gentamicin is not required
  - Vancomycin IV 1 g bd should be used as part of the initial antibiotic regime if the patient:
    — has an obvious catheter-related infection
      – rigors on flushing line
      – red and tender exit site
    — is known to be MRSA-positive
    — is in an institution where frequent *viridans streptococci* are found

- Alternative if allergic to vancomycin
  — Teicoplanin IV (400 mg bd for first 36 hours, then 400 mg od)
    – can also be considered for patients being treated at home
      • once daily dosing   • no dose monitoring
- Consider the addition of metronidazole IV 500 mg tds if the
  patient has:
  — diarrhoea   — abdominal pain
  — perianal sepsis   — dental/sinus infection
- Second line antibiotics and antifungals
  - Culture results are positive (only about 33%)
    — If a causative organism has been identified, modify antibiotic
      therapy as appropriate and continue use of broad spectrum
      antibiotics for at least 7 days
  - Patient remains unwell or febrile after 48 hours of IV antibiotics and
    blood culture results are negative
    — Repeat blood cultures each time patient spikes a fever
    — Discuss with microbiology team
    — Consider adding vancomycin 1 g IV bd for patients with a high
      probability of line infection
    — Consider starting antifungal treatment after 72 hours in patients
      who have:
      – been heavily pre-treated with chemotherapy
      – been neutropenic >14 days
      – had a previous suspected fungal infection
      – CXR infiltrates developed while on antibiotics
    — Antifungal treatment
      – amphotericin B
      – liposomal amphotericin B
      – voriconazole
      – caspofungin
    — Fungal infections
      – usually *Candida* or *Aspergillus*
      – have a high mortality if not treated early and effectively
      – very rarely isolated from blood cultures, some centres are
        using PCR to detect fungal antigens in the peripheral blood;
        however, antifungal therapy is usually commenced empirically
        after failure to respond to antibiotics
  - Patient becomes afebrile for >48 hours, and blood culture results
    are negative.
    — Consider changing to ciprofloxacin PO 500 mg bd for 7 days
    — Discharge may be considered when the neutrophil count is
      rising
- Antibiotic levels
  - Blood sample should be taken immediately before next dose is
    given (trough level)
  - If renal function is abnormal or previous levels have been raised,
    await result before giving antibiotic, otherwise give antibiotic once
    sample is obtained

- Serum levels should be checked
  - before every 5th dose
  - before every 3rd dose
    - if renal function is poor
    - previous levels have been raised
- Gentamicin levels are not required for standard first line treatment; if gentamicin is continued beyond two doses then monitoring of levels should be carried out
- Normal trough levels
  - Gentamicin <2 mg/l
  - Vancomycin 5–10 mg/l

Trials are ongoing to identify whether patients with low risk febrile neutropenia can be managed with oral antibiotics and early hospital discharge (ORANGE Trial).

Low risk febrile neutropenia can be defined according to a score ≥21 points on the Multinational Association for Supportive Care in Cancer (MASCC) index (see Table 12.2).

G-CSF
G-CSF in febrile neutropenia
- G-CSF should not routinely be used as adjunctive treatment with antibiotic therapy for patients with fever and neutropenia
- G-CSF should be considered in patients with fever and neutropenia
  - who are at high risk for infection-associated complications
  - have prognostic factors that are predictive of poor clinical outcomes
- High risk features include:
  - expected prolonged (>10 days) neutropenia
  - profound (<0.1×10^9/l) neutropenia
  - age >65 years
  - uncontrolled primary disease
  - pneumonia
  - hypotension
  - multi-organ dysfunction
  - invasive fungal infection
  - being hospitalized at the time of the development of fever
- G-CSF should be continued until reaching an absolute neutrophil count (ANC) of >1.5×10^9/l
- Doses
  - Filgrastim
    - 500 000 U/kg (5 g/kg) od SC
    - use prefilled syringe
      - 30×10^6 U (300 g)
      - 48×10^6 U (480 g)
  - Lenograstim
    - 19.2×10^6 units/m^2 od SC
    - <2 m^2: 33.6×10^6 unit (263 g) vial
    - >2 m^2: 13.4×10^6 unit (105 g) and 33.6×10^6 unit (263 g) vials

G-CSF in afebrile neutropenia
- G-CSF should not routinely be used for patients with neutropenia who are afebrile

G-CSF in primary prophylaxis
- Prevention of febrile neutropenia in patients with a >20% risk of febrile neutropenia, being treated with curative intent
- Risk of febrile neutropenia depends on a wide range of factors
  - Age
    — the risk of neutropenia following chemotherapy increases with age, consider chemotherapy dose reductions in older patients;
  - Conditions potentially enhancing the risk of serious infection:
    — poor performance status
    — poor nutritional status
    — the presence of open wounds
    — active infections
  - Disease characteristics
    — bone marrow compromise owing to involvement by tumour
    — extensive prior treatment
      - previous irradiation to the pelvis or other areas containing large amounts of bone marrow
      - history of recurrent febrile neutropenia while receiving earlier chemotherapy of similar or lesser dose intensity
    — advanced cancer
  - Myelotoxicity of the chemotherapy regimen
    — most commonly used regimens have a <20% risk of febrile neutropenia
    — high dose ifosfamide (>12 g/m^2)
    — BEP chemotherapy with etoposide doses of 166 mg/m^2 daily for 3 days
    — when available, alternative regimens offering equivalent efficacy, but not requiring G-CSF support, should be utilized

Table 12.2 MASCC index

Characteristic		Score
Burden of illness/symptoms	none or mild	5
	moderate	3
No hypotension		5
No COPD		4
Solid tumour/lymphoma or no previous fungal infection		4
No dehydration		3
Outpatient status at onset of fever		3
Age <60 years		2
Maximum possible score		**26**

- Dose-dense regimens
  — use of G-CSF allows a modest increase in dose density of
     chemotherapy regimens. Available data would suggest a survival
     benefit from the use of dose-dense regimens with G-CSF
     support in a few specific settings
    – node-positive breast cancer (TAC or FEC$_{100}$)
    – possibly non-Hodgkin's lymphoma
  — however, additional data in these settings are needed and these
     results cannot be generalized to other disease settings and
     regimens
  — many clinical trial protocols include G-CSF within the treatment
     regimen

G-CSF in secondary prophylaxis
- G-CSF is recommended for patients who experienced a neutropenic
  complication from a prior cycle of chemotherapy, in which a reduced
  dose may compromise disease-free or overall survival or treatment
  outcome
  - Examples of conditions that need to be treated on time without
    dose reductions to maximize potential cure are:
    — germ cell tumours
    — adjuvant breast cancer patients
    — lymphoma
    — Ewing's sarcoma
- In many clinical situations, dose reduction or delay may be a
  reasonable alternative (e.g. palliative treatment), as there is no
  evidence that dose maintenance or escalation improves clinically
  important outcomes
- Secondary prophylaxis results in:
  - fewer episodes of hospitalization for febrile neutropenia
  - greater dose intensity
  - but there is no evidence for improvement in:
    — survival   — toxicity
    — quality of life   — cost

G-CSF initiation, dosing, and duration
- G-CSF as prophylaxis should be given for 7–10 days, starting
  24–72 hours after the administration of myelotoxic chemotherapy
- G-CSF should be stopped at least 24 hours prior to any subsequent
  cycle of chemotherapy
- Doses
  - Filgrastim (see G-CSF in febrile neutropenia)
  - Lenograstim (see G-CSF in febrile neutropenia)
  - Pegfilgrastim
    — 6 mg SC single dose given 24 hours after completion of
       chemotherapy
    — Should not be used in patients <18 years or patients <45 kg

G-CSF prophylaxis in radiotherapy
- G-CSF should be avoided in patients receiving concomitant chemo-radiotherapy, particularly involving the mediastinum
- G-CSF may be considered in patients receiving radiotherapy alone if prolonged delays secondary to neutropenia are expected (rarely occurs)

Further reading

Klastersky, J., Paesmans, M., Georgala, A., Muanza, F., Plehiers, B., Dubreucq, L., Lalami, Y., Aoun, M. and Barette, M. (2006). Outpatient oral antibiotics for febrile neutropenic cancer patients using a score predictive for complications. *J. Clin. Oncol.* **24**: 4129–4134.

Smith, T.J., Khatcheressian, J., Lyman, G.H., Ozer, H., Armitage, J.O., Balducci, L., Bennett, C.L., Cantor, S.B., Crawford, J., Cross, S.J., Demetri, G., Desch, C.E., Pizzo, P.A., Schiffer, C.A., Schwartzberg, L., Somerfield, M.R., Somlo, G., Wade, J.C., Wade, J.L., Winn, R.J., Wozniak, A.J. and Wolff, A.C. (2006). 2006 Update of recommendations for the use of white blood cell growth factors: an evidence-based clinical practice guideline. *J. Clin. Oncol.* **24**(19): 1–19.

① Infections in the non-neutropenic patient

Infection can be a common occurrence in the cancer patient even in the absence of neutropenia and myelosuppression.

The reasons for this are multifactorial and include:
- Co-morbidity
  - Smoking
  - Alcohol
  - COPD
- Cancer factors
  - Cancer cachexia
  - Obstructing lesions
    - bronchial carcinoma
      - distal collapse/consolidation
    - bladder/prostate carcinoma
      - bladder outflow obstruction → UTI and pyelonephritis
    - cholangiocarcinoma/pancreatic carcinoma
      - ascending cholangitis
  - Disruption of local environment, enabling port of entry for pathogens
  - Impaired host defences
    - lymphoma
    - immunoparesis from myeloma
    - bone marrow infiltration by solid tumour
- Treatment factors
  - Steroids
    - immunosuppression
    - fungal infection
      - candidiasis
        - oral
        - oesophageal
        - vaginal
  - Disruption of normal mucosal barriers following treatment
    - chemotherapy
    - radiotherapy
  - Antibiotic therapy
    - risk of *Clostridium difficile* after any antibiotic, especially
      - cefuroxime
      - clindamycin
      - ciprofloxacin
    - antibiotic-resistant bacterial strains following prolonged antibiotic therapy
      - MRSA
      - VRE
    - candidiasis
      - oral
      - oesophageal
      - vaginal
  - Infected indwelling catheter/stent
    - central venous access device
    - Ommaya reservoir/shunt
    - urinary catheter
    - biliary stent
    - nephrostomy
    - ureteric stent

Infected central venous access devices (CVADs)

A large proportion of cancer patients now receive chemotherapy treatment through CVADs (Hickman, PICC, Groshong, Portocath). Cancer patients are at increased risk of infection, due to their disease and its treatment, and many of these infections are related to their CVADs.

Clinical features
- Pain and tenderness
  - at the site of insertion
  - proximally over vein/tunnelled line
- Swelling
- Erythema
- Discharge at site of insertion
- Pyrexia
- Rigors
  - within 30 minutes of flushing line
- Some patients develop some swelling, erythema, and tenderness around the insertion site within the first few days of insertion because of mechanical phlebitis, this will usually settle with anti-inflammatory drugs

Investigations
Bloods
- FBC
- Blood cultures
  - from all lumens of the CVAD
  - peripherally

Swab exit site if discharge present

Management
Antibiotics and removal of the CVAD device is the most successful management for eradicating the infection. Occasionally treatment with antibiotics alone may salvage the CVAD. Senior advice should be sought prior to removal of any CVAD.

Organisms
- Commonly Gram-positive cocci
- Skin commensals
  - Coagulase-negative *Staphylococci*
  - Diphtheroids
  - Blood cultures must be repeated prior to commencing antibiotics in patients with clinically non-infected CVADs and positive blood cultures growing commensals, to rule out contamination
- *Staphylococcus aureus*
  - Risk of metastatic complications
    — infective endocarditis
    — osteomyelitis
- *Enterococcus*

Antibiotics
- Until culture results are available
  - Vancomycin IV 1 g bd
  - Teicoplanin IV 400 mg bd for 36 hours, then 400 mg od
- If attempting to salvage CVAD, give antibiotics through the lumen(s) of the device
- When culture results are available, change to appropriate antibiotic
- Seek microbiology advice regarding length of treatment, according to
  - local protocol
  - whether CVAD has been removed
  - organism isolated
- Salvage is likely to fail if blood cultures remain positive 72 hours after commencing adequate antibiotics. Negative blood cultures must be documented prior to commencing further chemotherapy

Clostridium difficile infection
- Testing for *Clostridium difficile* toxin (CDT) should take place in all patients developing diarrhoea
  - within 2 months of a course of antibiotics
  - during an admission to hospital
- Proceed to an AXR if patient develops any signs of a systemic inflammatory response (~35%)
  - bowels open >6 times/day
  - HR > 90 bpm
  - temperature >37.5°C
- Discuss with gastroenterologist/colorectal surgeon/microbiologist if AXR reveals:
  - colonic diameter >5.5 cm
  - colonic mucosal oedema
- If CDT is positive, commence metronidazole PO 400 mg tds for 14 days
- In 20% of patients the diarrhoea will relapse after completion of metronidazole therapy
  - treat for a further 14–28 days with vancomycin PO 125 mg qds

Further reading

Tonna, I. and Welsby, P.D. (2005). Pathogenesis and treatment of *Clostridium difficile* infection. *Postgrad. Med. J.* **81**: 367–369.

① Myelosuppression

Cytotoxic chemotherapy targets rapidly dividing cells. The haematopoietic cells in the bone marrow are particularly susceptible, and virtually all chemotherapy regimens cause varying degrees of myelosuppression.

Different chemotherapy drugs have particular dispositions to target different cell lineages in the bone marrow, causing different patterns of myelosuppression (e.g. carboplatin commonly causes thrombocytopenia).

The average life span:
- red blood cell   120 days
- platelet   10 days
- white blood cell   1–2 days

This knowledge allows some prediction of the time course of anaemia, thrombocytopenia or leukopenia. However, some cytotoxic drugs can also caused delayed thrombocytopenia or leukopenia.

Anaemia
- Many patients receiving cytotoxic chemotherapy become anaemic
  - Multifactorial
    — absent nutritional stores
    — impaired marrow function
      – marrow infiltration by tumour
      – cumulative marrow suppression owing to previous treatment
    — anaemia of chronic disease
    — direct effect of current cytotoxic drug
  - Onset is usually insidious
- Particularly associated with:
  - Platinum chemotherapy
  - Cytarabine
  - Docetaxel
  - Paclitaxel
  - Topotecan

Causes, clinical features, investigation, and management
- See Anaemia 📖 p282

Thrombocytopenia
- Many patients receiving cytotoxic chemotherapy become thrombocytopenic
  - Particularly associated with:
    — Carboplatin
    — Mitomycin C
    — Dacarbazine
    — Lomustine
  - Delayed onset thrombocytopenia with a cumulative dose effect can occur with:
    — Mitomycin C
    — Fludarabine
    — Carmustine
    — Lomustine
    — Streptozocin

Causes, clinical features, investigation, and management
- See Thrombocytopenia 📖 p288

Leukopenia

- The most common cause of leukopenia in the cancer patient is that caused by current or previous cytotoxic chemotherapy; however, marrow infiltration by the cancer and other medications (e.g. carbimazole, clozapine, chlorpromazine, phenytoin) can also cause leukopenia.
- Neutrophils are particularly important in the host defence against bacterial and fungal infection, and therefore neutropenia is of most concern to the oncologist.
- Different chemotherapeutic agents cause differing degrees of myelosuppression, and therefore the risk and duration of neutropenia depends on the chemotherapy regime (i.e. the combination of chemotherapy drugs) as well as the doses given.
- The white cell count usually reaches a nadir 7–14 days post-chemotherapy, with recovery in a further 7–10 days. However, certain drugs commonly cause delayed neutropenia (up to 42 days post-chemotherapy).
  - Procarbazine
  - Mitomycin C
  - Carmustine
  - Lomustine
- Therefore all patients should be advised to consider themselves at risk from neutropenia from day 1 of their first cycle of chemotherapy until 4–6 weeks after their last cycle of chemotherapy. All patients must be advised of the risk of neutropenic fever and be encouraged to report any fevers or symptoms of infection via a 24-hour telephone contact number.
- Not all chemotherapy agents cause neutropenia, and therefore can, if necessary, still be given to a patient when they have become neutropenic.
  - Bleomycin
  - Vincristine
  - Tyrosine kinase inhibitors
    — Erlotinib (Tarceva)
    — Gefitinib (Iressa)
  - Monoclonal antibodies
    — Cetuximab (Erbitux)
    — Bevacizumab (Avastin)
    — Trastuzumab (Herceptin)
- Unlike anaemia and thrombocytopenia, uncomplicated leukopenia, however severe, does not always require treatment. A significant majority of patients receiving chemotherapy will become neutropenic between cycles, with no symptoms, and require no intervention. Neutropenia only becomes an important issue if the patient develops an infection (see Infections in the neutropenic patient p326).
- Simple precautions may reduce the risk of developing an infection whilst neutropenic.
  - If admitted to hospital, isolation in a side room is ideal.
  - Meticulous care of indwelling catheters with scrupulous aseptic technique when accessing line.
  - Although the most common source of infection is from commensal bacteria, patients should be advised to avoid people with obvious infections.

- Good dental hygiene and brushing with a soft brush.
- Use of sterilizing mouthwash, e.g. chlorhexidine.
- Regular handwashing by the patient and those with whom they come into contact.
- Prophylactic antibiotics (e.g. ciprofloxacin, levofloxacin) are not generally recommended in most trusts. Local protocol should be followed.
  - Studies by Cullen et al. (2005) and Bucaneve et al. (2005) have shown that the prophylactic use of levofloxacin reduces the incidence of fever, infections, and hospitalization, but not severe infections or death.
  - Any benefit must be balanced against the risk of the development of quinolone-resistant microorganisms.
  - They may be used with certain chemotherapy regimens:
    — docetaxel 100 mg/m^2.
    — anal chemoradiotherapy (mitomycin-C + 5-FU).
    — high dose chemotherapy.
  - Prophylactic co-trimoxazole (960 mg three times a week) is used when the risk of *Pneumocystis jiroveci* infection is high owing to prolonged neutropenia.
- Prophylactic fluconazole (50–400 mg PO od) should be prescribed to prevent oral *Candida* for patients expected to have severe neutropenia (<0.5 x 10^9/l) for more than 7 days. It should be stopped when neutrophil recovery (>0.5 x 10^9/l) occurs post-treatment. Fluconazole is effective against most *Candida* species, but has no activity against *Aspergillus*.
- Aciclovir is effective in the treatment and prophylaxis of herpes virus infection in neutropenic patients.
  - Aciclovir should not be used for primary prophylaxis.
  - HSV infection, or less commonly VZV infection, can occur in a neutropenic patient who has received chemotherapy and should be treated.
  - The treatment dose is 400 mg PO five times a day for 5 days. (10 mg/kg IV tds may be required in the setting of overwhelming infection).
  - Such patients may benefit from aciclovir secondary prophylaxis (200 mg PO tds) during subsequent courses of treatment.

References

Bucaneve, G., Micozzi, A., Menichetti, F., Martino, P., Dionisi, M.S., Martinelli, G., Allione, B., D'Antonio, D., Buelli, M., Nosari, A.M., Cilloni, D., Zuffa, E., Cantaffa, R., Specchia, G., Amadori, S., Fabbiano, F., Lambertenghi Deliliers, G., Lauria, F., Foà, R. and Del Favero, A., for the Gruppo Italiano Malattie Ematologiche dell'Adulto (GIMEMA) Infection Program. (2005). Levofloxacin to prevent bacterial infection in patients with cancer and neutropenia. *N. Engl. J. Med.* **353**(10): 977–987.

Cullen, M., Steven, N., Billingham, L., Gaunt, C., Hastings, M., Simmonds, P., Stuart, N., Rea, D., Bower, M., Fernando, I., Huddart, R., Gollins, S. and Stanley, A. for the Simple Investigation in Neutropenic Individuals of the Frequency of Infection after Chemotherapy +/− Antibiotic in a Number of Tumours (SIGNIFICANT) Trial Group. (2005). Antibacterial prophylaxis after chemotherapy for solid tumors and lymphomas. *N. Engl. J. Med.* **353**(10): 988–998.

:⚙: **Hypersensitivity reaction**

Any chemotherapy drug can potentially cause a hypersensitivity reaction. Generally these reactions are uncommon; however, some drugs are more commonly associated with hypersensitivity reactions.
- Paclitaxel (5%)
- Docetaxel (5%)
- Bleomycin
- Platinum-containing drugs
  - especially on re-challenging
    - classically the eighth dose of carboplatin

Hypersensitivity reaction may occur on:
- First exposure (pseudo-allergic)
  - mediated by massive histamine release from mast cells
- Subsequent exposure (type I hypersensitivity)

Infusion reaction
- Fever and chills
- Commonly occurs with:
  - First infusion of bisphosphonate
  - Bleomycin
  - Monoclonal antibodies
    - Cetuximab (Erbitux)
    - Trastuzumab (Herceptin)
    - Rituximab
    - Tositumomab (Bexxar)
    - Ibritumomab tiuxetan (Zevalin)
    - First dose infusion rate is reduced
    - Rituximab is premedicated with paracetamol and antihistamine
    - Hypersensitivity reaction is rare

Clinical features
Onset is usually within minutes of starting the infusion
- Flushing
- Urticarial rash and pruritus
- Dyspnoea and bronchospasm
- Hypotension and tachycardia
- Angio-oedema

Prevention
The incidence of hypersensitivity with taxanes is sufficiently high that routine premedication with steroids +/– antihistamines is required.

Docetaxel
- Dexamethasone 0.5–10 mg PO daily 12 hours and 6 hours before paclitaxel administration

Paclitaxel
- 30 minutes prior to administration of paclitaxel
  - Chlorphenamine 10 mg IV
  - Ranitidine 50 mg IV

Management
- Stop infusion
- Hydrocortisone IV 100 mg
- Chlorphenamine IV 10 mg
- Intravenous fluids
  - if required to maintain blood pressure
- High flow O_2
  - reduce O_2 to lowest possible rate to maintain O_2 saturation, if patient has previously received bleomycin
- Nebulized salbutamol 5 mg prn
- Patients should be monitored for at least 1 hour following a hypersensitivity reaction
- Senior advice should be obtained prior to subsequent chemotherapy
  - generally there is no cross-sensitivity between platinum drugs
    — consider substituting carboplatin for cisplatin and vice versa
  - premedication with dexamethasone and antihistamines, and slowing the rate of infusion may reduce the risk of further hypersensitivity reactions with subsequent cycles. If, despite this premedication, further hypersensitivity does occur the causative drug should not be used again

If patient has life-threatening anaphylaxis, also give:
- Epinephrine
  - 0.5 ml of 1:1000 (0.5 mg) IM
  - can be repeated every 5 minutes as required
  - monitor blood pressure, pulse and respiratory rate
  - if patient is peri-arrest give 5 ml of 1:10 000 (0.5 mg) by slow IV injection over 5 minutes
  - nebulized epinephrine (0.5 mg in 4 ml 0.9% saline) can be used for severe laryngeal oedema
- Aminophylline for bronchospasm
  - 250 mg IV over 15 minutes

ⓘ **Cardiotoxicity**

Chemotherapy-related cardiotoxicity can result in:
- Ventricular dysfunction and congestive cardiac failure
- Ischaemic events
- Arrhythmia
- Pericardial effusion
- Hypertension
- Infusion reaction-related hypotension
  - Monoclonal antibodies

Chemotherapy agents associated with cardiotoxicity
- Anthracyclines
  - Doxorubicin
  - Epirubicin
  - Mitoxantrone
- Monoclonal antibodies
  - Trastuzumab (Herceptin)
  - Bevacizumab (Avastin)
  - Cetuximab (Erbitux)
  - Rituximab (Rituxin)
- Paclitaxel
- 5-FU and capecitabine
- High dose cyclophosphamide
- High dose ifosfamide
- Interferon
- Interleukin-2
- Imatinib (Glivec)

Anthracycline-induced cardiotoxicity

Acute cardiotoxicity
- Onset 0–7 days post-anthracycline dose
- Thought to be the result of a catecholamine and histamine surge
- Uncommon
- May cause:
  - transient arrhythmia
  - myopericarditis
  - pericardial effusion
  - acute left ventricular failure
- Unrelated to dose, schedule or future development of chronic cardiotoxicity
- Management is symptomatic (See Cardiac masses 📖 p114)

Chronic cardiotoxicity
- Onset >1 month post-anthracycline, may not manifest for many years
- Incidence increases in a dose-related fashion, therefore for each anthracycline there is a maximum lifetime cumulative dose (MLCD)
  - Doxorubicin
    - 450 mg/m^2 with normal cardiac function
    - 400 mg/m^2 if cardiac dysfunction or mediastinal irradiation
    - Incidence of chronic cardiotoxicity
      - 550 mg/m^2 7% incidence
      - 600 mg/m^2 15% incidence
      - 700 mg/m^2 30–40% incidence
  - Epirubicin
    - 1000 mg/m^2 with normal cardiac function
    - 650 mg/m^2 if previous anthracycline or mediastinal irradiation
    - risk increases when dose >900 mg/m^2

- Mitoxantrone
  - 110 mg/m^2 with normal cardiac function
  - risk increases when dose >140 mg/m^2
- Liposomal anthracyclines appear to be less cardiotoxic
- A progressive irreversible cardiomyopathy owing to myocardial cell loss and fibrosis
- Results in:
  - Ventricular dysfunction and heart failure
  - Arrhythmias
- Risk factors for anthracycline-induced cardiomyopathy
  - Age >70 years
  - Cumulative dose
  - Mediastinal radiotherapy
  - Cardiac co-morbidity
  - Hypertension
  - Rate and schedule of drug administration
    - high peak dose increases cardiotoxicity
  - Concomitant cardiotoxic drugs
    - trastuzumab
    - bevacizumab
    - paclitaxel
- Radiotherapy to the heart at any time after anthracycline chemotherapy can cause a recall phenomenon, which may result in cardiac failure
- Monitoring
  - Patients at risk of anthracycline cardiotoxicity should have baseline investigations prior to commencing therapy
    - ECG
    - LVEF estimation
      - Echo
      - MUGA scan
      - Cardiac MRI
  - Patients should be considered for ongoing monitoring
    - during their treatment, if there are concerns regarding their cardiac function
      - in up to 4% of patients, the LVEF drops by >10% during anthracycline treatment
    - after completion of their treatment
- Management
  - Prevention is the best method to avoid chronic cardiotoxicity
  - Consider cardioprotectant
    - dexrazoxane
  - If there are concerns regarding cardiac function
    - consider alternative chemotherapy agents
    - reduce the dose of anthracycline
    - balance potential benefit versus risk of significant cardiac toxicity
    - avoid concurrent cardiotoxic drugs, e.g. trastuzumab
  - Drug treatment as for other types of cardiomyopathy
    - left ventricular dysfunction
      - ACE inhibitors
      - diuretics
      - beta blockers

— arrhythmias
  – beta blockers   – amiodarone
  – calcium antagonists

Trastuzumab-induced cardiotoxicity

- Trastuzumab is a monoclonal antibody, in clinical use for:
  - treatment of metastatic breast cancer
  - adjuvant treatment of breast cancer
- Obviously the risk benefit analysis is very different in these two settings, owing to the difference in treatment intention and life expectancy in the two groups
- The cardiotoxicity of trastuzumab in the metastatic breast cancer setting is less of an issue, and much of the work has been done in the adjuvant setting, although long term follow up data are still awaited
- Trastuzumab concomitantly with doxorubicin resulted in a 25% incidence of ventricular dysfunction (>10% decline in LVEF)
- The large adjuvant trastuzumab trials (HERA, NSABP trial B-31, NCCTG N9831) have used an anthracycline-based regimen as the control arm
  - HERA
    — LVEF <50% and reduction in LVEF of >10%
      – Control arm   2.3%
      – Trastuzumab arm   7.4%
    — Grade 3–4 cardiotoxicity or cardiac death
      – Control arm   0.0%
      – Trastuzumab arm   0.6%
  - NSABP trial B-31
    — Symptomatic cardiac events
      – Control arm   0.8%
      – Trastuzumab arm   4.3%
  - NCCTG N9831
    — Congestive cardiac failure
      – Control arm   0.2%
      – Trastuzumab arm   2.2–3.5%
    — Reduction in LVEF of >15%
      – Control arm   7.0%
      – Trastuzumab arm   14–17%
    — Cardiac death
      – Control arm   0.2%
      – Trastuzumab arm   0.2%
  - All results significant except for cardiac death in the NCCTG N9831
- Trastuzumab cardiotoxicity is generally reversible on discontinuation of the drug, with 70% of patients having full resolution of ventricular dysfunction within 6 months. There are no long term cardiotoxicity data available
- Risk of developing left ventricular dysfunction is dependent on pre-treatment LVEF and age (see Table 12.3)

Table 12.3 Risk of left ventricular dysfunction associated with trastuzumab treatment

		Risk of left ventricular dysfunction	
		<50 years of age	>50 years of age
Pre-treatment LVEF	50–54%	6.3%	19.1%
	55–64%	2.2%	5.2%
	>65%	0.6%	1.3%

Table 12.4 Rules for action in cardiac monitoring in asymptomatic patients on trastuzumab for adjuvant treatment of breast cancer

		Absolute reduction in LVEF		
		<10%	10–15%	>15%
LVEF during treatment	>55%	Continue	Continue	Hold
	50–55%	Continue	Hold	Hold
	<50%	Continue	Hold	Hold

- Monitoring
  - Baseline investigations prior to commencing trastuzumab
    — ECG
    — LVEF estimation
    – Echo   – MUGA scan
  - Trastuzumab treatment should not be offered if LVEF ≤55%, or patient has any of the following:
    — a history of documented congestive heart failure
    — high risk uncontrolled arrhythmias
    — angina pectoris requiring medication
    — clinically significant valvular disease
    — evidence of transmural infarction on ECG
    — poorly controlled hypertension
  - Echo or MUGA should be repeated every 3 months during trastuzumab treatment
  - Trastuzumab treatment should be suspended if the patient develops any symptoms of ventricular dysfunction or the LVEF drops by ≥10% from baseline and to <50% (see Table 12.4).
  - Repeat the LVEF assessment after 4 weeks
  - If criteria for continuation are met, restart trastuzumab
  - If two consecutive 'Holds' or a total of three 'Holds', discontinue trastuzumab

Ischaemic events

Many patients with cancer have risk factors for ischaemic heart disease.

5-Fluorouracil and capecitabine

- 5-FU-based therapy is rarely associated with angina and myocardial infarction
- Thought to be caused by coronary artery vasospasm
- The risk is increased in patients with coronary artery disease
- Patients should be advised of the risk and consented for ischaemic events
- Angina or past history of myocardial infarction is not a contraindication to 5-FU-based therapy, although 5-FU should be avoided if possible in patients with active ischaemic heart disease
- Patients should have a baseline ECG prior to commencing 5-FU-based therapy
- If chest pain develops during 5-FU-based therapy, a clear history, ECG and troponin blood test are vital to determine the likelihood of an ischaemic cause
- If ischaemia is the most likely diagnosis, 5-FU-based therapy should be discontinued and advice obtained from a cardiologist regarding optimal management of the ischaemic heart disease
- If ischaemia is felt to be unlikely, 5-FU-based therapy can be cautiously continued
- Management of an ischaemic event follows standard guidelines as for angina and myocardial infarction in the non-cancer patient

Arrhythmias

- May occur with:
  - Paclitaxel
  - Anthracyclines
  - 5-FU
  - Cisplatin
  - Rituximab
  - Trastuzumab
- The majority of chemotherapy-associated arrhythmias occur during or soon after infusion of the chemotherapy, are short-lived, asymptomatic, and do not require any intervention
- Any ventricular or supraventricular arrhythmia may occur
  - paclitaxel is particularly associated with bradycardia
- In patients with no prior history of cardiac problems, routine cardiac monitoring during chemotherapy administration is not necessary
- Any patient developing an arrhythmia must be assessed for cardiovascular compromise
- If a patient develops symptomatic arrhythmia, they should receive treatment (see Cardiac masses 🔲 p114)
- If further cycles of chemotherapy are appropriate
  - the patient should be discussed with a cardiologist
  - these should be deferred until the patient has become stable on anti-arrhythmia medication
  - cardiac monitoring should be used for future chemotherapy administration

Bevacizumab-induced cardiotoxicity

- Hypertension
  - Severe hypertension (>200/110 mmHg) in up to 5% of patients
  - Risk of:
    - — hypertensive encephalopathy
    - — subarachnoid haemorrhage
- Arterial thromboembolism in up to 5% of patients
  - Thrombotic stroke
  - Transient ischaemic attack
  - Myocardial infarction
  - Angina
- Cardiac failure
  - Increased risk in patients given anthracyclines previously or concurrently

Further reading

Ferguson, C., Clarke, J., and Herity, N.A. (2006). Ventricular tachycardia associated with trastuzumab. *N. Engl. J. Med* **354**: 648–649.

Piccart-Gebhart, M.J., Procter, M., Leyland-Jones, B., Goldhirsch, A., Untch, M., Smith, I., Gianni, L., Baselga, J., Bell, R., Jackisch, C., Cameron, D., Dowsett, M., Barrios, C.H., Steger, G., Huang, C-S., Andersson, M., Inbar, M., Lichinitser, M., Láng, I., Nitz, U., Iwata, H., Thomssen, C., Lohrisch, C., Suter, T.M., Rüschoff, J., Sütö, T., Greatorex, V., Ward, C., Straehle, C., McFadden, E., Dolci, M.S. and Gelber, R.D., for the Herceptin Adjuvant (HERA) Trial Study Team. (2005). Trastuzumab after adjuvant chemotherapy in HER2-positive breast cancer. *N. Engl. J. Med.* **353**: 1659–1672.

Romond, E.H., Perez, E.A., Bryant, J., Suman, V.J., Geyer, C.E., Davidson, N.E., Tan-Chiu, E., Martino, S., Paik, S., Kaufman, P.A., Swain, S.M., Pisansky, T.M., Fehrenbacher, L., Kutteh, L.A., Vogel, V.G., Visscher, D.W., Yothers, G., Jenkins, R.B., Brown, A.M., Dakhil, S.R., Mamounas, E.P., Lingle, W.L., Klein, P.M., Ingle, J.N. and Wolmark, N. (2005). National Surgical Adjuvant Breast and Bowel Project trial [B-31] and the North Central Cancer Treatment Group trial [N9831]. Trastuzumab plus adjuvant chemotherapy for operable HER2-positive breast cancer. *N. Engl. J. Med.* **353**: 1673–1684.

Shan, K., Lincoff, M.A. and Young, J.B. (1996). Anthracycline-induced cardiotoxicity. *Ann. Intern. Med.* **125**: 47–58.

Trastuzumab for the adjuvant treatment of early-stage HER2-positive breast cancer. NICE technology appraisal guidance 107 (2006). www.nice.org.uk

! **Pulmonary toxicity**

Chemotherapy drugs may cause:
- Acute pneumonitis
- Pulmonary fibrosis

Chemotherapy drugs that may cause pulmonary toxicity.
- Bleomycin
  - toxicity seen in 3–7% of patients
  - dose-related
  - avoid cumulative dose >400 000 U
- Mitomycin C
- Busulphan
- Melphalan
- Cyclophosphamide
- Methotrexate
- Gemcitabine
- Cytarabine
- Carmustine
- Lomustine

Risk factors for pulmonary toxicity

- Age
  - Bleomycin, HR 2.3 if >40 years
- Pulmonary disease
  - COPD
  - Emphysema
- Previous thoracic radiotherapy
- High cumulative dose
  - Bleomycin, HR 3.5 if >300 000 U
- Renal impairment
  - Bleomycin, HR 3.3 if GFR <80 ml/minute
- High FiO_2 increases the risk of bleomycin pulmonary toxicity
  - If a patient receiving bleomycin becomes hypoxic, use the lowest FiO_2 to maintain adequate oxygenation

Clinical features

Pulmonary toxicity is evident by the development of new respiratory symptoms or a change in lung appearance on serial imaging. Symptoms usually develop over several weeks or months. If symptoms develop over minutes or hours, a hypersensitivity reaction is likely.
- Dyspnoea
- Non-productive cough
- Hypoxia
  - increases with exercise
- Fatigue
- Fever
- Tachypnoea
- Tachycardia
- Bibasal crepitations

Investigations
Imaging
- CXR
  - reticulonodular pattern
  - may be normal
- HRCT chest
  - ground-glass opacification
  - fibrosis

- pleural effusion

Pulmonary function tests (PFTs)
- Restrictive ventilatory pattern
  - ↓ absolute vital capacity
  - $FEV_1/FVC > 80\%$
- Reduced gas transfer (T_{LCO}, K_{CO})
  - most sensitive test for early detection of pulmonary toxicity

Differential diagnosis
- Opportunistic infection
- Lymphangitis carcinomatosis
- Pre-existent parenchymal lung disease
  - Idiopathic pulmonary fibrosis
  - Drugs
    — amiodarone
    — sulfasalazine
    — nitrofurantoin
    — penicillamine

Monitoring
- PFTs and CXR should be carried out prior to commencing bleomycin therapy
- Serial PFTs and CXRs to detect any change in pulmonary status

Management
- Withdrawal of the implicated drug
- Prednisolone 40 mg PO od
  - taper dose over subsequent 3–6 months
  - no strong evidence for benefit
- Methylprednisolone IV and pentoxifylline have also been tried

Many patients will improve clinically (and radiologically); however, the majority will be left with a permanent deficit in gas transfer. The clinical impact of this deficit depends crucially on the patient's pre-treatment lung function and respiratory reserve.

If a patient needs a general anaesthetic, the anaesthetist must be informed of their previous bleomycin treatment.

⊙ **Neurotoxicity**

The peripheral, central, and autonomic neurological systems may be differentially affected by a number of chemotherapeutic agents. Most of this toxicity is reversible; however, some agents may cause irreversible neurotoxicity.

The development of neurotoxicity is usually dose-dependent.
- Cumulative dose
- High dose treatment

Chemotherapy agents that may cause neurotoxicity

Vinca alkaloids
- Vincristine>vinblastine>vinorelbine
- Associated with cumulative dose
  - vincristine dose limited to 2 mg per cycle of treatment.
- Peripheral neuropathy
- Autonomic neuropathy
- Cranial nerve palsy → jaw pain
- Recurrent laryngeal nerve palsy → vocal cord dysfunction
- Generally reversible, although symptoms may persist for 3–4 years

Platinum drugs
Cisplatin
- Peripheral neuropathy
  - cumulative dose >400 mg/m^2
  - generally reversible, symptoms may persist for 6–12 months
- Ototoxicity
  - tinnitus is reversible
  - high frequency hearing loss is often irreversible
  - consider audiometry to monitor hearing loss
  - associated with high dose >100 mg/m^2 and fast rate of infusion
  - care with concomitant ototoxic drugs, e.g. furosemide

Oxaliplatin
- Acute pharyngolaryngeal dysaesthesia
  - within hours of drug administration, often triggered by exposure to cold
  - subjective sensation of:
    — dysphagia — jaw spasm
    — dyspnoea — chest tightness
    — abnormal tongue sensation
  - usually lasts for a matter of seconds or minutes
  - reduced by slowing rate of subsequent infusions
- Peripheral sensory neuropathy
  - 85–95% of patients
  - dysaesthesia and/or paraesthesia of extremities
  - triggered by exposure to cold
  - associated with cumulative dose
  - generally reversible, although symptoms may persist for 6–12 months

Taxanes
Paclitaxel and docetaxel
- Peripheral and autonomic neuropathy
  - generally reversible, although symptoms may persist for 6–12 months
  - associated with both high doses and cumulative dose
    - paclitaxel
      - single dose >175 mg/m^2 and cumulative dose 725 mg/m^2
    - docetaxel
      - single dose >100 mg/m^2 and cumulative dose >400 mg/m^2

Ifosfamide
- Encephalopathy

Intrathecal chemotherapy
Methotrexate and cytarabine
- Can cause:
  - aseptic meningitis
    - headache
    - meningism
    - fever
    - photophobia
    - nausea and vomiting
    - starts 1–2 days after treatment, peaks on the second or third day, and usually resolves by day 5
    - treat with a 5- day course of dexamethasone PO
  - leukoencephalopathy
    - especially if patient has also had cranial radiotherapy

Peripheral neuropathy
Peripheral neuropathy is the most common toxicity associated with chemotherapy and is particularly associated with:
- Cisplatin
- Paclitaxel
- Vincristine
- Docetaxel
- Oxaliplatin

Risk factors
- Dose
- Diabetic neuropathy
- Previous or concurrent use of neurotoxic drugs

Clinical features
- Progressive sensory paraesthesia
  - glove and stocking distribution
- Dysaesthesia
- Absent deep tendon reflexes
- Loss of proprioception
- Loss of motor function (with vincristine)

Management
- The only effective management is discontinuation of the causative drug
- It is associated with cumulative dose; therefore continued administration of drug will cause progression of symptoms

- Carboplatin is less neurotoxic than cisplatin and it may occasionally be appropriate to substitute carboplatin
- Peripheral neuropathy is generally reversible; however, it may take 6–12 months for symptoms to resolve entirely

Autonomic neuropathy

Autonomic neuropathy is particularly associated with vincristine and the taxanes.

Clinical features
- Paralytic ileus
- Constipation
- Urinary retention
- Bradycardia
- Postural hypotension

Management
- Supportive management
  - metoclopramide PO 10–20 mg tds may improve intestinal motility
- It is associated with cumulative dose; therefore to prevent progression of symptoms the causative drug should be discontinued

Ifosfamide encephalopathy

Thought to be due to the ifosfamide metabolite chloroacetaldehyde.

Risk factors
- High doses of ifosfamide
- Renal dysfunction
  - reduced clearance of chloroacetaldehyde
- Large pelvic mass
- Hypoalbuminaemia
- Concurrent sedative drugs
  - opioids
  - benzodiazepines

Clinical features
- Somnolence
- Ataxia
- Disorientation
- Agitation
- Vivid dreams
- Hallucinations
- Seizures
- Coma

Prevention
- Calculate risk of encephalopathy using nomogram before commencing each cycle of ifosfamide (see Fig. 12.1)
- If risk >80%, ifosfamide should not be given
- If risk >20% give prophylactic methylthioninium chloride (methylene blue) PO 50 mg tds, starting on day 1 of treatment, and continuing for 24 hours after completion of ifosfamide administration

Management
- Stop ifosfamide infusion
- Methylthioninium chloride IV 50 mg tds, until resolution of encephalopathy. Prophylactic methylthioninium chloride should then be used for all subsequent cycles
- Consider haloperidol for agitation

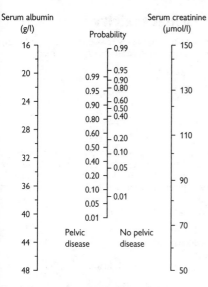

Fig. 12.1 Ifosfamide encephalopathy nomogram.

- The probability of developing ifosfamide encephalopathy can be predicted using this nomogram.
- The probability is predicted from:
  - Serum albumin (g/l)
  - Serum creatinine (μmol/l)
  - Presence of pelvic disease
    — Primary malignancy
    — Metastatic disease Philadelphia.

Further reading

Donegan, S. (2001). Novel treatment for the management of ifosfamide neurotoxicity: rationale for the use of methylene blue. *J. Oncol. Pharm. Prac.* **6**(4): 153–165.

Fischer, D.S., Knobf, M.T., Durivage, H.J. and Beaulieu, N.J. (2003). The *Cancer Chemotherapy Handbook*, 6th edn. Mosby.

⊙ **Gastrointestinal toxicity**

The epithelium of the GI tract is constantly regenerating. Chemotherapy targets rapidly dividing cells and therefore GI toxicity is common.
- Gastrointestinal toxicity
  - Oral mucositis (stomatitis)
  - Nausea and vomiting
    — see Nausea and vomiting 📖 p38
  - Diarrhoea
    — see Diarrhoea 📖 p48

Oral mucositis

Disruption of the dividing stem cell population prevents production of cells to replace cells shed from the surface. The average life span of an oral mucosal cell is about 7–10 days. Therefore mucositis generally develops within a week of receiving chemotherapy and normally recovers within 2–3 weeks.
- May result in:
  - Pain
  - Difficulty eating
    — decreased nutritional intake
  - Secondary infection
    — bacterial   — fungal
    — viral
    — particularly important if patient neutropenic
  - Loss of taste sensation

Oral mucositis is one of the most common side effects of chemotherapy, being present at some level in 40–75% of cases.
- Chemotherapy drugs that commonly cause oral mucositis
  - Anthracyclines   • Taxanes
    — Doxorubicin   — Docetaxel
    — Epirubicin   — Paclitaxel
  - Antimetabolites   • Cyclophosphamide
    — Methotrexate   • Etoposide
    — 5-FU
    — Capecitabine

Risk factors
- Pre-existing oral conditions
  - periodontal disease
  - dental caries
- Poor oral hygiene   • Xerostomia
- Poorly fitting dentures   • Smoking
- Poor nutrition   • Alcohol consumption
- Poor oral care post-chemotherapy
- Chemotherapy drug, dose, and regime

Prevention of oral mucositis
- Optimize dental hygiene
    - Brush teeth at least twice daily with a soft toothbrush and fluoride toothpaste
    - Ensure dentures are cleaned regularly, soak dentures overnight
    - Rinse mouth twice daily with 0.9% saline
    - Corrective dental work may need to be carried out prior to commencing chemotherapy

Treatment of oral mucositis
- Dry mouth
    - Regular sips of water
    - Sucking ice cubes
    - Artificial saliva
    - Sugar-free chewing gum
- Dry lips
    - Emollients
- Pain
    - Topical treatment
        — Benzydramine 0.15% (Difflam) mouthwash 15 ml qds
            - may cause stinging, so can be diluted 15 ml benzydramine with 15 ml water
        — Choline salicylate oral gel 8.7% (Bonjela) prn
        — Gelclair prn
        — Carmellose sodium (Orabase)
            - mechanical protection
            - Adcortyl in orabase (corticosteroid)
        — Aspirin 300 mg gargle q4h
            - should not be swallowed to avoid systemic absorption
        — Local anaesthetic
            - 5% viscous lidocaine
    - Systemic treatment
        — Use analgesics as per the WHO analgesic ladder (see Pain 📖 p2)
            - NSAIDs (soluble)
                - anti-inflammatory effect
            - Morphine sulphate liquid
                - severe mucositis may require morphine SC
- Infection
    - Mouthwash
        — Chlorhexidine 0.2% bd
            - it may cause stinging, so can be diluted 10 ml chlorhexidine with 10 ml water
        — Hexetidine (Oraldene) 0.1% 15 ml bd
    - Viral
        — Aciclovir 200 mg PO five times a day, for 5 days.
    - Candidiasis
        — Nystatin oral suspension 100 000 U PO qds for 7 days
        — Fluconazole 50–100 mg PO od for 7–14 days
    - Bacterial
        — Metronidazole 400 mg PO tds
        — Flucloxacillin 250–500 mg PO qds
- For a coated tongue use effervescent vitamin C

⑦ **Hepatotoxicity**

Liver function is crucial to the normal functioning of the body as it is vital in the metabolism and elimination of waste products, including the clearance of certain chemotherapeutic drugs.

Liver dysfunction in cancer patients is a common feature, due to:
- primary liver disease
- hepatic metastases
- toxic effect of chemotherapeutic agents

Chemotherapy drugs may cause:
- Acute hepatitis
  - Often presents as asymptomatic elevation in LFTs
    — Capecitabine
    — Carboplatin
    — Carmustine
    — Cytarabine
    — Docetaxel
    — Etoposide
    — Gemcitabine
    — Imatinib
    — Irinotecan
    — Hepatic artery infusion of 5-FU
    — Lomustine
    — Methotrexate
    — Mitoxantrone
    — Oxaliplatin
    — Paclitaxel
    — Pemetrexed
    — Vincristine
    — Interferon
- Veno-occlusive disease
  - High dose conditioning chemotherapy pre-bone marrow transplant (BMT)
- Hepatic fibrosis
  - Long term methotrexate

Monitoring

Bloods
- LFTs
  - commonly causes a raised ALT/AST with normal bilirubin
  - before starting chemotherapy and with each subsequent cycle

Elevation in LFTs during chemotherapy may be due to:
- Chemotherapy-induced hepatotoxicity
- Other drugs
  - Many commonly used drugs can be associated with hepatotoxicity
    — fluconazole
    — antibiotics
    — NSAIDs
    — calcium antagonists
    — tamoxifen
    — oral hypoglycaemics
    — haloperidol
    — allopurinol
- Progressive malignant disease
  - Hepatic metastases
  - Porta hepatis lymphadenopathy

Management
- Consider stopping any other drug that may be contributing to the hepatotoxicity
- Most chemotherapy-induced acute hepatitis is mild and transient, and the chemotherapy agent can often be continued
- Fulminant hepatic failure is very rare
- If hepatotoxicity is progressive the chemotherapy agent should be stopped. This decision should be made by senior members of the team, after consideration of:
  - treatment intent
  - other options for treatment
  - degree of hepatotoxicity

Hepatic veno-occlusive disease
- See Stem cell transplant 📖 p301

Dose reduction in hepatic dysfunction
Liver dysfunction can lead to increased chemotherapy drug toxicity.
- Reduction in hepatic drug metabolism and biliary excretion.
- Hypoalbuminaemia can alter protein binding of cytotoxic drugs.

Dynamic tests of liver function are not widely used. Liver biochemistry tests reflect liver damage rather than liver function. Therefore most dose adjustments are empirical. Local protocols should be followed.

Drugs that require dose reduction in the presence of elevated LFTs.
- Anthracyclines
  - doxorubicin
  - epirubicin
- Taxanes
  - paclitaxel
  - docetaxel
- Etoposide
- Irinotecan
- Vinca alkaloids
  - vincristine
  - vinblastine
  - vinorelbine

ⓘ **Haemorrhagic cystitis**

Haemorrhagic cystitis is a rare complication of treatment with ifosfamide or high dose cyclophosphamide (>1.5 g/m^2). The ifosfamide metabolite acrolein is directly toxic to the bladder epithelium, resulting in inflammation, ulceration, and haemorrhage.

Clinical features
- Onset is usually during, or shortly after completing, administration of ifosfamide or cyclophosphamide
- Dysuria
- Frequency
- Haematuria
  - microscopic
    - >3 RBC per high powered field
  - macroscopic

Prevention
- Adequate hydration (2 l/m^2/day) to maintain good urine output
- Mesna
  - It is excreted by the kidney and binds to acrolein in the urine to form a non-toxic thioether
  - It also reduces the metabolism of ifosfamide to acrolein
  - It has no effect on the chemotherapeutic efficacy of ifosfamide or cyclophosphamide
  - It must be administered (bolus or infusion) before the first dose of ifosfamide or cyclophosphamide and continued after the last dose
    - it has a short half life compared to ifosfamide and cyclophosphamide
    - it must be present in the urine before acrolein comes into contact with the urothelium
  - Mesna dose for ifosfamide infusions
    - Pre-ifosfamide: 20% of ifosfamide dose as IV bolus
    - With ifosfamide: 100% of ifosfamide dose as IV infusion
    - Post-ifosfamide: 60% of ifosfamide dose as IV infusion over 12 hours (longer if ↓GFR)
  - Mesna dose for bolus ifosfamide
    - 60% of ifosfamide dose as IV infusion

Management
- If macroscopic haemorrhagic cystitis develops
  - Stop infusion of ifosfamide or cyclophosphamide
  - Increase intravenous hydration
  - If risk of clot retention insert a 22-F three-way irrigation catheter and commence bladder irrigation
  - If bleeding continues, discuss with urologist regarding further intervention, e.g. cystoscopy

① **Nephrotoxicity**

A number of chemotherapy drugs are directly or indirectly nephrotoxic. Many chemotherapy drugs are predominantly excreted by the kidneys, and any increase in renal impairment can result in reduced excretion → increased [cytotoxic drug] → increased toxicity. Some drugs are nephrotoxic and renally excreted, and there is therefore the potential for a vicious cycle of progressive nephrotoxicity. Nephrotoxicity may cause irreversible renal failure, and therefore close monitoring is vital.

Chemotherapy drugs which may cause nephrotoxicity:
- Cisplatin
  - proximal and distal tubular damage
- Ifosfamide
  - proximal tubular damage
- High dose cyclophosphamide
  - SIADH
- High dose methotrexate
  - proximal and distal tubular damage
- Mitomycin C
  - haemolytic uraemic syndrome (rare)
- High dose carmustine/lomustine
  - glomerular and tubular damage
- Streptozocin
  - tubular damage

Risk factors for nephrotoxicity

- Age >70 years
- Diabetes mellitus
- Renovascular disease
- Hydronephrosis
- Renal impairment (↓GFR)
- Dehydration
  - chemotherapy-related diarrhoea
  - chemotherapy-related vomiting
- Concurrent use of nephrotoxic drugs
- Dose of nephrotoxic chemotherapy

Clinical features

- Often the patient is asymptomatic
- When renal impairment is significant
  - malaise
  - anorexia
  - nausea and vomiting
  - dyspnoea
  - pruritus
  - drowsiness
  - confusion
  - arrhythmias
  - seizures

Investigations and monitoring

Bloods

- U&Es
- Mg^{2+}, Ca^{2+}, phosphate
- The creatinine clearance must be calculated before administration of:
  - any nephrotoxic drug
  - any drug that requires dose adjustment in the presence of renal impairment

Various methods exist for creatinine clearance calculation; follow local protocol for method and frequency of calculation.

- Creatinine clearance calculation prior to first cycle with subsequent monitoring by serum creatinine prior to every cycle
- Creatinine clearance calculation prior to every cycle

Creatinine clearance (GFR) calculations

- Cockcroft and Gault

$$GFR \text{ (ml/minute)} = \frac{((140 - age) \times k \times weight \text{ (kg)})}{serum\ creatinine\ (\mu mol/l)}$$

where $k = 1.23$ (male), 1.05 (female)

- 24-hour urine collection with paired serum creatinine
- $[^{51}Cr]$-EDTA creatinine clearance

The development of renal impairment during chemotherapy must not automatically be attributed to the chemotherapy agent, and should be investigated appropriately (see Acute renal failure 📖 p268)

Management

- Close monitoring of renal function allows early identification of nephrotoxicity and institution of measures to control it.
  - stop all other nephrotoxic drugs (e.g. NSAIDs, ACE inhibitors, gentamicin).
  - ensure adequate hydration.
- Any deterioration in renal function is important as it may herald further deterioration if the nephrotoxic drug is continued.
- The only effective measure to prevent further deterioration in renal function is to stop the causative drug.
- The decision whether to continue with the nephrotoxic agent should be made by senior members of the team, after consideration of
  - treatment intent.
  - other options for treatment.
  - degree of renal compromise.
- Ideally, renal impairment is detected at an early stage; however, patients may progress to acute renal failure and should be managed appropriately (see Acute renal failure 📖 p268).

Prevention of cisplatin nephrotoxicity

Cisplatin is a commonly used chemotherapeutic agent and is significantly nephrotoxic.

- Every patient receiving cisplatin should:
  - Receive hydration before and after treatment to minimize the risk of nephrotoxicity
    - 0.9% saline with K^+ and Mg^{2+} supplementation
      - cisplatin is associated with hypokalaemia and hypomagnesaemia
  - Have a urine output of >100 ml/hour during cisplatin administration and post-hydration
    - If urine output is <100 ml/hour:
      - when cisplatin is due to be administered further IV 0.9% saline should be given
      - during post-hydration give:
        20–40 mg furosemide PO/IV or 200 ml mannitol 10% IV
  - If patient is in positive fluid balance >2 litres 8 hours after completion of post-hydration, give 20–40 mg furosemide PO/IV or 200 ml mannitol 10% IV.

Dose reduction in renal impairment

Certain renally excreted chemotherapy drugs require dose adjustment in the presence of renal impairment.

- Bleomycin
- Cisplatin
- Carboplatin
- Carmustine
- Lomustine
- Melphalan
- Ifosfamide
- Methotrexate
- Fludarabine
- Capecitabine
- Etoposide
- Irinotecan
- Topotecan

Follow local protocol for dose adjustment. Adjustment is usually empirical according to GFR (see Table 12.5).

- An exception is carboplatin

  Dose (mg) = Target AUC x (GFR+25)

Table 12.5 Clinical interpretation of creatinine clearance

GFR (ml/min)	Clinical interpretation
>50	Acceptable renal function for most drugs
30–50	Mild-moderate renal impairment
<30	Severe renal impairment

⑦ **Skin toxicity**

Skin toxicity following chemotherapy and biological therapy can vary from mild to extreme.

Any chemotherapy drug may cause skin toxicity; however, certain drugs are more commonly associated with skin toxicity.

- 5-FU
- Capecitabine
- Liposomal doxorubicin
- Bleomycin
- EGFR inhibitors
  - Erlotinib (Tarceva)
  - Gefitinib (Iressa)
  - Cetuximab (Erbitux)
- Docetaxel
  - significant nail changes
- Methotrexate

Palmar–plantar erythrodysaesthesia

Palmar–plantar erythrodysaesthesia (PPE) most commonly affects the hands and feet. It is a syndrome of tender erythematous plaques and desquamation. There is often associated swelling, pain, tenderness to touch, and dysaesthesia.

- Commonly occurs with:
  - Capecitabine (up to 50% of patients)
  - 5-FU
  - Liposomal doxorubicin

Management

- Regular emollients
- Pyridoxine 50 mg PO tds until PPE resolved
- Dose reduction
- Delay subsequent cycle to allow recovery
- Discontinue drug

EGFR inhibitor-associated rash

It has a pustular/papular inflammatory appearance; it resembles acne vulgaris (although with a different aetiology and pathology). It particularly affects the face, head and upper torso.

- It is common
  - Erlotinib (Tarceva)   68–75%
  - Gefitinib (Iressa)   43–54%
  - Cetuximab (Erbitux)   88–90%
- It is mostly mild to moderate but can be severe, leading to dose reduction, dose interruption or treatment cessation
- A correlation between rash incidence/severity and clinical outcome has been reported
- The occurrence of rash is dose-related

- It commonly appears within the first 2 weeks of treatment
- In some patients the rash may gradually resolve despite continued treatment
- Referral to a dermatologist should be considered if the rash is of uncharacteristic appearance or distribution

Associated features
- Pruritus
- Dry skin
- Erythema
- Paronychial inflammation
- Secondary infection
  - Signs may be masked in:
    - — neutropenic patients   — patients on steroids
  - *Staphylococcus aureus*
    - — impetigo appearance
      - – yellow/brown crust   – oozing of fluid
  - Cellulitis
  - HSV/VZV

Management
- Cover with make-up
  - dermatologist approved cover-up
- Regular emollients to prevent and alleviate skin dryness
- Avoid strong sunlight or use high factor sunscreen (SPF>15)
- Do not use topical acne medications
  - topical retinoids   • benzoyl peroxide
- Analgesia as required
  - increased pain may be a sign of secondary infection
- Use antihistamines as required to help with pruritus
- Secondary infection
  - Oral antibiotics
    - — minocycline
      - – also has weak anti-inflammatory effect
      - – good activity against *Staphylococcus aureus*
  - Topical antibiotics
    - — topical clindamycin
    - — topical mupirocin
      - – if *Staphylococcus aureus* cultured or clinical diagnosis of impetigo
  - If antibiotic resistance is suspected, culture the pustules to determine the bacterial strain before treating
- Dose reduction or cessation of therapy is also a management option

Further reading

Pérez-Soler, R., Delord, J.P., Halpern, A., Kelly, K., Krueger, J., Massuti Sureda, B., Von Pawel, J., Temel, J., Siena, S., Soulières, D., Saltz, L. and Leyden, J. (2005). HER1/EGFR inhibitor-associated rash: future directions for management and investigation. Outcomes from the HER1/EGFR inhibitor rash management forum. *The Oncologist* **10**: 345–356.

☼ Extravasation

Extravasation is the incorrect delivery of a cytotoxic agent into the sub-dermal or subcutaneous tissues surrounding the administration site.

The degree of tissue damage depends on the type, concentration, and quantity of drug extravasated.

Chemotherapy agents are classified according to their tissue damaging capabilities (see Table 12.6).

- Vesicant
  - An agent that has the potential to cause pain, inflammation, blistering, and irreversible tissue damage, including necrosis and loss of motor function and mobility
- Exfoliant
  - An agent that is capable of causing inflammation and skin damage, but is less likely to cause tissue damage
- Irritant
  - An agent that causes pain and inflammation at the administration site, but rarely results in irreversible tissue damage
- Inflammatory agents
  - An agent capable of causing mild to moderate inflammation
- Neutral
  - An agent that does not cause inflammation or damage

Risk factors for extravasation

- Multiple cannulation/venepuncture sites
  - avoid needle insertion distal to recent (<24 hours) venepuncture site
- Position
  - avoid siting cannula
    — in antecubital fossa
    — crossing joints
    — overlying vital structures
      – nerves   – tendons
    — in previously irradiated sites
- Co-morbidity
  - thrombocytopenia   • lymphoedema
  - peripheral vascular disease   • Raynaud's disease
- Fragile veins
  - elderly patients   • cachectic patients

Clinical features

- Pain, burning, stinging around cannula site
- Erythema or swelling around cannula site
- Signs of poor flow via the cannula
  - resistance   • reduced flow rate
  - inadequate flashback of blood

Table 12.6 Classification of cytotoxic agents

Vesicant	Exfoliant	Irritant	Inflammatory agent	Neutral
Carmustine	Cisplatin	Carboplatin	5-FU	Bleomycin
Doxorubicin	Docetaxel	Etoposide	Methotrexate	Cyclophos-phamide
Epirubicin	Liposomal doxorubicin	Irinotecan	Pemetrexed	Cytarabine
Mitomycin C	Oxaliplatin			Fludarabine
Mitoxantrone	Topotecan			Gemcitabine
Paclitaxel				Ifosfamide
Vinblastine				Interferon
Vincristine				Interleukin-2
Vinorelbine				Melphalan
				Rituximab
				Trastuzumab

Prevention

- Safe positioning of cannula
- Regular check on cannula site and flow during chemotherapy infusion
- Vesicant drugs should be administered first
- Bolus vesicant drugs should be administered through a fast running drip
- Patient education
  - Patient to inform staff immediately if they experience any symptoms suggestive of extravasation during drug administration

Management

- All chemotherapy units should have an 'Extravasation policy' and an 'Extravasation kit'
- Follow local policy
- The basic principles of treatment include removing and neutralizing the effects of the extravasated drug
  - Stop the infusion
  - Aspirate as much of the drug as possible from the extravasation site via the cannula
  - Summon the doctor and collect the extravasation kit
  - Mark the area and remove the cannula
  - Apply cold pack regularly for 24 hours
    - exceptions (apply warm pack)
      - vinca alkaloids
      - oxaliplatin

- Follow specific local extravasation guidelines for specific antidotes
- Apply hydrocortisone cream 1% bd
- Elevate limb
- Call plastic surgical team if vesicant drug has been extravasated
- Document the extravasation in the patient's notes
- Review the patient at 24 hours and 7 days, as a minimum
- If chemotherapy is to be continued, where possible avoid using the extravasated limb

Radiotherapy-related emergencies

⑦ Introduction to radiotherapy side effects

Radiotherapy treatment will usually cause side effects. These may range from mild and reversible to life-threatening effects. Severe side effects are likely to be more acceptable to those patients being treated curatively. For patients receiving radiotherapy with palliative intent we must ensure that the radiotherapy side effects do not negate the benefit we are hoping to achieve.

Radiotherapy side effects are generally predictable, and can be divided into two phases.

- Acute effects
  - Seen in tissues that rapidly regenerate
    — epidermal layer of skin
    — bone marrow
    — gastrointestinal epithelium
  - Onset days to weeks after beginning of therapy
    — depends on length of time taken for a cell to develop from a stem cell to a fully differentiated cell
  - Rapidly repaired by stem cells
  - Usually self-limiting and reversible
- Late effects
  - Seen in slowly proliferating tissues
    — kidney
    — lung
    — heart
  - Onset months to years
    — usually a fibrotic reaction
  - May slowly improve with time, but the damage is never completely repaired

The severity of the reaction depends on:
- Volume of tissue treated
- Dose delivered
  - Total dose
  - Dose per fraction
  - Length of time over which dose is delivered
- Tissue sensitivity
- Co-morbidity
  - Inflammatory bowel disease
  - Connective tissue disease
  - Diabetes mellitus
- Chemotherapy
  - Previous
  - Concurrent

If side effects encountered are more severe than anticipated, consider:
- Radiation sensitivity syndromes
  - Ataxia telangiectasia
  - Fanconi's anaemia
  - Gardner's syndrome
  - Usher's syndrome
- Infection
- Co-administration of drugs
- Tumour progression/relapse

Managing side effects
Prevention
- Treatment planning
  - Identify organs at risk (OAR)
  - Shield OAR where possible
- Protective drugs
  - Amifostine

Monitoring
- Patient education
- Regular reviews during therapy

Intervention
- Early recognition and treatment of acute side effects is important to avoid patients deteriorating during their therapy such that they require gaps in their treatment course.
  - Gaps in therapy result in reduced chance of disease control, owing to rapid repopulation.

Further reading
Emami, B., Lyman, J., Brown, A., Coia, L., Goitein, M., Munzenrider, J.E., Shank, B., Solin, L.J. and Wesson, M. (1991). Tolerance of normal tissue to therapeutic irradiation. *Int. J. Radiat. Oncol. Biol. Phys.* **21**: 109–122.

Faithful, S. and Wells, M. (2003). *Supportive Care in Radiotherapy.* Churchill Livingstone.

Hall, E.J. and Giaccia, A.J. (2005). *Radiobiology for the Radiologist,* 6th edn. Lippincott, Williams and Wilkins.

Late Effects of Normal Tissues Consensus Conference. San Francisco, California, August 26–28, 1992. (1995) *Int. J. Radiat. Oncol. Biol. Phys.* **31**(5): 1035–1364.

Steel, G.G. (2002). Basic clinical radiobiology 3rd edn. Hodder Arnold.

⑦ **Skin toxicity**

Acute skin toxicity has become less frequent with the advent of skin sparing megavoltage radiotherapy treatment machines. However, it does remain a significant problem in patients receiving irradiation to:

- Breast/chest wall
- Head and neck
- Anus
- Vulva
- Rectum
- Non-melanomatous skin cancer

The severity of the skin reaction can be exacerbated by concomitant chemotherapy. Previous administration of an anthracycline may also exacerbate radiotherapy skin toxicity, and anthracyclines given after radiotherapy may result in a 'recall' of the previous skin reaction in prior sites of radiation.

Clonogenic stem cells located in the basal layer of the epidermis normally divide to replace superficial cells shed from the skin surface. These cells are rapidly proliferating and so are very sensitive to radiation-induced damage. Loss of these clonogenic cells results in reduced re-population and ultimately loss of integrity of the skin.

Stem cell loss starts to occur at 20–25 Gy, so skin changes are visible by the second or third week of therapy. Moist desquamation results from sterilization of clonogenic stem cells from the basal layer. Small areas heal by regeneration from the basal layer; however, larger areas require stem cells to migrate in from the surrounding epidermis. Moist desquamation usually heals within 4 weeks of completing radiotherapy; however, large areas may take longer.

Clinical features

Mild erythema and dry desquamation
Seen in 80% of patients.
- Dry skin
- Scaly
- Itchy

Moist desquamation
Seen in 10–15% of patients.
- Blistering
- Peeling
- Sloughing

Necrosis
Very rare.

Risk factors
- Intrinsic
  - Areas where skin rubs together
    - axilla
    - infra-mammary
    - perineum
    - inguinal
  - Co-morbidity
    - general skin condition
    - nutritional status
    - smoking
    - alcohol
  - Age
  - Ethnicity

- Extrinsic
  - Dose
    - — total dose (>50 Gy)
    - — hyperfractionation
    - — dose per fraction (>2 Gy/#)
  - Beam
    - — kilovoltage photons
    - — electrons
      - - deliver 85–95% of the dose to the skin, megavoltage photons deliver 20% of the dose to the skin
  - Beam tangential to skin
  - Concomitant chemotherapy
  - Use of bolus
  - Patient use of inappropriate skin products
    - — perfumed products
    - — alcohol-containing skin products
    - — zinc- or silver-containing creams
      - - anusol
      - - flamazine

Management

Erythema and dry desquamation

- Gentle washing
  - mild, non-perfumed soaps and shampoos
  - lukewarm water
- Avoid friction
  - gently pat dry
  - wear loose natural fibre clothing
- Use moisturizer
  - aqueous cream applied liberally daily after therapy
  - start after first fraction
- Dry shave with an electric razor
- Protect skin from extremes of temperature
- Avoid
  - perfumes
  - deodorants
  - make-up
  - cleansers
  - toners
  - all can be irritant and may exacerbate the erythema
  - powders
    - — cause skin dryness and may produce a build-up effect by blocking hair follicles and sweat glands, thus exacerbating the reaction
- 1% hydrocortisone cream
  - good for itching
  - may mask infection
  - does not reduce the progression to desquamation
- Antihistamine for itch

Moist desquamation

- Antiseptic agents
  - Little benefit over saline irrigation
  - Provides transient antiseptic effect
  - Increased risk of sensitivity reactions
  - Povidone–iodine (Betadine)
  - Proflavine cream

- Silver sulfadiazine (Flamazine)
  - contains silver, so should only be used once radiotherapy is completed
- Simple dressings
  - Provide the ideal wound healing environment (moist and clean)
  - Skin reactions occur mainly in areas where dressings are not easily applied
  - Need to be:
    - readily conformable
    - able to absorb serous leakage without macerating the adjacent normal skin
    - easily removable
      - without removing or disturbing granulation
      - to avoid a bolus effect during radiotherapy
  - May need to change dressings once or twice a day
  - Hydrogels
    - easily applied
    - conformable
    - rehydration and cooling properties
    - they have no adhesiveness and therefore need secondary dressings to keep in place
      - foam dressing, e.g. Mepilex
    - the secondary dressing also serves to reduce evaporation and keep the hydrogel moist
    - examples
      - Intrasite conformable   – ActiForm cool
  - Hydrocolloids
    - good for light–moderate exudative wounds
      - patchy moist desquamation
    - disadvantage is that can be very adhesive and risk removing granulating tissue
    - examples
      - Granuflex   – ActivHeal hydrocolloid
  - Alginates
    - good for confluent moist desquamation or fungating wounds
    - converts to a hydrophilic dressing on contact with the wound
    - very absorbent, may dry out skin too much
    - encourages granulation
    - they have no adhesiveness and therefore need secondary dressings to keep in place
      - foam dressing, e.g. Mepilex
    - examples
      - Sorbsan   – ActivHeal alginate
- Analgesia
  - Use analgesics as per the WHO analgesic ladder (see Pain ☐ p2)
  - Regular NSAIDs are particularly useful
- Treatment of any secondary infection
  - Topical metronidazole 0.8% gel (Metrotop) bd
  - Flucloxacillin 500 mg PO qds for 7 days

ⓘ **Oral mucositis**

Mucositis is an acute side effect of radiotherapy to the head and neck.
- Squamous cancers of the upper aerodigestive tract
- Salivary gland malignancies
- Lymphomas

It is caused by loss of stem cells from the basal epithelial layer. This results in reduced epithelial cell replacement, ultimately producing ulceration and a breakdown of the mucosal barrier of the oropharyngeal cavity. Damaged cells release cytokines which induce inflammation.

It usually starts by 12–14 days after the start of treatment, and usually settles within 2–4 weeks after completion of radiotherapy. Radiation oral mucositis may rarely persist for up to 8 weeks, significantly longer than chemotherapy-induced mucositis.

Clinical features
- Pain
  - difficulty eating
- Bleeding from inflamed mucous membranes
  - rarely severe
- Sialadenitis
  - usually transient
- Xerostomia
  - dry mouth
  - development of dental caries
- Taste alteration

Risk factors
- Volume of upper aerodigestive tract treated
  - mucositis can be mild in irradiation of unilateral neck lymph nodes
  - mucositis is often severe when large volumes are irradiated, as in the treatment of nasopharyngeal carcinoma
- Dose (>2 Gy/#)
- Concomitant chemotherapy
  - 5-FU
- Secondary infection
  - viral
    - HSV
  - bacterial
  - fungal
    - Candida

Management
- Careful oral hygiene by atraumatic cleansing of the oral mucosa
  - Brush teeth at least twice daily with a soft toothbrush and fluoride toothpaste
  - Ensure dentures are cleaned regularly, soak dentures overnight
  - Rinse mouth frequently with 0.9% saline

- Pain
  - Topical treatment
    - mucosal coating agents
      - choline salicylate oral gel 8.7% (Bonjela) prn
      - gelclair prn
      - carmellose sodium (Orabase)
        - adcortyl in orabase (corticosteroid)
      - sucralfate suspension 1 g qds
    - mouthwash
      - benzydamine 0.15% (Difflam) 15 ml every 1½ to 3 hours
        - it may cause stinging, so can be diluted 15 ml benzydamine with 15 ml water
      - aspirin 300 mg gargle q4h
        - should not be swallowed to avoid systemic absorption
    - local anaesthetic
      - 5% viscous lidocaine
  - Systemic treatment
    - use analgesics as per the WHO analgesic ladder (see Pain 📖 p2)
      - NSAIDs (soluble)
        - anti-inflammatory effect
      - morphine sulphate liquid
        - severe mucositis may require morphine SC
- Maintain lubrication
  - regular sips of water
  - sucking ice cubes
  - artificial saliva
  - sugar-free chewing gum
- Infection
  - Mouthwash
    - chlorhexidine 0.2% bd
      - it may cause stinging, so can be diluted 10 ml chlorhexidine with 10 ml water
    - hexetidine (Oraldene) 0.1% bd
  - Viral
    - aciclovir 200 mg PO five times a day, for 5 days
  - Candidiasis
    - nystatin oral suspension 100 000 U PO qds for 7 days
    - fluconazole 50–100 mg PO od for 7–14 days
  - Bacterial
    - metronidazole 400 mg PO tds
    - flucloxacillin 250–500 mg PO qds
- Nutritional state
  - Careful assessment by a dietician prior to starting treatment and regular review during radiotherapy is vital to optimize the patient's nutritional intake.
  - Patients frequently need nutritional supplementation and may need feeding via NG or PEG feeding tubes.
  - Placement of a PEG feeding tube prior to radiotherapy should be considered in patients:
    - requiring treatment to a significant volume of the oropharynx
    - with a poor pre-treatment nutritional state

⑦ **Cardiotoxicity**

Radiotherapy is commonly used to treat malignancy in the thorax in both a curative and palliative manner. The heart is therefore often irradiated during radiotherapy treatment to:

- Breast
- Lung
- Oesophagus
- Lymphoma

Radiotherapy treatment can result in:
- Pericardial disease
  - Acute pericarditis
    — usually occurs in the first year after radiotherapy
    — clinical features
      - fever   – ECG changes
      - pleuritic chest pain
    — management
      - NSAIDs
  - Pericardial effusion
    — usually asymptomatic
    — usually if >60% of heart has received radiation
  - Constrictive pericarditis
- Coronary artery disease
  - Angina and myocardial infarction
    — usually occurs many years (>15 years) after radiotherapy
- Valvular dysfunction
- Acute cardiomyopathy
  - Rare
  - >45 Gy to whole heart
  - Increased risk if previous anthracycline chemotherapy

① **Radiation pneumonitis**

Radiotherapy is commonly used to treat malignancy in the thorax in both a curative and palliative manner. The lungs are therefore often an organ at risk for radiotherapy treatment.

- Breast
- Lung
- Oesophagus
- Lymphoma

Acute effects of radiation to the lung

- Up to 60% of patients may experience some symptoms within 24 hours of palliative radiotherapy (8–10 Gy/#)
  - chest pain   45%
  - fevers/rigors/sweating   35%
  - in 70% of patients these symptoms last less than 2 hours

Radiation pneumonitis

Radiation has a direct (in-field) toxic effect on the lung parenchyma.

- In the acute phase this causes:
  - pneumocyte damage
  - reduction in surfactant production
  - an alveolar and interstitial inflammatory response
- Clinical chest signs usually become evident 6 weeks to 6 months after radiotherapy, when:
  - alveolar fluid is present
  - alveolar collapse occurs
- Clinically evident radiation pneumonitis occurs in 5–15% of patients receiving thoracic radiotherapy
- Up to 60% of patients will have asymptomatic radiological changes of radiation pneumonitis
- Over time (months to years) progression to irreversible fibrosis may occur
  - the presence and severity of acute alveolitis is not predictive for lung fibrosis
  - lung fibrosis may be associated with a further decline in gas transfer and a reduction in vital capacity/operating lung volumes

Bilateral alveolitis following radiotherapy (independent of field) has also been described and is likely to be an immunologically mediated process.

Clinical features

- Dry cough
- Breathlessness
- Systemic features
  - fever
  - malaise
- Tachypnoea
- Hypoxia

Risk factors for symptomatic radiation pneumonitis

The degree of symptomatic radiation pneumonitis depends to a great extent on the function of the non-irradiated lung. Any area of lung receiving >20 Gy will be rendered functionless. Many patients have cardiopulmonary co-morbidity that means any reduction in the volume of functioning lung results in significant symptoms. Lung function tests should be considered for all patients receiving radiotherapy to their thorax to ensure that there is 'respiratory reserve' to tolerate the treatment.

- Volume of lung treated to more than 20 Gy (V_{20})
  - If V_{20} >35% of total lung volume there is a significant risk of life-threatening radiation pneumonitis
- Fractionation
- Concomitant chemotherapy
- Pre-treatment lung function
  - Ideally >50% predicted
    - FEV_1 — gas transfer factor
- Co-morbidity
  - Pre-existing lung disease
    - COPD   — pulmonary fibrosis
    - connective tissue disease
  - Smoking

Investigations

Imaging
- CXR
  - May be normal in the acute phase
  - May see perivascular shadowing and patchy alveolar infiltration (weeks)
  - Characteristically changes:
    - do not follow
      - anatomical boundaries
      - usual patterns seen in other diseases
    - reflect treatment fields
      - often having straight edges
- HRCT chest
  - Abnormalities range from patchy ground-glass opacification to consolidation
  - May diagnose other conditions
    - progressive malignancy   — opportunistic infection
    - lymphangitis carcinomatosis
  - See Fig. 13.1

Lung function tests
It is most useful to compare pre- and post-treatment lung function tests, because of the potential confounding by pre-existent lung pathology, e.g. COPD.
- Reduced operating lung volumes
  - body plethysmography
- Reduced gas transfer (T_{LCO}, K_{CO})

Bronchoscopy
- Bronchoalveolar lavage may show a non-specific inflammatory infiltrate
  - It is rarely helpful in the diagnosis of radiation pneumonitis

Lung biopsy
- This can be:
  - Percutaneous
  - Transbronchial
- Rarely needed in practice; however, can be useful to exclude other causes if the HRCT is not diagnostic
  - Lymphangitis carcinomatosis
  - Idiopathic pulmonary fibrosis
  - Opportunistic infection
- Accurate diagnosis of other conditions may be more difficult once steroid treatment has been commenced

Management
- Steroids
  - reduce the inflammatory component, but have no effect on the development of late pulmonary fibrosis
  - prednisolone 40 mg PO od for 4 weeks followed by a gradual reducing regime over 3–6 months
  - observe carefully for relapse of symptoms after withdrawal of treatment
  - use pulmonary function tests to help monitor response/progression
- Antibiotics
  - systemic features (e.g. fever, malaise) may be due to radiation pneumonitis; however, may also be due to a coexisting infection
  - amoxicillin 500 mg PO tds for 5 days
  - clarithromycin 250 mg PO bd for 5 days
- Oxygen
- Investigational drugs
  - amifostine
  - pentoxifylline
- Lung fibrosis
  - this is irreversible
  - management
    — symptomatic support
    — home oxygen may be required
  - referral to a respiratory physician may be beneficial

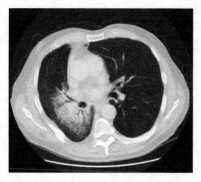

Fig. 13.1 CT scan showing interstitial fibrotic reaction consistent with radiation fibrosis in a patient 3 months post CHART for right lower lobe non-small cell lung cancer. Note volume loss in the right hemithorax.

⑦ **Neurotoxicity**

Neurological toxicity is one of the most feared and serious complications of radiotherapy. It can have a huge impact on quality of life, ranging from paraesthesia to paralysis or neuropsychiatric effects.

Late neurotoxicity is usually predictable, irreversible, and progressive; therefore prevention of late neurotoxicity is paramount. The risk of late neurotoxicity should be minimized by appropriate radiotherapy treatment planning, taking into account the known risk factors.

Acute effects
- Caused by:
  - tissue swelling
  - transient demyelination
- Usually short lived
- Risk factors
  - large volumes treated
  - dose per fraction (>2 Gy/#)

Late effects
- Caused by:
  - demyelination
  - vascular damage with resulting ischaemia
- Usually permanent
- Risk factors
  - dose per fraction >2 Gy
  - dose >50 Gy
  - use of chemotherapy
    — previous or concurrent
    — intrathecal or intravenous
  - hyperfractionation
    — especially myelopathy

Brachial plexopathy
- Seen in patients being treated for breast cancer or lymphoma receiving radiotherapy to:
  - axilla
  - supraclavicular fossa

Acute plexopathy
- Onset may be during radiotherapy or up to 4 weeks after completing radiotherapy

Clinical features
- Numbness of the digits
- Weakness of the biceps and shoulder girdle

Management
- Intervention is not usually needed
- Corticosteroids may accelerate the resolution of symptoms

Late plexopathy
- Onset occurs months to years after therapy
  - median onset 10–12 months
- Risk increases with doses >60 Gy (in 2 Gy/#).

Clinical features
- Paraesthesia
- Weakness
  - especially small muscles of hand
  - can progress to paralysis
- Pain
  - occurs late in course of condition
  - commonly neuropathic

Investigations
- MRI to exclude tumour infiltration
- Nerve conduction studies

Management
- Analgesia
  - use analgesics as per the WHO analgesic ladder (see Pain 🕮 p2)
  - consider early use of adjuvant analgesics for neuropathic pain
  - TENS machine
- Nerve block
- Rehabilitation
- Occupational therapy
- Physiotherapy

Myelopathy
- Seen in patients receiving radiotherapy with fields overlapping the spine
  - Head and neck tumours
  - Lymphoma
  - Lung cancer
  - Oesophageal cancer
  - Craniospinal irradiation
  - Retroperitoneal sarcoma
  - Spinal intramedullary tumours
  - Spinal cord compression
  - Lymph nodes
    - mediastinal
    - para-aortic

Acute myelopathy
- Onset is usually 2–6 months after completing therapy
- It is transient and self-limiting
  - usually <6 months
- It is not predictive for development of late myelopathy
- Caused by transient demyelination in the posterior columns and lateral spinothalamic tracts

Clinical features
- Lhermitte's phenomenon
  - electric shock-like sensation radiates down the spine on flexion of the neck
- No neurological signs

Investigations
Usually no investigation is required, unless there are atypical features.
- MRI
  - exclude tumour infiltration
  - may show demyelination
- Vitamin B_{12} level
  - to exclude deficiency

Management
- Reassurance
- Adjuvant analgesia is occasionally needed
  - gabapentin   • carbamazepine

Late myelopathy
- Bimodal distribution of onset
  - 12–14 months and 24–28 months
- Usually irreversible and often progressive
- It is due to a combination of demyelination and vascular changes
- Risk increases with:
  - dose >45 Gy (2 Gy/#)   • dose >2 Gy/#

Clinical features
- Usually insidious but occasionally acute onset
- Pattern depends on:
  - anatomical location
    — spinal level
  - extent of damage
    — complete or partial
    — transverse myelopathy
- Combination of:
  - sensory dysfunction
    — paraesthesia   — dysaesthesia
    — loss of proprioception
  - motor dysfunction
    — weakness   — paraplegia
  - autonomic dysfunction
    — sphincter control

Investigations
- MRI
  - exclude tumour infiltration causing spinal cord compression
  - will show:
    — demyelination   — cord swelling
  - image the whole CNS to exclude systemic demyelinating conditions
    — multiple sclerosis
- Vitamin B_{12} level
  - to exclude deficiency
- CSF
  - raised protein and lymphocytes

Management
- See late plexopathy

Encephalopathy
- Seen in patients receiving cerebral radiotherapy

Acute encephalopathy
- Onset occurs during or shortly after completion of therapy
- Due to cerebral oedema induced by the disruption of the blood–brain barrier

Risk factors
- Dose (>2 Gy/#)
- Whole brain irradiation

Clinical features
- Raised intracerebral pressure
  - headache
  - nausea
  - drowsiness
- Neurological deficits
- Fever

Management
- Corticosteroids
  - dexamethasone 4–8 mg PO bd
    — reduce the dose as symptoms resolve

Subacute encephalopathy (somnolence syndrome)
- Onset 1–6 months after completion of radiotherapy
- Occurs following whole brain irradiation

Clinical features
- Somnolence
- Irritability
- Apathy
- Headache

Management
- May settle spontaneously over weeks to months
- Corticosteroids may reduce the duration of somnolence syndrome

Late encephalopathy
Radiation necrosis
Occurs 1–3 years after completion of radiotherapy.
Caused by damage of small vessels in the high dose volume resulting in coagulative necrosis.
- Clinical features
  - Seizures
  - Raised intracranial pressure
  - Focal neurological deficits
    — motor
    — sensory
- Risk factors
  - Dose
    — dose per fraction >2 Gy/#
    — total dose >55 Gy
  - Total volume of brain irradiated
  - Concomitant chemotherapy
  - Age of patient

- Investigations
  - MRI
    - contrast-enhancing mass with associated oedema
  - MRI spectroscopy
    - to differentiate necrosis from recurrent tumour
  - PET
    - to differentiate necrosis from recurrent tumour
- Management
  - Corticosteroids
    - high dose dexamethasone 8–16 mg PO bd
  - Surgical debulking
    - allows steroid tapering
    - to exclude recurrent tumour

Leukoencephalopathy
Occurs 1–2 years after completion of therapy.
- Risk is increased by:
  - Doses >55 Gy
  - Intrathecal chemotherapy
    - methotrexate   — cytarabine
  - Age
    - elderly   — children <2 years
- Clinical features
  - In adults
    - lethargy   — confusion
    - personality changes   — dementia
    - memory deficits
  - In children
    - neurocognitive impairment
      - memory deficits   – behavioural problems
      - learning disabilities
    - avoid cranial irradiation in children <2 years, in an attempt to minimize neurocognitive impairment
- Management
  - Supportive care

Endocrinopathies
- Hypothalamic and pituitary dysfunction is seen in 70–80% of patients at 10 years after cranial radiotherapy.
- Biochemical changes are evident long before endocrinopathies are clinically apparent.
  - Surveillance, with regular blood tests, is therefore vital.
- Patients should receive appropriate hormone replacement and referral for management by an endocrinologist should be considered.

⑦ Osteoradionecrosis

Osteoradionecrosis is a serious late effect, usually occurring 1–2 years after completion of radiotherapy. Osteoradionecrosis most commonly affects the mandible after radical radiotherapy to the buccal cavity (1–9% after external beam radiotherapy and 2–40% after brachytherapy), but it can be seen at other sites.

Risk factors
- Dose
  - >66 Gy to the bone
- Fractionation
  - Hypofractionation
    - >2 Gy/#
  - Hyperfractionation
    - interfraction interval <6 hours
- Brachytherapy
  - May produce very high local doses if the implant is adjacent to bone
- Poor dental hygiene
- Co-morbidity
  - Poor nutrition
  - Alcoholism

Causes
- Loss of osteoblasts and osteoclasts
  - Hypocellular tissue that has a very limited capacity for remodelling or repair
- Disruption of the microvasculature
  - Hypoxic tissue

The resulting devitalized bone is therefore very prone to damage.
- Trauma
  - Tooth extraction
- Infection

Clinical features
- Non-healing wound
- Pain
- Swelling
- Pathological fracture

Differential diagnosis
- Bone metastasis
- Osteomyelitis

Investigations
Imaging
- CT/MRI
  - Visualize the extent of the problem
  - Exclude recurrent disease
- Bone scan
  - To visualize osteoradionecrosis and rule out multiple bone metastases

Management

Optimal management requires a truly multidisciplinary approach.

Prevention

- Dental review
  - Prior to radiotherapy
    - any extractions needed must be performed 10–14 days prior to starting radiotherapy
    - aggressive caries control in restorable teeth
    - periodontal scaling
    - consider initiation of (lifelong) fluoride treatment
  - On completion of radiotherapy
    - regular 6-monthly dental reviews
    - maintain optimal dental hygiene
    - early detection of potential problems
    - any dental extractions needed should be performed in a specialist unit
      - minimal trauma
      - prophylactic antibiotics
      - hyperbaric oxygen therapy can be considered pre- and post-extraction in high risk cases

Intervention

Conservative management

- Optimize nutritional status
  - dietician input
- Careful superficial debridement
- Regular saline irrigation
- Antibiotics if evidence of superficial infection
  - amoxicillin 500 mg PO tds
  - metronidazole 400 mg PO tds
- Hyperbaric oxygen therapy promotes healing by maximizing tissue oxygen tension
- Pentoxifylline 400 mg PO tds may help in resistant cases
- Outcome
  - 40–50% resolve
  - 10–30% stabilize
  - 25–35% progress

Surgical intervention

- Needed in resistant or very extensive cases
- Aim to:
  - resect damaged, non-viable tissue
  - remove infective foci
  - reconstruct with vascularized bone grafts
- Patient will need preoperative and postoperative hyperbaric oxygen therapy

① **Gastrointestinal toxicity**

The GI tract is vulnerable to the effects of radiotherapy as it contains many rapidly proliferating cells.

Oesophagitis

The oesophagus is often irradiated during treatment of:
- Oesophageal tumours
- Lymphomas
- Lung tumours

Oesophagitis is often the key dose limiting toxicity of radiation to this region.
- Onset usually occurs after 20 Gy
  - 2 weeks of conventionally fractionated therapy
- May last for up to 6 weeks after completion of radiotherapy

Clinical features
- Substernal burning
- Odynophagia
- Dysphagia

Risk factors
- Dose and fractionation
  - Total dose
  - Dose per fraction
- Length and volume of oesophagus treated

Management
- Pain control
  - Barriers
    — Sucralfate suspension
    — 1 g qds, 1 hour before meals
  - Analgesics
    — Use analgesics as per the WHO analgesic ladder (see Pain 📖 p2)
    — Regular NSAIDs are particularly useful because of the inflammatory component of radiation oesophagitis
    — Liquid/soluble formulation
- Antacids
  - PPI to minimize acid reflux which exacerbates symptoms
- Dietary
  - Bland, soft foods
  - Nutritional supplements may be needed
- Ensure there is no coexistent *Candida* infection
  - If symptoms are severe consider empirical treatment with fluconazole 50–100 mg PO od for 7–14 days

Nausea and vomiting
See Nausea and vomiting 📖 p38.

Diarrhoea
See Diarrhoea 📖 p48.

Proctitis

Radiation proctitis can occur during radiotherapy for pelvic malignancies.

- Rectal
- Prostate
- Bladder
- Gynaecological

Damage to the rectal mucosa usually starts after 30–40 Gy (3–4 weeks of therapy).

Clinical features

- Diarrhoea
- Rectal urgency
- Tenesmus
- Rectal bleeding

Management

- Diarrhoea
  - see Diarrhoea 📖 p48
- Pain
  - use analgesics as per the WHO analgesic ladder (see Pain 📖 p2)
  - regular NSAIDs are particularly useful because of the inflammatory component of radiation proctitis
  - steroid enemas reduce inflammation
    — use if patient develops tenesmus or rectal bleeding
    - proctofoam HC bd (can be used up to qds)
    - predfoam 20 mg bd
  - perianal discomfort or exacerbation of haemorrhoids
    — proctosedyl ointment bd (apply morning and night)
    — lidocaine gel/ointment (instillagel)
    - externally or PR
    - may cause stinging initially
  - limited evidence for sucralfate enemas being effective

Late gastrointestinal toxicity

- Oesophageal
  - benign strictures
  - motility dysfunction
  - persistent ulceration and bleeding
    — must distinguish from recurrent tumour
- Small/large bowel
  - bowel obstruction
  - perforation
  - bleeding
    — radiation telangiectasia
  - chronic proctitis
  - fistula
    — enterocolic
    — colovesical
    — colovaginal

The diagnosis of late GI toxicity should be a diagnosis of exclusion. If a patient presents with symptoms following radiotherapy, the patient should be investigated fully, particularly to rule out recurrent or secondary malignancy, before the symptoms are attributed to a late radiotherapy effect.

⑦ **Radiation hepatitis**

Radiation to the liver may cause acute veno-occlusive pathology.

The clinical features and abnormal LFTs usually appear 4–8 weeks after completion of the radiotherapy.

The risk of radiation hepatitis increases when doses exceed 30 Gy (1.8–2 Gy/#) to the whole liver. Higher doses can be given to smaller volumes of the liver. If radiotherapy is given concurrently with chemotherapy, severe radiation hepatitis can be seen at lower radiation doses.

Clinical features

- Fatigue
- Rapid weight gain
- Abdominal swelling
- RUQ pain
- Ascites
- Hepatomegaly
- Jaundice is rare

Investigations

Bloods

- LFTs
  - ALT/AST
    — moderately raised (2–3x normal)
  - Bilirubin
    — normal or minimally raised

Imaging

- CT
  - No characteristic CT findings
  - Excludes progressive malignancy
- MRI

Management

Generally self-limiting.

Progressive and potentially fatal in a minority of patients.

- Supportive measures
  - paracentesis
  - diuretics
- Limited data to support using:
  - steroids
  - anticoagulants

Late hepatotoxicity

If the dose to the liver is >25 Gy, fibrosis may develop as a late effect.

Conformal radiotherapy should be used to minimize the volume of liver receiving a dose >25 Gy to minimize late hepatotoxicity.

⑦ **Radiation cystitis**

Damage to the urothelium may be:
- Intentional
  - Treatment of bladder cancer
- Inevitable because of close anatomical proximity in the treatment of pelvic malignancies
  - Prostate
  - Rectal
  - Gynaecological

Radiation cystitis is seen in up to 80–90% of patients having pelvic radiotherapy. It usually develops after 2–3 weeks (20–30 Gy). It is caused by:
- Irritation of the bladder urothelium
- Bladder outflow obstruction owing to prostatic swelling

Clinical features

Overlap of obstructive and irritant features.
- Dysuria
- Frequency
- Incontinence
- Nocturia
- Haematuria
  - rare

Dysuria and frequency may last for many weeks after the therapy has finished, whilst incontinence and nocturia have usually settled within 4 weeks of completion of the therapy.

Risk factors
- Dose
- Fractionation
- Volume treated
- Prior surgery/chemotherapy
- Co-existing infection
  - also exacerbates symptoms and delays recovery

Management

Prevention
- Regular and careful screening for urinary tract infection
  - treat infection with appropriate antibiotics
  - prophylactic antibiotics offer no benefit
- Cranberry juice reduces frequency of infection by:
  - reducing bacterial adhesion to urothelium

Symptomatic relief
- α blockers
  - reduce obstruction from the swollen prostate by relaxing smooth muscle at the bladder neck
  - Tamsulosin 400 µg PO od
  - caution in:
    - renal impairment
    - hepatic dysfunction
    - concomitant antihypertensive drugs
    - cardiac disease
  - side effects
    - dry mouth
    - blurred vision
    - headaches
    - drowsiness
    - hypotension
    - erectile dysfunction
- Antimuscarinic drugs
  - relax urinary smooth muscle and reduce bladder contractions
  - Tolterodine 2 mg PO bd
  - side effects
    - dry mouth
    - blurred vision
    - constipation
    - drowsiness
- Analgesia
  - use analgesics as per the WHO analgesic ladder (see Pain 📖 p2)
  - regular NSAIDs are particularly useful because of the inflammatory component of radiation cystitis
- Good fluid intake
  - keeps urine dilute thus making it less irritant
  - reduce fluid intake in the evenings, to minimize nocturia
- Sodium citrate/potassium citrate
  - mild alkalinization of the urine
  - may relieve the discomfort of radiation cystitis
  - proprietary brands available

Late urological toxicity

Bladder fibrosis results in reduced bladder volumes, resulting in frequency and nocturia. Telangiectasia can result in ongoing haematuria. Full urological investigation is required to rule out recurrence of the primary malignancy. Urethral strictures may also develop as a late toxicity.

Moral, legal, and ethical emergencies

⚠ **Cardiopulmonary resuscitation**

A cardiac or respiratory arrest is a medical emergency that quickly renders a patient incompetent. In the absence of clear instruction to the contrary, the default position for an attending medical and nursing team is to commence cardiopulmonary resuscitation (CPR); however, this may not be reasonable in a patient in the terminal phase of their illness, or for whom the burdens of intervention clearly outweigh the potential benefits. Owing to the need for immediate intervention, there is a danger that this balance of burden to benefit will not be as carefully considered as it would for other medical interventions.

As a treatment CPR has a low success rate and carries high morbidity, especially in the context of metastatic cancer. As cancer becomes more advanced this issue needs to be carefully and proactively considered in the light of the extent of the cancer, the potential for response to further treatment, the patient's own wishes and their perception of their quality of life. If the potential burden of CPR exceeds the potential benefit then a 'do not attempt resuscitation' (DNAR) order should be considered.

- Potential benefits of CPR
  - To prolong life that is of a quality acceptable to the patient
  - To allow time for active management of reversible pathology
- Potential burdens of CPR
  - A distressing and undignified death
  - Extension of life that is so short or of such poor quality that it is not of value to the patient or their family
  - Permanent neurological impairment
    — especially if CPR is delayed or prolonged
  - Trauma related to CPR
    — sternal or rib fractures
      - especially if there are bony metastases
    — splenic rupture

Effectiveness of CPR

- All patients in a hospital setting
  - Re-establishment of cardiac output 41%
  - Survival to discharge 13%
    — It is most effective in people with a reversible medical condition who have a witnessed disturbance of heart rhythm in a hospital setting
    — It is least effective when:
      - the arrest is unwitnessed
      - the attempt at CPR is prolonged
      - there is co-morbid disease
        - pneumonia
        - sepsis
        - renal failure
        - heart failure
        - metastatic cancer

- Cancer patients spending 50% or more of their time in bed have a survival to discharge of only 2–3%
- Cancer patients suffering a cardiac arrest owing to pre-existing medical conditions unresponsive to treatment have a survival to discharge of only 0–2%

Legal and ethical issues

- Professional responsibility regarding CPR is the same as for any other treatment.
- Decisions must be informed by the Human Rights Act 1998.
  - The right to life (Article 2)
  - The right to be free from inhuman or degrading treatment (Article 3)
  - The right to receive information (from Article 10)
- Patients cannot insist on a treatment that the doctor believes is not in their best interests.
- Patients have a right to refuse any treatment, including CPR, and an Advance Decision to this effect, whether written as a specific document or as a record of the patient's wishes in the medical notes, is legally binding as long as the patient was mentally competent when it was made.
  - See The Mental Capacity Act 2005 📖 p406.

Cardiorespiratory arrest in a cancer patient

- If no CPR decision is documented
  - If the patient is not terminally ill and the wishes of the patient are unknown then CPR should always be attempted.
  - If a patient is clearly dying from irreversible pathology then the moral imperative is to prevent unnecessary harm and CPR should be withheld.
  - CPR must not be attempted if it is contrary to the recorded, sustained wishes of a competent and informed adult patient (see The Mental Capacity Act 2005 📖 p406).

Decision-making

Decisions on CPR are best made in advance as part of overall care planning, and should, if possible, involve the whole health care team. Proactive decision-making is in the best interests of the patient to ensure appropriate treatment in the event of cardiorespiratory arrest.

Factors relevant to the decision will include:
- The likely clinical outcome of CPR.
- The prognosis from current pathology.
- Options for further active treatment of the cancer.
- The patient's perception of what constitutes an acceptable quality of life.
- The patient's wishes as regards further active management and CPR.
- Cancer patients who survive CPR will often require ICU support. If ICU support would be inappropriate, then a DNAR order should be considered.

Where the balance of benefit to burden of CPR is genuinely uncertain then the patient's wishes become paramount.

If a patient insists on a request for CPR against the advice and explanation of the health care team then there is no moral obligation on the team to provide this treatment if they feel that it is against the patient's best interests. Careful documentation of all discussions with the patient is vital in this situation. A second opinion may be needed in this situation, with transfer of care if appropriate.

Decisions regarding CPR must be reviewed regularly and in the light of changes in the patient's condition and wishes.

Discussion with patients regarding CPR

- Discussions around CPR involve sensitive and skilled communication and should be conducted by senior and more experienced members of the medical team.
- If patients indicate that they do not wish to pursue a discussion on CPR then this should be respected and documented.
- Discussion regarding CPR can be distressing for the patient and this must be weighed against the potential benefit of discussion for the individual patient.
- CPR is best discussed as part of a consideration of available treatment options and overall care planning.
- It is very easy for the concepts of CPR and 'active management' to become confused and they must be clearly differentiated. Patients must be reassured that a DNAR order does not imply withdrawal of active treatment, and all other treatment and care appropriate for the patient will continue to be considered and offered.
- Patients may want close friends and relatives to be involved in the discussion regarding CPR; however, refusal by a competent patient to allow information to be disclosed to family or friends must be respected.
- Patients and relatives may have unrealistic expectations about the nature and likely success of CPR, and this may need to be sensitively explored.
- Objective discussion of CPR is difficult in the emotionally charged context of breaking bad news and may simply add to the patient's distress.
- It is not helpful to discuss CPR with the patient in a way that suggests that they have a choice when the medical team has already decided that CPR is not a treatment they would be prepared to give.

Recording and communicating decisions
All discussions and decisions regarding CPR must be carefully documented and communicated to all health care professionals involved in the ongoing care of the patient.

The entry in the medical records must:
- Date the decision
- Give reasons for decision

To improve communication to other members of the healthcare team it is also very useful to document the suitability of future intervention.
- Artificial nutrition and hydration
- Intravenous antibiotics
- Non-invasive ventilation
- Dialysis
- HDU/ICU

Further reading

Decisions relating to cardiopulmonary resuscitation. A joint statement from the British Medical Association, the Resuscitation Council (UK) and the Royal College of Nursing. January 2002. www.bma.org.uk. J. Med Ethics 2007 27, 312–318.

Ethical Decision-Making in Palliative Care: Cardiopulmonary Resuscitation (CPR) for People who are Terminally Ill. The National Council for Palliative Care Ethics Working Party. Revised version Jan 2002.

Human Rights Act 1988 www.opsi.gov.uk

⑦ The Mental Capacity Act 2005

The Mental Capacity Act 2005 came into force in England and Wales on 1st April 2007. It provides a statutory framework to empower and protect vulnerable people who are not able to make their own decisions.

Key principles
- A presumption of capacity.
  - Every adult has the right to make his, or her, own decisions and must be assumed to have capacity to do so unless it is proved otherwise.
  - Capacity relates to a specific decision at a specific time.
  - For a patient to prove capacity to make decisions about their ongoing treatment, they should be able to:
    — Understand information about their condition and treatment.
    — Remember this information.
    — Deliberate about the therapeutic choices posed by the information.
    — Believe that the information applies to them.
  - If there is uncertainty regarding assessment of capacity a second opinion should be sought.
- The right for individuals to be supported to make their own decisions.
  - People must be given all appropriate help before anyone concludes that they cannot make their own decisions.
- Individuals must retain the right to make what might appear to be eccentric or unwise decisions.
- Best interests
  - Anything done for, or on behalf of, people without capacity must be in their best interests.
  - This must take account of any previously expressed or written statements made by the person in relation to their wishes, feelings, beliefs and values, and the views of carers, close family members, and close friends.
  - If there is uncertainty regarding a person's best interests a second opinion should be sought.
- Least restrictive intervention
  - Anything done for, or on behalf of, people without capacity should be the least restrictive of their basic rights and freedoms. If the patient may regain capacity at a future date, consideration must be given to deferring the decision until such a time.

Designated representative
Lasting powers of attorney
- The act allows a person to appoint a 'lasting power of attorney' to act on their behalf, in their best interest, if they should lose capacity in the future.

- This person will have authority to make decisions relating to financial, health, and welfare decisions.
  - Refusing treatment
    - including CPR
  - Consenting to treatment
- Lasting powers of attorney must be registered with the Public Guardian.
- The Public Guardian should be notified, and may act to overrule lasting powers of attorney, if there are concerns as to their suitability or decision-making.

Court-appointed deputies

- The Court of Protection may appoint a deputy to take decisions on welfare, healthcare, and financial matters as authorized by the Court, but they will not be able to refuse consent to life-sustaining treatment.

Independent Mental Capacity Advocate

- A person, who lacks capacity but has no one to speak for them, will have an Independent Mental Capacity Advocate (IMCA) appointed to support them.
- The IMCA makes representations about the person's wishes, feelings, beliefs and values, at the same time as bringing to the attention of the decision-maker (e.g. doctor) all factors that are relevant to the decision.
- Doctors treating a patient who has not appointed a lasting power of attorney, must take account of the representation of the IMCA; however, the final decision rests with the consultant. The IMCA cannot make the decision on behalf of the person lacking capacity, but may challenge the decision-maker on behalf of the person lacking capacity if necessary.

Advance Decision to refuse treatment

- People may make a decision in advance to refuse treatment if they should lose capacity in the future.
- People cannot make an Advanced Decision to refuse basic care
  - washing
  - clothing
- Healthcare professionals must act in accordance with a valid, applicable Advance Decision.
- For an Advance Decision to apply to any treatment which a doctor considers necessary to sustain life, the decision must
  - be in writing.
  - be signed and witnessed.
  - state that the decision stands 'even if life is at risk'.

Further reading

The Mental Capacity Act 2005 www.opsi.gov.uk

Resuscitation guidelines

Adult basic life support

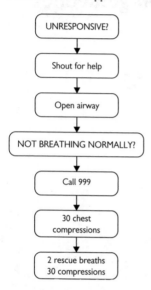

Adult advanced life support algorithm

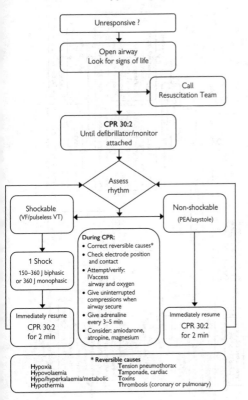

Tachycardia algorithm (with pulse)

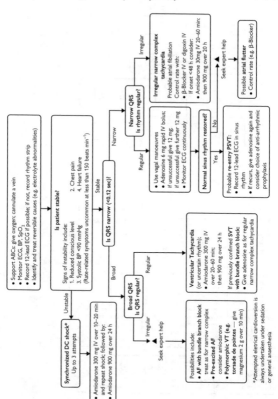

Bradycardia algorithm
(includes rates inappropriately slow for haemodynamic state)

If appropriate, give oxygen, cannulate a vein, and record a 12-lead ECG

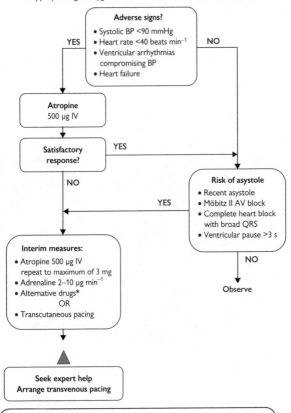

Adverse signs?
- Systolic BP <90 mmHg
- Heart rate <40 beats min⁻¹
- Ventricular arrhythmias compromising BP
- Heart failure

YES

NO

Atropine
500 μg IV

Satisfactory response?   YES

NO

Risk of asystole
- Recent asystole
- Möbitz II AV block
- Complete heart block with broad QRS
- Ventricular pause >3 s

YES

NO

Interim measures:
- Atropine 500 μg IV repeat to maximum of 3 mg
- Adrenaline 2–10 μg min⁻¹
- Alternative drugs*
  OR
- Transcutaneous pacing

Observe

Seek expert help
Arrange transvenous pacing

*Alternatives include:
   Aminophylline
   Isoprenaline
   Dopamine
   Glucagon (if beta blocker or calcium channel blocker overdose)
   Glycopyrrolate can be used instead of atropine

Index